AF430882

Elementary
Pharmacoinformatics

Elementary
Pharmacoinformatics

T. Durai Ananda Kumar

M.Pharm.,

Sr. Assistant Professor,
Dept of Pharmaceutical Chemistry,
Gokaraju Rangaraju College of Pharmacy,
Nizampet, Hyderabad-500 090. India.

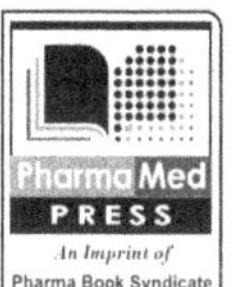

PharmaMed Press
An imprint of Pharma Book Syndicate

A Unit of BSP Books Pvt. Ltd.
4-4-316, Giriraj Lane,
Sultan Bazar, Hyderabad - 500 095.

© 2014, *by Publisher*

Published by

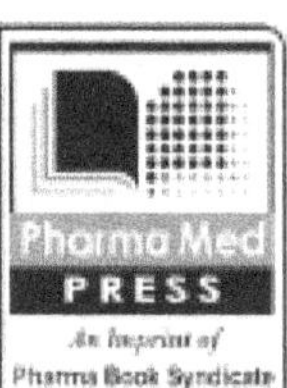

PharmaMed Press

An imprint of Pharma Book Syndicate

A Unit of BSP Books Pvt. Ltd.
4-4-316, Giriraj Lane, Sultan Bazar, Hyderabad - 500 095.
Phone: 040-23445605, 23445688; Fax: 91+40-23445611
E-mail: info@pharmamedpress.com

ISBN: 978-93-85433-66-5 (HB)

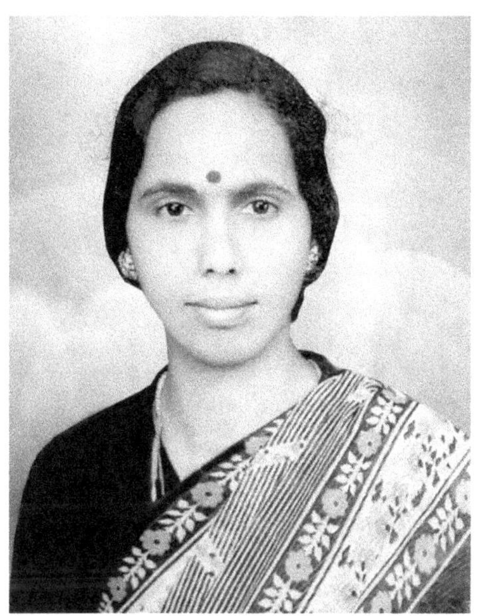

(L) Smt SN Muthulakshmi

ஈன்ற பொழுதின் பெரிதுவக்கும் தன்மகனைச்
சான்றோன் எனக்கேட்ட தாய்   .....குறள்

The mother, hearing her son's merit

Delights more than when she begot   ....Kural

FOREWORD

The integration of chemistry and computers on one side and their applications for unearthing the biological processes in relation to drugs is an achievement by no means small and has bestowed with Nobel Prize-2013. The high profile areas, namely molecular biology, organic-medicinal chemistry, pharmacology and information technology, all converged to provide fruitful scope for the exploring and evaluating the drug discovery. Therefore, this area is dearer to the scientists and academicians alike. The genomics and proteomics pooled a large amount of biological data, which can be utilized in drug design process.

Pharmacoinformatics has been attracting the attention of the policy makers as a subject of current importance. Thus, it has been incorporated into the curriculum of several universities. At present, no book is available in the market. This maiden effort made by Mr. T. Durai Ananda Kumar is very commendable and helpful to the beginners as well as practicing medicinal chemists. Mr. T. Durai Ananda Kumar had spent 7 years on teaching and conducting practicals on this area and applied to the students and continuously verified the veracity of the contents several times, with dedication. With this edition, the information is made available to the students at large across India. I have no hesitation to place on record that this book immensely benefits the students.

The book consists of four parts spreading through 29 chapters covering both theoretical and practical concepts. The first part covers the different databases, their structure and applications as it becomes the heart of Pharmacoinformatics. The second part deals with pharmacy automation services both in hospitals and community pharmacies. The third part mainly devoted to conventional and modern drug research aspects giving special emphasis on rational drug design. The fourth part elaborates the homology modeling techniques in a very concise manner. It includes both theory and experiments for practicals and practice.

This book certainly a companion for students of B. Pharmacy and M. Pharmacy (Pharmaceutical chemistry and pharmacology specializations), in addition to biotechnology and other scientists wish to enter this thrust area, Pharmacoinformatics.

Hyderabad
17-10-2013

Prof. C. V. S. Subrahmanyam,
M. Pharm, PhD.,
Principal,
Gokaraju Rangaraju College of Pharmacy,
Bachupally, Hyderabad-500 090

PREFACE

With the blessing of my mother (L) Smt. S.N. Muthulakshmi, father Mr. D. Thirumoorthy, teachers and well wishers I present this book entitled "Elementary Pharmacoinformatics" to the active academic and research community.

Pharmacoinformatics is an informatics based discipline, concerned with the information on drugs and related substances, discovery and development of drugs using high performance computing and graphic tools. Informatics improves the quality health care of patients through barcode verification and electronic modification administration record (eMAR). This process is known as 'pharmacy automation' and provides accuracy and efficiency in medication usage. Rational design of new chemical entities (NCEs) through computer aided drug design (CADD) is an emerging approach (mechanistic approach). Bioinformatics, study of information content and flow in biological systems has profound application in pharmaceutical and diagnostic concerns. It plays major role in the identification of new drug targets with the help of molecular biology and bio-physical techniques (X-ray and NMR spectroscopy techniques).

The high demand for the user-friendly, elementary level book on 'pharmacoinformatics' stimulated this project. The driving force behind this project has been the persuasion and constant encouragements from the student community. This book covers principles and applications of health informatics, cheminformatics and bioinformatics.

The main objective of this material is to provide a comprehensive overview of the current advances and *in silico* strategies used in drug information and drug design. The following features of the material reflects the objectives

- Systematic approach and simple language
- Neat and self explanatory diagrams
- Proceeding for the entry level student
- Emphasis on molecular level approach of drug design strategies
- The application section provides opportunity to have hands on experience

It is considered appropriate to begin with a stepwise introduction to topics that are necessary for the easier understanding. The text is divided in to four parts and described in 29 chapters.

Part 1: Information Databases: This section describes the different types of database and their significance in pharmacoinformatics.

Part 2: Patient centric pharmacoinformatics: The role of informatics and pharmacist in the health care of patients is described in this section.

Part 3: Drug discovery: Traditional to modern drug discovery processes are detailed and emphasis is given to computer aided drug design.

Part 4: Bio-informatics: The utility of bioinformatics in drug design process is explained with application section in user-friendly manner.

The book avoids the use of high level descriptions to convert the subject interesting. It is not necessary to read the manuscript strictly in chapter order. The greatest care was taken to avoid the errors, if any appear please do light upon it. Certainly improvements are needed; hence users are requested to record their suggestions. I hope that, this material will be of immense benefit to the learning community of pharmacy, bio-technology, biomedical engineering and other interdisciplinary fields.

The love and support my wife Mrs. M. Sudha, consistently offered were the most important elements in seeing the project to a satisfactory conclusion.

I offer my sincere thanks to Prof (Dr) C.V.S. Subrahmanyam, Principal, Gokaraju Rangaraju College of Pharmacy, Hyderabad for his suggestions and encouragements. I express my exquisite thanks to Mrs. N. Swathi, Senior Assistant Professor, for sharing her views and constructive suggestions. I extend my sincere gratitude to Dr. G. Gangaraju, President, and Mr. G.V.K. Rangaraju, Vice-President, Gokaraju Rangaraju Educational Society for the learning atmosphere provided. I am grateful to a number of friends and students, who helped me as reviewers.

Over the past 6 years many students helped developing the quantum of information and I appreciate their inputs. My special thanks are due to student friends Mr. D. Gowtham Reddy, Ms V. Lakshmi Indira and Mr. S. Varun Raj for their valuable contributions in different phases of this project. This work has been influenced from literatures, books and related materials by many authors.

I gratefully acknowledge Mr. I. Laxman Rao, Librarian and Mr. V. V. Rajan Raju, Library Assistant for their constant help in library phase. I would like to thank Mr. A. Santhosh, BSP Books (P) Ltd, Hyderabad. who helped in many ways to keep the project moving forward. My sincere thanks to Mr. Anil Shah, Director, BSP Books (P) Ltd, Hyderabad, for the co-operation extended in attending to neatness and correctness of the material.

-Author

CONTENTS

PHARMACOINFORMATICS 1

INFORMATION DATABASES 5

CHAPTER 1

DATABASES

CHAPTER 2
DATA MINING

CHAPTER 3
SEARCH MACHINES

PATIENT CENTRIC PHARMACOINFORMATICS

CHAPTER 4
DRUG INFORMATION

CHAPTER 5

PHARMACY AUTOMATION

DRUG RESEARCH 65

CHAPTER 6

DRUG DISCOVERY

CHAPTER 7

DRUG DEVELOPMENT

CHAPTER 8

DRUG DESIGN

CHAPTER 9

QUANTITATIVE STRUCTURE ACTIVITY RELATIONSHIP (QSAR)

CHAPTER 10

VIRTUAL SCREENING

CHAPTER 11

TARGET IDENTIFICATION

CHAPTER 12

MOLECULAR MODELING

CHAPTER 13

DOCKING

CHAPTER 14

ARGUSLAB

BIOINFORMATICS **175**

CHAPTER 15

BIOLOGICAL DATABASES

CHAPTER 16

BIOPHYSICAL TECHNIQUES

CHAPTER 17

MOLECULAR BIOLOGY

CHAPTER 18

HOMOLOGY MODELING

CHAPTER 19

SEQUENCE SIMILARITY

CHAPTER 20

DOT MATRIX

CHAPTER 21

DYNAMIC PROGRAMMING

CHAPTER 22

HEURISTIC METHOD

CHAPTER 23

SEQUENCE COMPARISON METHODS

CHAPTER 24

PHYLOGENETIC ANALYSIS

CHAPTER 25

GENE PREDICTION

CHAPTER 26

SCORING SYSTEM

CHAPTER 27

3D STRUCTURE PREDICTION USING SWISS MODEL

CHAPTER 28

MOLECULAR VISUALIZATION

CHAPTER 29

RECEPTORS

Symbols

Log P:	Partition coefficient
Es:	Steric substituent constant
π:	Hansch substitution constant
f:	Fragmentation constan
R_m:	Chromatographic R_m value
σ:	Hammett substituent constant
σ_1:	Inductive substitutive constant
σ^*:	Taft's substitution constant
F:	Field-Inductive constant
σ_1:	Inductive substituent constant
E_{str}:	Energy of stretching
E_{bend}:	Bond length change
$E_{torsion}$:	Change in the conformation
εE_{cou}:	Electrostatic attraction
E_{vdW}:	Vander waals force
K_ϕ:	Torsional barrier constant
ϕ:	Actual torsional angle
ϕ_{offset}:	Unstrained bond angle
K_θ:	Angle bending force constant
θ:	Actual bond length
$\hat{H}$:	Hamiltonian
Ψ (sigh):	Wave function
E:	Total energy
U:	Potential energy
K:	Kinetic energy

Abbreviations

AAPCC:	American association of Poison Control Centers
ADMs:	Automated Dispensing Machines
ADEPT:	Antibody Directed Enzyme Prodrug Therapy
ADR:	Adverse Drug Reaction
AM1:	Austin Model 1
ANSI-SPARC:	American National Standard Institute - Standards Planning and Requirements Committee
ASN.1:	Abstract Syntax Notation
BAC:	Bacterial Artificial Chromosomes
Bio-PERL:	Biological Practical Extraction and Report Language
BLAST:	Basic Local Alignment Search Tool
BLOSUM:	BLOcks SUbstitution Matrix
CADD:	Computer Aided Drug Design
CAID:	Chi Automatic Interaction Detection
CART:	Classification and Regression Trees
cDNA:	Circular DNA
CDSS:	Clinical Decision Support System
CG:	Conjucate Gradient
CNDO:	Complete Neglect of Differential Overlap
CODIS:	Combined DNA Index System
CPOE:	Computerized Provider Order Entry, Computerized Physician Order Entry
CPK:	Corey-Pauling-Koltun
dNTP:	Deoxy Nucleoside Tri Phosphate
ddNTP:	Dideoxy Nuceoside Tri Phosphate
DBMA:	Database Management System
DCL:	Data Control Language
DDBJ:	DataBank of Japan

DDL:	Data Definition Language
DICs:	Drug Information Centers
DOE:	Design of Experiments
DML:	Data Manipuation Language
DP:	Dynamic Programming
DQL:	Data Query Language
DSS:	Decision Support Systems
EBI:	European Bioinformatics Institute
EHR:	Electronic Health Record
EHT:	Extended Huckel Theory
EMBL:	European Molecular Biology Laboratory
EMBOSS:	European Molecular Biology Open Software Suite
EMM:	Electronic Material Management
E-Value:	Expectation Value
EST:	Expanded Sequence Tags
FASTA:	FAST Approximation
FBI:	Federal Bureau of Investigation
F*ISH:*	Fluorescent *In Situ* Hybridization
FMO:	Frontier Molecular Orbital theory
GCG:	Genetics Computer Group
GDEPT:	Gene Directed Enzyme Prodrug Therapy
GI:	Gene Identity number
GPAT:	Genetic Prodrug Activated Therapy
GPCR:	G-Protein Coupled Receptors
HBA:	Hydrogen Bond Acceptors
HBD:	Hydrogen Bond Donors
HIS:	Hospital Information Systems
HIT:	Health Information Technology
HTS:	High Throughput Screening
HGP:	Human Genome Project

HOMO:	Highest Occupied Molecular Orbital
HM:	Homology Modeling
HMM:	Hidden Markov Model
HSP:	High Scoring Segment Pair
IDIS:	Iowa Drug Information Service
IGM:	Internet Grateful Med
IPA:	International Pharmaceutical Abstract
ISH:	*In Situ* Hybridization
IUB:	International Union of Biochemistry
LFER:	Linear Free Energy Relationship
LGIC:	Ligand (transmitter) Gated Ion Channels
InfLibNet:	Information and Library Network
KDD:	Knowledge Discovery in Databases
LUMO:	Lowest Unoccupied Molecular Orbital
MDM:	Mutation Data Matrix
MDS:	Molecular Dynamic Simulations
MEDLARS:	MEDical Literature Analysis and Retrieval System
MeSH:	Medical Subject Heading
MIPS:	Munich Information Center for protein Sequences
MMDB:	Molecular Modeling Database
MNDO:	Modified Neglect of Differential Overlap
MSA:	Multiple Sequence Alignment
MSP:	Maximum Segment Pair
MPSS:	Massively Parallel Signature Sequencing
NBRF:	National Biomedical Research Foundation
NCBI:	National Center for Biotechnology Information
NCIDD:	National Criminal Investigation DNA Database
NDC:	National Drug Control
NF:	Normal Form
NJ:	Neighbor Joining method PSI-BLAST

OPAC:	Online Public Access Catalog
NSCP:	Non-Specific Conformational Perturbation
OPRP:	Open Reading Frames Prediction
PACS:	Picture Archiving and Communication System
PASS:	Prediction of Activity Spectra for Substances
PAM:	Percentage of Acceptable point Mutation, Point Accepted Mutation, Percent Accepted Mutation.
PAGE:	Poly Acrylamide Gel Electrophoresis
PCILO:	Perturbation Configuration Integration using Localized Orbital
PCR:	Polymerase Chain Reaction
PDB:	Protein Data Bank
PERL:	Practical Extraction and Report Language
PHI-BLAST:	Pattern Hit Initiated BLAST
PIR:	Protein information Resource
PM3:	Parameterised Model 3
PTC:	Pharmacy and Therapeutics Committee
PTM:	Post Transitional Modifications
PSI-BLAST:	Position-Specific Iterated BLAST
QSAR:	Quantitative Structure Activity Relationship
QSTR:	Quantitative Structure Toxicity Relationship
RCSB:	Research Collaboratory for Structural Bioinformatics
RDD:	Rational Drug Design
RDMS:	Relational Database Management System
rDNA:	recombinant DNA
RFID:	Radio Frequency Identification
RMSD:	Root Mean Square Deviation RO5: Rule of Five
RP-HPLC:	Reverse Phase HPLC
RP-TLC:	Reverse Phase Thin Layer Chromatography
SAR:	Structure Activity Relationship

SABF:	Spatial Arrangement of Backbone Fragments
SBDD:	Structure Based Drug Design
SCOP:	Structural Classification of Proteins
SCP:	Specific Conformational Perturbation
SD:	Steepest Descent Method
SGIC:	Second Messenger Gated Ion Channels
SMRT:	Single Molecule Real Time sequencing
SP:	Sum of Pairs
SIB:	Swiss Institute of Bioinformatics
SAM:	S-Adenosyl Methionine
SnRNP:	Small nuclear Ribo Nucleo Proteins
SOUL:	Software for University Library
STAT:	Signal Transducers and Activators of Transcription
SQL:	Structured Query Language
TOPKAT:	Toxicity Prediction by Komputer Assisted Technology
TOXNET:	Toxicology Data Network
TPSA:	Total Polar Surface Area
UFF:	Universal Force Field
UPGMA:	Unweighed Pair Group Method with Arithmetic mean
VDEPT:	Virus Directed Enzyme Prodrug Therapy
VGIC:	Voltage Gated Ion Channels
YAC:	Yeast Artificial Chromosomes
2DBPS:	2D Barcode Prescription System

Pharmacoinformatics

Drug discovery warrants a multidisciplinary approach such as molecular biology, chemistry, toxicology, pharmaceutical sciences and computational technology. The increased recognition of information technology in drug discovery is witnessed by bioinformatics and cheminformatics. Modern drug discovery requires systems that have the ability to access and manipulate large quantities of data quickly and easily. Integration of technological advancements with bioinformatics and cheminformatics leads to the field pharmacoinformatics, it refers to the interface of technology with the practice of pharmacy. Pharmacoinformatics has become important tool in evolving new drug development.

Pharmacoinformatics Aspects

Basically pharmacoinformatics involves two main aspects.

1. Service aspect
2. Scientific aspect

Service aspect: Service oriented pharmacoinformatics is more patient centric, involves in drug distribution and drug information services. The main applications of this field includes

1. Use of barcodes in preparation and dispensing/delivery of medications and pharmacy departmental applications
2. e-Prescribing
3. Automated dispensing machines (ADMs)
4. Healthcare informatics
   - Electronic health record (EHR) systems
   - Hospital information systems (HIS)
   - Decision Support Systems (DSS)
5. Toxicoinformatics

Scientific aspect: Scientific aspect of pharmacoinformatics deals with the drug discovery, drug development and drug design activities using *in silico* techniques.

Information Technologies

Pharmacoinformatics includes many emerging information technologies such as

- Bioinformatics
- Genome informatics
- Proteome informatics
- Chemoinformatics
- Chemical reaction informatics
- Toxicoinformatics
- Immunoinformatics

Bioinformatics: National center for Biotechnology Information (NCBI) defines, Bioinformatics as a field of science in which biology, computer science and information technology merge into a single discipline. It has profound application in pharmaceutical and diagnostic concerns and plays major role in the identification of new drug targets with the help of molecular biology and bio-physical techniques (X-ray and NMR spectroscopy techniques).

Genome informatics: Genome informatics, encompasses the various methods and algorithms for analyzing and extracting biologically relevant information from the rapidly growing biological and essential sequence databases. Genome informatics came into existence with the initiation of human genome project (HGP). Genome informatics is helpful in drug discovery process, and the main functions are the optimisation of target selection, unveiling the complexity of gene expression and resolving the genetic variation at the genomic and cellular level.

Proteome informatics: The principle application of proteome informatics include discovery of diagnostics, targets and naturally occurring protein therapeutics, target validation, drug candidate selection, mode of action studies and toxicology.

Cheminformatics: Cheminformatics deals with the information of the molecules and utilizes systems and scientific methods to store, retrieve, and analyze the immense amount of molecular data. Starting from the lead identification through various phases of drug development, cheminformatics has become an integral part of the drug-discovery process (rational drug design).

Chemical reaction informatics: Chemical reaction informatics plays an important role in the field of pharmacoinformatics. Chemical reaction informatics enables chemist to explore synthetic pathways, design and record completely new experiments from scratch or by beginning with reactions found in the reaction databases. There are currently 15-20 million reactions in a wide variety of chemical reaction databases (CASReact, ChemReact, CrossFire Plus, etc).

Toxicoinformatics: Toxicoinformatics predicts the toxicity of chemical molecules in biophase. There are essentially two basic approaches being used in toxicoinformatics

1. Based on modeling Structure Activity Relationship (SAR)
2. Rule based methods.

TOPKAT, MULTICASE, COMPACT, etc are some of the useful databases. TOPKAT (Toxicity Prediction by Komputer Assisted Technology) uses Quantitative Structure Toxicity Relationship (QSTR) regression models developed using electrotopological descriptors like electronic properties (charge, electron density, residual electronegativity, effective polarisability), connectivity descriptors, shape descriptors (kappa shape indices) and substructure descriptors from a library of 3000 molecular fragments. Carcinogenicity, mutagenicity, skin and eye irritation, acute inhalation toxicity and skin sensitization can be calculated from these databases.

Immunoinformatics: Immunoinformatics facilitates the understanding of immune function by modeling the interactions among immunological components. Major immunoinformatics developments include

- Immunological databases
- Sequence analysis and structure modeling of antibodies
- Modeling of the immune system
- Simulation of laboratory experiments
- Statistical support for immunological experimentation
- Immunogenomics, etc.

In future, these technological developments are expected to grow both in terms of their reliability and scope. Thus, this emerging pharmacoinformatics technology is becoming an essential component of pharmaceutical sciences.

INFORMATION DATABASES

An information system is a combination of computer hardware and software, organizes the data into information and enables the analysis of information to produce knowledge. The database system is a collection of related information and can be accessed through database management systems.

Manual paper-based systems are the traditional databases, and are associated with several problems such as storage requires large filling cabinet, data duplication, loss or damage and involves time consuming search. Computerized databases were developed to overcome the above mentioned problems.

These databases find applications in health care for patient care recording, surveillance of patient status and treatment advise. The databases were also assists research community in drug design and related clinical procedures. MEDLINE, International pharmaceutical abstract, Chemical abstract, Protein databank and Binding database are the few note worthy databases, used in pharmacoinformatics.

CHAPTER 1

DATABASES

Database is heart of pharmacoinformatics, provides adequate and updated information. In everyday life, we are in the need of information ranging from basic information to scientific information. Print and electronic indices (books and journals) developed to retain the published information, which facilitates quick identification of relevant information.

Technically database can be defined as

1. Physical collection of logically related records (data).
2. Collection of database files and each database file is a collection of records.

Four classes of databases known are

Archieval - It accepts data as it is and most are public. eg: GeneBank

Curated - Mostly private

Public

Private

1.1 Types of Databases

Three major types of pharmacoinformatics databases are known and are

1. Pharmaceutical databases
    (a) Literature database
    (b) Chemical database
2. Biological databases
    (a) Structure databases
    (b) Sequence databases

3. Relational databases
   (a) Structured Query Language (SQL)
   (b) Practical Extraction and Report Language (PERL)

1.2 Components of Databases

Database has two main components

1. Field: Each piece of information in a database is called field, which means the smallest unit in a database. In database there can be five categories of fields, they are:

   - Numeric
   - Character
   - Logic
   - Memo
   - Date

2. Record: All the related events of particular field constitute a record, which is a collection of logically related fields.

1.3 Database Schema

The overall description of a database is called as database schema and 3 types of schemas are known.

1. Internal schema: It contains definitions of the stored records and specifies how the data is stored.

2. External schema: It describes external views of the data, there are many external schema for the given database. It excludes irrelevant data as well as data which the user is not authorized to access.

3. Conceptual schema: It describes the types of data stored in database and relationships between them.

1.3.1 Database Architecture

- The database architecture defines the nature of the data and structure of the data.

- The database architecture specifies, set of rules and processes that dictate how data should be stored in a database and how data is accessed by components of a system.

- The database architecture includes data types, relationships and naming conventions. It describes the organization of all database objects and their working methodologies. It affects integrity, reliability, scalability and performance of database.

1.3.2 ANSI-SPARC 3 Level Architecture

American National Standard Institute - Standards Planning And Requirements Committee (ANSI - SPARC) is an abstract design standard for Database Management System (DBMS). Most commercial DBMS are based on this system.

1. It allows independent customized user views – each user should be able to access the same data.

2. It hides the physical storage details from users.

3. The database administrator should be able to change the database storage structure without affecting the user views.

4. The internal structure of the database should be able to changes to the physical aspects of the storage.

The database administrator should be able to change the conceptual or global structure of the database without affecting the users.

1.3.3 Data Redundancy

Identical data stored in two or more files are known as data redundancy.

Dependencies between attribute (column) causes data redundancy. It occurs in database systems which have a field that is repeated in two or more tables. It leads to data anomalies and corruption, hence should be avoided. Database normalization prevents redundancy by making use of proper foreign keys.

1.4 Database Applications

- Redundancy can be reduced
- Data inconsistencies can be avoided
- Allows data sharing and data migration between systems
- Provides security restriction
- Data integrity can be maintained
- Balances conflicting requirements.

1.5 Database Management System (DBMS)

The stress is given to creation as well as management of database. Database management involves creating, modifying, deleting and adding data in files and using this data to generate reports or answer the queries.

The software allows to perform these functions easily are called as database management system (DBMS). DBMS attempt to make the physical data non-redundant and also optimizes resource utilization. The windows based database available in the market is MS ACCESS, which is a part of Microsoft windows.

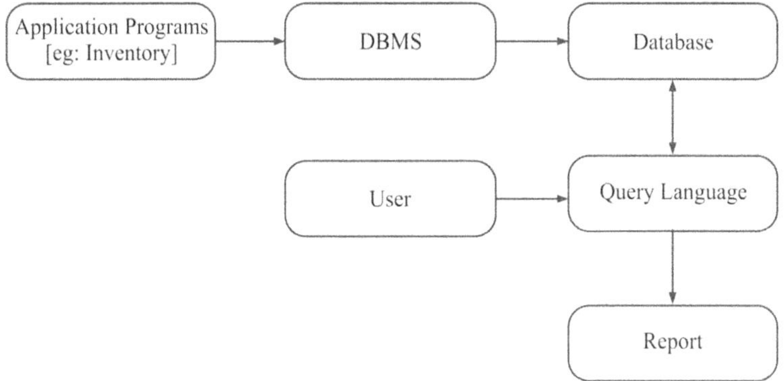

Fig. 1.1 Schema represents DBMS approach.

DBMS allows inserting, updating, deleting and processing of data. Some of the important DBMS are Oracle, Ingress, Sybase, Dbase 3+, Foxpro, MS access, Dataease, Dataflex, Advanced revelation., etc. Primary tasks of DBMS are:

- Database development: Define and organize the contents, relationships and structure of the data needed to build s database.
- Database interrogation: It involves information retrieval and report generation. End users can selectively display information, produce reports and documents.
- Database maintenance: It helps in adding, deleting, updating, correcting and protecting the data in a database.
- Application development: It is used to develop prototypes of data entry careens queries, forms, reports, tables and lebels for a prototype application / use 4th Generation Language (4GL) or application generator to develop program codes.

Benefits of DBMS

1. The amount of data redundancy in stored data can be reduced.
2. Data inconsistencies can be removed.
3. Stored data can be shared by a single or multiple users.
4. Standards can be set and followed.

5. Data integrity can be maintained.
6. Security of data can be implemented.
7. Data independence can be achieved.

1.6 Relational Database Management System

A relational database matches data by using common characteristics found within the data set. The resulting groups of data are organized and much easier for people to understand. Such a grouping uses the relational model / schema and this database is called as relational database. The soft ware used to do this grouping is called as relational database management system (RDMS).

1.7 Normalization

Database normalization is a critical part of good database architecture, which ensures data integrity and avoids data redundancy.

1.8 Relationship

Database relationship creates a history for the tables. A properly normalized database has a well-organized hierarchy. For each relationship between two tables, one table is the parent and one table is the child. For example, a patient table may be the parent of prescription detail table.

1.9 Primary and Foreign Keys

Database relationships are embodied through primary keys in parent tables and foreign keys in child tables.

- Primary key is a field in a table whose value uniquely identifies each record and defines relationship within a database.
- Foreign key is a field in a table that refers to parent records in another table. It need not have unique values in the referencing relation.

1.10 Elements of DBMS

- Data Definition Language (DDL): It provides link between logical and physical views of the database. It is used to define the physical characteristics of each record and fields.

- Data Manipulation Language (DML): It provides techniques for retrieval, sorting, display and deletion of data/records.

- Data Query Language (DQL): It allows retrieving data from the database and imposing ordering upon it.

- Data Control Language (DCL): It controls the access to data and to the database.

1.11 Relational Databases

A relational database uses relationally two-dimensional tables to store different pieces of information inside tables and nothing more. All operations on data are done on the tables themselves or produce other tables as a result. A relational database contains one or many tables, which is a basic storage structure of relational database management system (RDMS).

1.11.1 Relational Database Terminology

Relational database theory uses set of mathematical terms, which are roughly equivalent to Structured Query Language (SQL) database terminology.

Relational term	SQL equivalent
Realtion, base	table
Derived	view, query result, result set
Tuple	Row
Attribute	coloumn

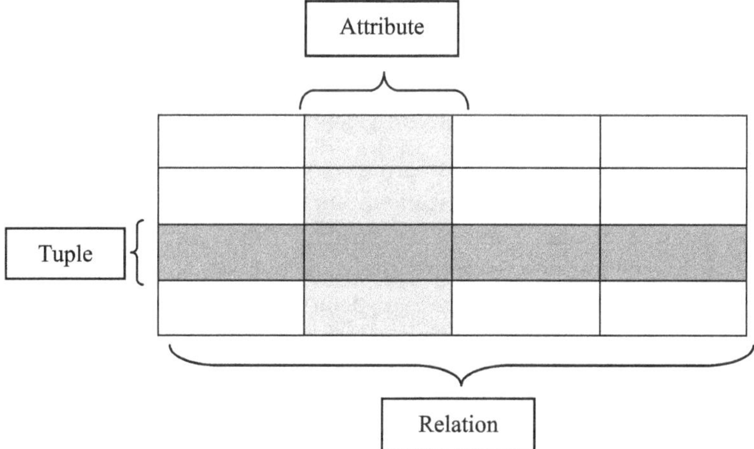

A table is set of rows and columns. Each row is set of column with only one value for each. All rows from the same table have the same set of columns. The row from a relational table is analogous to a record, and the columns to a field. Relational database serve in two ways.

1. Retrieving subset of its column.
2. Retrieving subset of its row.

1.12 Rules Governing Relational Database

CODD rules and Normalization rules are the two important rules which governs the functions of relational database.

1.12.1 Codd Rules

They specify set of rules that relational database must comply in order to be relational.

Rule 1 - The information rule

All data should be presented to the user in table form. Data are represented only one way; as values within columns within rows

1. The basic requirement of the relational database
2. Simple, consistent and versatile.

Rule 2 - Guarranteed access rule

All data should be accessible without ambiguity. This can be accomplished through a combination of the table name, primary key and column name.

1. Every value can be accessed by providing table name, column name and key.
2. All data are uniquely identified and accessible via this identity.

Rule 3 - Systematic insert, update and delete

All fields should be allowed to remain empty. This involves the support of a null value, which is distinct from an empty string or a number with a value of zero. This can't apply to primary keys. In addition, most database implementations support the concept of a nun-null field constraint that prevents null values in a specific table column.

Rule 4 - Dynamic on-line catalogue

A relational database must provide access through the same tools that are used to access data. This is usually accomplished by storing the structure definition within special system tables. Catalog can be queried by authorized users as part of the database.

Rule 5 - Comprehensive data sublanguage rule

The database must support at least one clearly defined language that includes functionality for data definition, data manipulation, data integrity and database transaction control. All commercial relational databases use forms of the standard SQL as their supported comprehensive language.

1. Used interactively and embedded within programs.
2. Supports data definition, data manipulation, security, integrity constraints and transaction processing.

Rule 6 - View updating rule

Data can be presented to the user in different logical combinations, called views. Each view should support the same full range of data manipulation that direct-access to a table has available. In practice, providing update and delete access to logical views is difficult and is not fully supported by any current database.

Rule 7 - High-level insert, update and delete

Data can be retrieved from a relational database in sets constructed of data from multiple rows and or multiple tables. This rule states insert, update and delete operations should be supported for any retrievable set rather than just for a single row in a single table.

Rule 8 - Physical data independence

The user is isolated from the physical method of storing and retrieving information from the database. Change can be made to the underlying architecture without affecting the user access.

Rule 9 - Logical data independence

Data should not change when logical structure changes. Users and programs are independent of the logical structure of the database.

Rule 10 - Integrity independence

SQL should support constraints on user input that maintain database integrity. All databases do preserve two constraints through SQL.

Rule 11 - Distribution independence

A user should be completely unaware of whether or not the database is distributed.

Rule 12 - No subversion rule

There should be no way to modify the database structure other than through the multiple row database language.

Codd's ZERO rule

The system be able to manage databases entirely through its relational capabilities, no matter what additional capabilities the system may support.

1.12.2 Normalization

Normalization is the process of simplifying the relationship between data elements in the records.

Title	Author name 1	Author name 2	ISBN	Subject	Pages	Publishers
PHP and MySQL Web Development	Luke Welling	Laura Thomson	0672317842	PHP, MySQL	867	Sams
MySQL tutorial	Luke Welling	Laura Thomson	0672317845	MySQL	300	Sams

This table is not very efficient with storage. The names of the authors are too long, contains many characters. The repetition of their names will occupy more storage space, and there is chance for entering their name with spell mistake. This leads to less efficient searching and gives results missing with some data. Normalization helps in this regard to reduce the redundant data, to improve storage efficiency, data integrity and scalability.

Normalization is a step by step decomposition of complex records into simple records and are carried out

1. To structure the data between tables so that data maintenance is simplified.
2. To allow data retrieval at optimal speed.
3. To simplify data maintenance through updates, inserts and deletes.
4. To reduce the need to restructure tables as new application by rationalization arise.
5. To improve the quality of design for an application by rationalization of table data.

Normalization decomposes data into two dimensional tables, eliminates any relationship in which table data does fully depend upon the primary key of a record and contains transitive dependencies. The database community developed series of guidelines called as normal forms. They are

- First normal form (1 NF)
- Second normal form (2 NF)
- Third normal form (3 NF)
- Fourth normal form (4 NF)
- Fifth normal form (5 NF)
- Domain / key normal form (DKNF)
- Sixth normal form (6 NF)

First normal form (1 NF)

The above table contains two (more than one) author field and contains more than one piece of information. This complicates the search operation and First normal form helps in overcoming these problems by modifying the table. 1NF involves the removal of redundant data from horizontal rows and ensures that there is no duplication of data in the table. 1NF creates separate tables for each group of related data and identify each row with a column or set of columns.

Normalized by 1NF

Title	Author	ISBN	Subject	Pages	Publishers
PHP and MySQL Web Development	Luke Welling	0672317842	MySQL	867	Sams
PHP and MySQL Web Development	Laura Thomson	0672317842	PHP	867	Sams
MySQL tutorial	Laura Thomson	0672317845	MySQL	300	Sams
MySQL tutorial	Luke Welling	0672317845	MySQL	300	Sams

In this case author and subject columns are reduced into one. Splitting the table into author table, subject table and book table will improves the normalization process.

Author ID

Author ID	First name	Last name
1	Luke	Welling
2	Laura	Thomson

Author table is splitted into two columns in order to store little information in each coloumn. Each table has a primary key, which connects all the tables when querying the data. A primary key must be unique (no two books will be given same ISBN number).

Subject table

Subject ID	Subject
1	MySQL
2	PHP

Book Table

ISBN	Title	Pages	Publisher
0672317842	PHP and MySQL Web Development	867	Sams
0672317845	MySQL Tutorial	300	Sams

Second normal form (2 NF)

Second normal form deals with redundancy of data in vertical columns. In this table publisher column contains repeating data. Second normal form breaks this table and creates separate publisher information table.

ISBN	Title	Pages	Publisher
0672317842	PHP and MySQL Web Development	867	Sams
0672317845	MySQL Tutorial	300	Sams

Normalised Table

Publisher ID	Publisher
1	Sams

1. 2NF meets all the requirements of the first normal form.

2. It removes subsets of data that apply to multiple rows of a table and places them in separate tables.

3. 2NF creates relationships between these new tables and their predecessors through the use of foreign keys.

Third normal form (3 NF)

3NF looks for data which is not dependent on the primary key and remove those columns.

1.13 Scripting Languages

Every computer architecture has its own 'machine language' such as FORTRAN, C, C++. A disadvantage of compilers is, whenever modification is made to source code, it must be recompiled before it can run. The computer scripts offer an 'alternative strategy', scripting languages, use interpreters instead of compilers. Python, Ruby and PERL are some of the popular scripting languages useful in pharmaco-informatics.

> **Script – What you give an actor ?**
>
> **Program – What you give an audience ?**

PERL - Practical Extraction and Report Language

PERL is a high level but easy to use programming language and available for most operating systems. It makes easy things easier and hard things possible where as professional programming languages make all things equally difficult. Using PERL series of complex tasks can be reduced to a single statement. PERL is preferred for processing sequence analysis and database management.

Bio-PERL

A popular tool-kit developed as a collection of integrated PERL modules for transforming and manipulating sequence data and annotations, accession remote databases and parsing output from programs such as BLAST, FASTA etc. Bio-PERL also facilitates local execution of programs from the EMBOSS suite. Bio-PERL modules save time and effort.

Applications of Bio-PERL

- Bioperl provides access to sequence data and transforming formats of databases
- Bioperl assists in sequence similarity search
- Bioperl creates and manipulates sequence alignment
- Bioperl is useful in searching structures of genome
- Bioperl develops machine readable annotations

Sequence analysis: Parsing and annotation is useful in the analysis of simple patterns and Bioperl provides mechanisms for parsing and running.

BLAST parsing: Parsing NCBI, WuBlast, bl2seq and psi-blast can be done through the bioperls modules

- Bio::Tools::Blast
- Bio::Tools::Bplite
- Bio::Tools::BPbl2seq
- Bio::Tools::BPpsilite

BLAST running: Running BLAST locally and remotely is built-in to bioperl through the modules

- Bio::Tools::Run::StandAloneBLast
- Bio::Tools::Run::RemoteBlast

Multiple sequence alignment parsing: Multiple sequence alignment are also staple of bioinformatics research. Bioperl offers the Bio::AlignIO system for reading and writing MSA reports produced by a variety of sources include ClustalW and CCG.

ClustalW and TCoffee: Parsing ClustalW and CCG can be done through the bioperls modules

- Bio::Tools::Run::Alignment::Clustal
- Bio::Tools::Run:: Alignment::TCoffee

Gene prediction and parsing: Genscan and Mzef produce Bio:: SeqFeature::GeneStructure for gene prediction and parsing

1.14 Structured Query Language (SQL)

Structured Query Language (SQL) has been a command language, provides an interface to relational database systems. In common usage of SQL also encompasses Data Manipulations Language (DML), for INSERTs, UPDATEs, DELETEs and Data Definition Language (DDL), used for creating and modifying tables and other database structures.

A relational database uses, relationally or two-dimensional tables to store different pieces of information inside tables and nothing more. All operations on data are done on the tables themselves or produce other tables as the result. A relational database contains one or many tables, which is a basic storage structure of relational database management system (RDMS). Each row is set of column with only one value for each.

All rows from the same table have the same set of columns. The row from a relational table is analogous to a record, and the columns to a field. Relational database serves in two ways

> ➢ Retrieving subset of its column.

> ➢ Retrieving subset of its row.

S. No	Medicine name	Category	Cost	Expiry date

Properties

1. It can be accessed and modified by executing Structured Query Language (SQL) statements.

2. It contains a collection of tables with no physical pointers and uses a set of operators.

3. A single row or table representing all data required for a particular medicine, each row in a table should be identified by a primary key, which allows no duplicate key / values.

4. A column or an attribute contains the medicine name.

5. The serial number identifies a medicine in the table. In this example, the serial number column is designated as primary key.

6. A primary key must contain value and the value must be unique.

7. A column containing cost value is a foreign key which defines how table relate to each other.

8. A field may have no value in it, this is called a null value.

9. A field can be found at the intersection of row and column, there can be one value in it.

General guideline for executing SQL commands

- SQL commands may be on one / many line.

- Clauses are usually placed on separate lines.

- Tabulation can be used.

- Command words can't be split across lines.

- SQL commands are not case sensitive.

- Place a semi-colon (;) at the end of the last clause.

SQL features

- SQL can be used by a range of users, including those with little or no program knowledge.
- It is non procedural language.
- It reduces the amount of time required for creating and maintaining systems

SQL rules

1. It starts with a verb, each verb is followed by number of clauses and a space ( ) separates clauses.
2. A comma (,) separates parameters without a clause.
3. A semicolon (;) is used to end SQL statements.
4. Statement may be split across lines but keywords may not.
5. Lexical units such as identifiers, operator names, literals are separated by one or more spaces or other delimiters that will not be confused with the lexical unit.
6. Reserved words cannot be used as identifiers unless enclosed with double quotes.
7. Identifier can contain up to 30 characters and must start with an alphabetic character.
8. Character and date literals must be enclosed within single quotes.
9. Numeric literals can be represented by simple values.
10. Scientific notation as 2×10^5.
11. Comments may be enclosed between /*and*/ symbols and may be multi line.
12. Single line comments may be prefixed with a – symbol.

Components of SQL

Data definition language (DDL): It is set of SQL commands used to create, modify and delete database structures but not data.

Examples:

Create: To create objects / tables in the database.

Alter: Alter the structure of the database.

Drop: Delete objects from the database.

Truncate: Remove all records from a table, including all spaces allocated for the records are removed.

Data Manipulation Language (DML): It is area of SQL that changing data within the database.

Examples:

Insert: Insert records (database) into a table

Update: Updates existing data within a table.

Delete: Deletes specified records from a table, the space for the records remain.

Call: Call a PL/SQL or Java program.

Explain Plan: Explain access path to data.

Lock: TABLE control concurrency.

Data Control Language (DCL): It is the component of SQL statement that control access to data and to the database.

Examples:

Commit: Save work done

Save Point: Identify a point in a transaction to which we can roll back

Rollback: Restore database to original since the last COMMIT

Set Transaction: Change transaction options like what rollback segment to use.

Grant /Revoke: Grant or take back permissions to or from the oracle users.

Data Query Language (DQL): It is the component of SQL statement that allows retrieving data from the database and imposing ordering upon it.

Example

Select: Retrieve data from the database.

Using CREATE command

```
SQL> create table database(sno number(2),name varchar(5),fname varchar(5),place varchar(6),contact n
umber(10));

Table created.
```

Using INSERT command

```
SQL> insert into database values(&sno,'&name','&fname','&place',&contact);
Enter value for sno: 21
Enter value for name: arun
Enter value for fname: g
Enter value for place: hyd
Enter value for contact: 9876543210
old   1: insert into database values(&sno,'&name','&fname','&place',&contact)
new   1: insert into database values(21,'arun','g','hyd',9876543210)

1 row created.
```

Using "/" helps adding next set of data (record) without writing new insert command

```
SQL> /
Enter value for sno: 22
Enter value for name: kumar
Enter value for fname: g
Enter value for place: sec
Enter value for contact: 8796423121
old   1: insert into database values(&sno,'&name','&fname','&place',&contact)
new   1: insert into database values(22,'kumar','g','sec',8796423121)

1 row created.

SQL> /
Enter value for sno: 23
Enter value for name: kumar
Enter value for fname: g
Enter value for place: hyd
Enter value for contact: 9854232110
old   1: insert into database values(&sno,'&name','&fname','&place',&contact)
new   1: insert into database values(23,'kumar','g','hyd',9854232110)

1 row created.
```

Using SELECT command

```
SQL> select * from database;

       SNO NAME  FNAME PLACE     CONTACT
---------- ----- ----- ------ ----------
        21 arun  g     hyd    9876543210
        22 kumar g     sec    8796423121
        23 kumar g     hyd    9854232110
```

Using SELECT command

```
SQL> select name, place from database;

NAME  PLACE
----- ------
arun  hyd
kumar sec
kumar hyd
```

Using DISTINCT command

```
SQL> select distinct place from database;

PLACE
------
hyd
sec
```

Using AND command

```
SQL> select * from database where name='kumar' and fname='g';

       SNO NAME  FNAME PLACE    CONTACT
---------- ----- ----- ------ ----------
        22 kumar g     sec    8796423121
        23 kumar g     hyd    9854232110
```

Using OR command

```
SQL> select * from database where name='kumar' or fname='m';

       SNO NAME  FNAME PLACE    CONTACT
---------- ----- ----- ------ ----------
        22 kumar g     sec    8796423121
        23 kumar g     hyd    9854232110
        24 mani  m     hyd    9876453423
```

Using DELETE command

```
SQL> delete from database where sno=23;

1 row deleted.

SQL> select * from database;

       SNO NAME  FNAME PLACE    CONTACT
---------- ----- ----- ------ ----------
        21 aruna g     hyd    9876543210
        22 kumar g     sec    8796423121
        24 mani  m     hyd    9876453423
        25 msdhu g     bply   8746453533
```

Using TRUNCATE command

```
SQL> truncate table database;

Table truncated.

SQL> select * from database;

no rows selected
```

Truncate command removes data only and retains the constructed table, so that data can be added further.

```
SQL> insert into database values(&sno,'&name','&fname','&place',&contact);
Enter value for sno: 26
Enter value for name: meena
Enter value for fname: r
Enter value for place: kply
Enter value for contact: 8797967564
old   1: insert into database values(&sno,'&name','&fname','&place',&contact)
new   1: insert into database values(26,'meena','r','kply',8797967564)

1 row created.
```

Using SELECT command

```
SQL> select * from database;

       SNO NAME  FNAME PLACE    CONTACT
---------- ----- ----- ------ ----------
        26 meena r     kply   8797967564
```

Using DROP command

```
SQL> drop table database;

Table dropped.
```

Drop command completely removes the constructed table along with stored data.

```
SQL> insert into database values(&sno,'&name','&fname','&place',&contact);
Enter value for sno: 27
Enter value for name: ravi
Enter value for fname: r
Enter value for place: hyd
Enter value for contact: 9877676662
old   1: insert into database values(&sno,'&name','&fname','&place',&contact)
new   1: insert into database values(27,'ravi','r','hyd',9877676662)
insert into database values(27,'ravi','r','hyd',9877676662)
            *
ERROR at line 1:
ORA-00942: table or view does not exist
```

## CHAPTER 2

DATA MINING

Data mining is the process of extraction of hidden predictive information from large databases. It is a powerful new technology with great potential to help companies focus on the most important information in their data warehouses. It is related to the sub area of statistics called exploratory data analysis, which has similar goals and relies on statistical measures. It is also closely related to artificial intelligence called knowledge discovery and machine learning.

Data mining is the process of discovering valid, novel, understandable and potentially useful patterns in data. Data mining include data collection, data cleaning, data engineering, algorithm engineering, algorithm running, result evaluation and knowledge utilization. Data mining process can be grouped in to

1. Supervised: discovers predictive pattern

2. Unsupervised: Provides relationship between data's

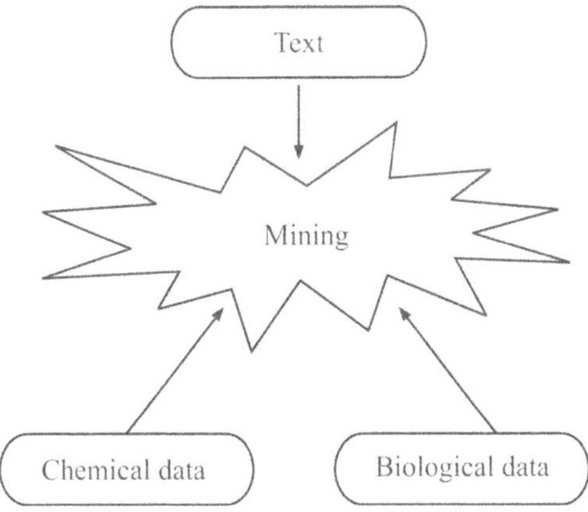

Fig. 2.1 Types of data mining.

2.1 Data Mining Tasks

It commonly involves four classes of tasks.

- Clustering: A process of discovering similar groups and structures in the data without using known structures in the data.

- Classification: An attempt to classify molecules based on the presence and absence of pharmacophore is typical example for this type.

- Regression: An attempt to find a function, which models the data with the least error.

- Association rule learning: Searches for relationships between variables and is also known as market basket analysis.

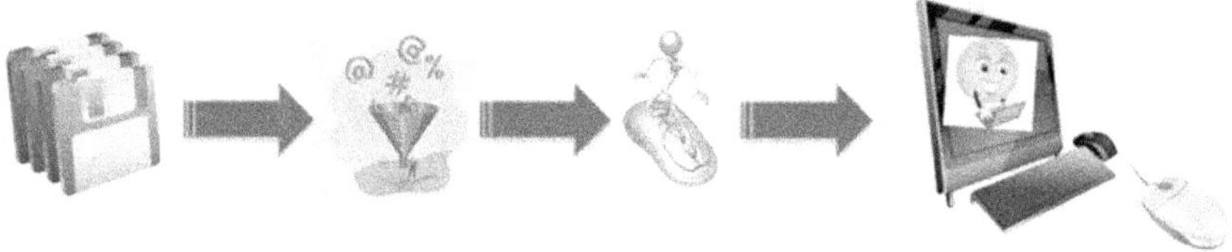

Fig. 2.2 Process of data mining.

2.2 Data Mining Techniques

The most commonly used techniques in data mining are

- Artificial neural networks: Non-linear predictive models that learn through and resemble biological neural networks in structure.

- Decision trees: Tree-shaped structures that represent sets of decisions to generate rules for the classification of a dataset. Specific decision tree methods include classification and regression Trees (CART) and Chi Automatic Interaction Detection (CAID).

- Genetic algorithms: Optimization techniques that use process such as genetic combination, mutation and natural selection in a design based on the concepts of evolution.

- Nearest neighbor method: A technique that classifies each record in a dataset based on a combination of the classes.

2.3 Knowledge Discovery in Databases (KDD)

Knowledge discovery in databases (KDD) is a branch of data mining. The number and the size of databases are rapidly growing because of the large amount of data obtained and this growth exceeds human capacities to analyze the databases. KDD facilitates the automatic searching of large volume of data and it is the non-trivial extraction of implicit, previously unknown and potentially useful information from databases. Typical tasks of KDD includes:

1. Clustering
2. Classification / regression
3. Empirical discovery: The discovery of associations / deviations in spatial databases.

Essential elements of KDD

- Efficiency and accuracy.
- High-level language.
- Automated learning.

Applications

1. It is used in information retrieval process.
2. It enables new patterns discovery process.

2.4 Data Mining Applications

Data mining is widely used in the fields of engineering, bioinformatics, genetics, medicine and education.

- Bioinformatics software tools derives genes/proteins involved in particular disease and identifies therapeutic targets through computer analysis of biological data.
  - ProFunc: predicts protein function from 3D structure.
  - Pocket-Finder: a binding pocket detection algorithm.
  - Q-siteFinder: a new method of ligand binding site prediction.
  - P-CATS (Prediction of CATalytic residueS in proteins): predicts the catalytic residues in proteins from the atomic coordinates.
- Data mining in genetics:
  - It helps in understanding the mapping relationship between the inter-individual variation in human DNA sequences and variability in disease susceptibility.
  - It finds outs how the changes in an individual's DNA sequence are related with the risks of developing common diseases such as cancer.
  - It helps in the diagnosis, prevention and treatment of the diseases (multifactor dimensionality reduction).

- Data mining in adverse drug reaction surveillance:
  - It is used to screen drug safety issues in the WHO global database and produces a report of suspected adverse drug reactions.
- Data mining in educational research:
  - It is utilised to identify the factors leading students to reduce their learning capabilities.
- Subject-based data mining:
  - It uses an initiating datum to determine how other information's are related to the initiating datum.

2.5 Bibliographic Databases

Bibliographic database is the specialized database designed for handling bibliographic references. They are also known as personal information systems, bibliographic reference managers, or personal bibliographic software. These systems help in three essential research tasks.

1. Building a database of references to journal articles, books and other research publications, using both manual and electronic input methods.
2. Searching the created database by author, subject, journal name and other criteria.
3. Generating a list of selected references from the database in a format required for publication.

2.5.1 Database Structure

- It accommodates unlimited number of records and creates more than one database.
- Records in one database can be copied or moved to other databases.
- Numerous input forms for different citation formats (e.g., journals, theses) are allowed.
- Customizable field displays and records can be sorted based on field type (e.g., date, author, journal title).
- Imports records downloaded from external indexes, catalogs and from word processor files.
- Detects duplicate records and performs spell check of records.
- Edits records individually or globally and creates authority lists for selected fields.

2.5.2 Applications

- Formats references in multiple bibliographic styles to meet the requirements of scholarly publications.

- Creates independent bibliographies organized by subject.

- Exports references in different file formats for use in other programs.

- Creates course reserve list and reading lists for students.

- Maintains faculty publication lists, catalogs special collections and reprint collections.

- Maintains bibliographies of references in research areas of personal interest.

- Creates and maintains a reference database shared across a network.

2.6 Library Catalogue

A library catalogue is a register of all bibliographic items found in a library or network of libraries. It describes WHAT the library owns, tells WHERE the items are stored and shows HOW to get those items. Library catalogue gives access to physical items (books, CDs, etc) and electronic resources. Many libraries have replaced card catalogue with online public access catalog (OPAC) for the purpose of saving space for other use, such as additional shelving.

2.6.1 Types

- Author catalogue: Sorted alphabetically according to the authors or editors names.

- Title catalogue: Sorted alphabetically according to the title of the entries.

- Dictionary catalogue: A catalog in which all entries (author, title, subject, series) are interfiled in a single alphabetical order.

- Keyword catalogue: Sorted alphabetically according to some system of keywords.

- Mixed alphabetic catalogue forms: Contains mixed author / title, or an author / title / keyword catalogue.

2.6.2 Cataloguing Rules

It allows consistent cataloguing of various library materials. It clarifies how to find an entry and how to interpret the data in an entry. The larger a collection, the more elaborate cataloguing rules are needed. Cataloguing rules prescribe:

- Which information from a bibliographic item is included in the entry?
- How this information is presented on a catalogue card or in a cataloguing record?
- How the entries should be sorted in the catalogue?

2.6.3 Online Public Access Catalogue (OPAC)

The card catalog has been effectively replaced by Online Public Access Catalogue (OPAC). OPAC need not be sorted, the user can choose author, title, keyword or systemic order. OPAC offer many advantages over card catalogue such as space saving, accessible to visually impaired and wheel chair bound people.

CHAPTER 3

SEARCH MACHINES

On-line databases can be utilized for information search through search engines. In 1994, one of the first web search engine, the World Wide Web Worm (WWWW) had an index of 110,000 web pages and web accessible documents. As of November, 1997, the top search engines claim to index from 2 million (WebCrawler) to 100 million web documents. It is foreseeable that by the year 2020, a comprehensive index of the Web will contain over a billion documents. Search engines crawl the Web and log the words from the web pages they find in their databases. Using a search engine without a clear search strategy is like trying to find a particular book in the stacks of a library. Search engines vary in size, accuracy, features, and flexibility. The program (CGI, server module or separate server) that accepts the request from the URL, searches the index, and returns the results page

3.1 Types of Search

Sequential and binary search are the two major types of search.

- Sequential search: It is the most straightforward and elementary search and also known as linear search. A search for data that compares each record in a file (or each items in a list) one after the other. Finding a specific item from the book in first instant is difficult and it requires sequential search (alphabet sorting).

- Binary search: It locates the position of the item in a sorted array and is also known as half interval search. Looking for the specific item approximately half way is the best example of this kind. If the query starts with alphabet 'S', then the first half of the book need not to be viewed.

Search machines bring relevant information after going through number of operations. They are as follows:

- Key word searching: Using appropriate keyword will exclude irrelevant pages.

- Refining the search: Search machines provide refined search through Boolean operators (AND, OR, NOT, + and – .

- Relevancy ranking: In most search machines the result page appears with hits according to their relevancy.

- Meta tags: Web page author can decide the keywords to index the document.

- Concept based searching: Concept based search try to determine what the query mean exactly. The query heart apart from coronary, stroke, cholesterol and arteriosclerosis also returns hits on love, and passion.

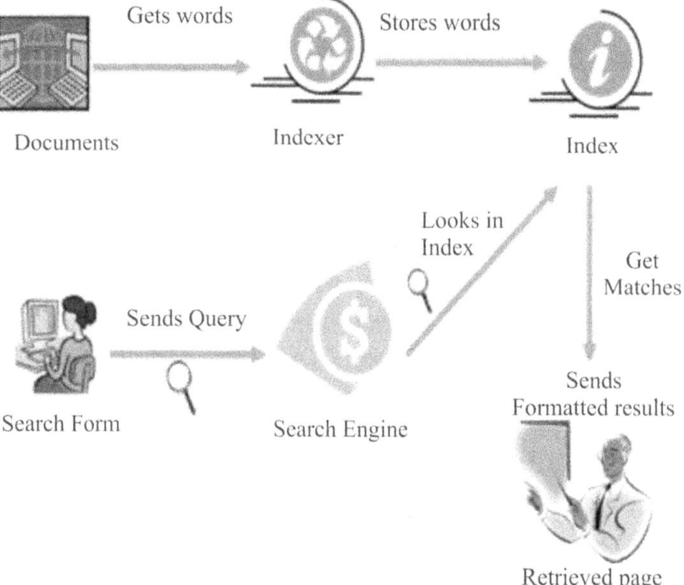

Fig. 3.1 Process of information search.

3.2 Search Strategies

Search machines retrieves the information from the databases, indexer collects key words and store them in index. Once the query is submitted machine matches the key word of the query to the index key words and rank them according to their previous browsing.

Strategy 1 (keyword/phrase search in all fields)

- Removes stopwords, stems the remaining words and searches for the words in all searchable fields

- Punctuation marks and stopwords are replaced with the Boolean AND, but the words in between are retained as phrases.

Strategy 2 (subject headings search)

- The first approach was to identify the best matching headings.
- The second approach was to identify exact matches.

3.3 Search Algorithms

Algorithms are set of rules that precisely define sequence of operations. They are deeply concerned with the process of sorting and searching the data, which provides an ideal framework for the application to information retrieval. Many computer programs contain algorithms that specify instructions for calculation, data processing and automated reasoning. Different kinds of algorithms used are

Soundex algorithm: It is based on the six phonetic human speech sounds and it includes:

- Bilabial: Sound produces with both the lips.
- Dental: Articulated with the tip or blade of the tongue against / near the upper front teeth.
- Labiodental: Utter with the participation of the lip and teeth.
- Alveolar: Articulated with the tip of the tongue touching or near the teeth ride.
- Velar: Formed with the back of the tongue touching or near soft palate, the velar 'k' of 'kill' cool.
- Glottal: The interruption of the stream during speech by closure of the glottis.

Metaphone algorithm: It is alternative to soundex algorithm and it reduces the word to a 1-4 character code using relatively simple phonetic rules. It ignores all the occurrences of vowels after the leading letter, but retaining the same when they come as an initial. It reduces alphabet to 16 consonant sounds viz B, X, S, K, J, T, F, H, L, M, N, P, R, O, W and Y, where the 'sh' is represented as X and zero as 'th' sound.

Phonex: The word is derived from metaphone and soundex and it gives only 36.37 % correct matches.

Stemming algorithm: It converts a word to root. Conversion of plurals to singulars and derivation of verb from the gerund is the best example of this algorithm.

3.4 Search Guidelines

A search engine is not a human, it is a program that matches the words given on the web. So describe the need with as few terms as possible, because each additional word limits the results. Choose descriptive words, the more unique the word the more likely to get good results.

Search basics

- Phrase search: Several words in the query (implicit *and*) fragments the sentence and increases the number of results. So putting double quotes (" ") around a set of words, helps considering the word in exact order without any change.
- Search within specific website: Specifying the exact website improves the search.
- Synonyms: The tilde ~ in front of a word (no space after the tilde) considers the synonyms.
- Terms to exclude: Minus sign (-) immediately before a word (without space) ignores that word containing page.
- AND function: AND (in upper case) in front of each word includes two or more prescribed words.
- Fill in the blanks: The * or wildcard, helps finding unknown term(s).
- Plus (+): Plus (+) sign immediately before word matches that word precisely and ignores synonyms.
- Alternative spelling: OR operator (in capital) in front of the query allows alternative words in the search.
- Prepositions: Ignore prepositions like 'the', 'a', and 'for'.
- Punctuation: Punctuation in popular word having particular meaning are not ignored (examples include dollar sign, underscore sign, etc.).

3.5 Search Engines

Some of the important search engines are listed below

- Google   www.google.com
- Bing   www.bing.com
- Yahoo   www.yahoo.com
- Altavista   www.altavista.com

Google: www.google.com

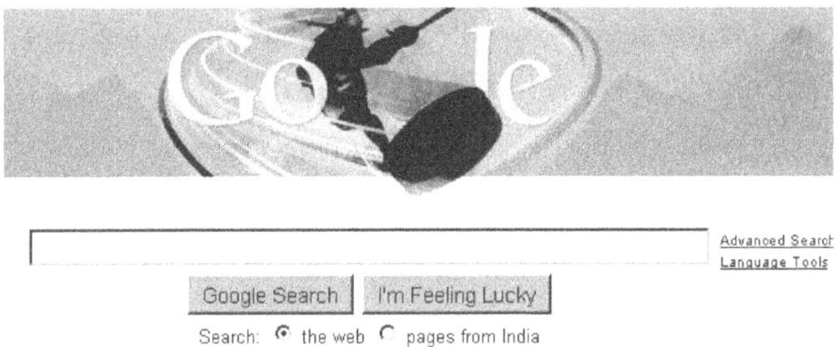

Typing key words and click on search button instantly generates results. The keywords should go from the general to the more particular to retrieve relevant information pages. Usage of syntax, ignoring capitals and typing in lower case may improve the search strategy. Google has a in-built spelling checker. To be certain of finding the phrase place 'to be or not to be' in double inverted commas ("   ") or use the exact phrase space in advanced search. The advanced search option can be used to specify the file format of result i.e *.doc, *.ppt, *.pdf and *.html.

The result page contains the following components

1. The title: The title of the webpage.
2. The snippet: The algorithmic attempt to extract the part of the page most relevant to the page.
3. The URL: The web page address.
4. Cached link: A link to the earlier version of the web page (it can be used if the page wanted is not available).

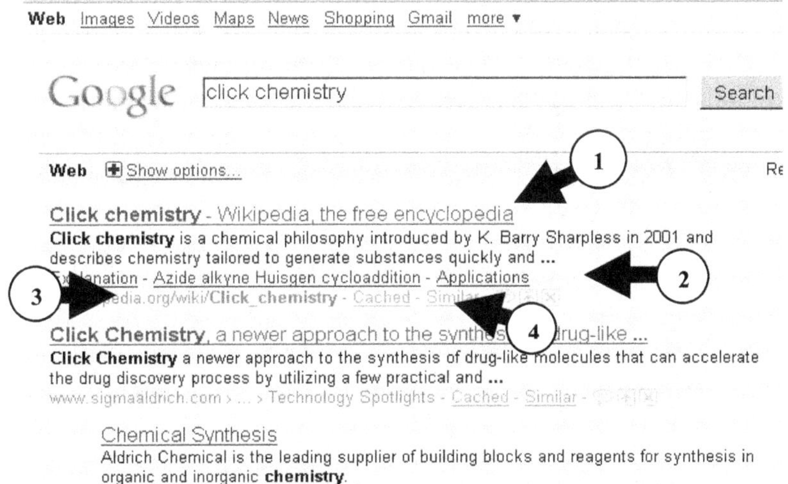

Google Scholar

Google Scholar provides a simple way to broadly search for scholarly literature across many disciplines and sources.

Features

- Explores related works, citation, authors and publications.
- Identifies recent development in any area of research.

Search tips for Google Scholar

1. Finding recent papers: Using "since year", "sort by date" options (left sidebar) helps in finding newer articles.
2. Locating full text article: Using "FindIt@Harvard" and "PDF" present in right of the search result and "all versions", "related articles" / "cited by" options enables one to find full text article.
3. Use secondary sources like "Wikipedia" to pick up the correct terminologies (correct term for "over weight" is "padiatric hyper-alimentation")

Bing Search (Microsoft Network): http://www.bing.com

Bing (formerly Live Search, Windows Live Search, and MSN Search) is a web search engine from Microsoft. It is based on a partnership between Microsoft and the local PBL network. Three design goals are set in the development of Bing are delivering great results; delivering a more organized experience; and simplifying tasks and providing insight. All these leads to faster and more confident decisions. It provides features such as best match, deep links (allowing more insight) and preview (provide a better sense of the related site's relevancy). It also includes explore pane, web groups, related searches and quick tabs. In being results will be displayed in the order of presented in order of popularity.

PATIENT CENTRIC PHARMACOINFORMATICS

Patient centric pharmacoinformatics focus on the adverse drug events (ADEs). It streamlines and improves the accuracy and efficiency of the medication use. Drug information services and pharmacy automation are the major discipline which provides quality health care.

Major health risks are mainly due to the improper use and administration of drugs. Drug information provides critically examined and relevant information of any aspect of drug use. Hospital patient care also an important risk factor for medication errors. Improving patient care through automation is an emerging technology, which improves quality care of patients. Technologies such as computerised physician order entry (CPOE), telemedicine, electronic reminders, barcode verification and electronic medication administration record (eMAR) helps in reducing ADEs.

## CHAPTER 4

DRUG INFORMATION

Drug information is the provision of unbiased, well-referenced and critically evaluated up-to-date information on any aspect of drug use. It includes written and oral information about medicines and pharmacotherapy, in response to a request from health care providers, organisations, committees and patients. The provision of accurate and timely drug information is a salient part of rational drug therapy. This promotes the safe and effective use of medicines. Proper use of medications requires critically evaluated relevant information for physicians, nurses and patients.

- **Drug information:** It refers to overall pharmacy service/ pharmaceutical care process.

- **Medicine information:** It highlights the functions related to medicinal drugs rather than drugs of abuse.

- **Poison information:** It provides information on the toxic effects of an extensive range of chemicals, plants and animal toxins.

4.1 Development of Drug Information

Pharmacists are ideally placed to provide drug information to the health professionals and the consumers. Development of drug information centers (DICs) and drug information specialists are the important step in clinical pharmacy concept. The DIC is involved directly and indirectly in patient care and act as a monitor of its characteristics. The DIC should provide professional services to support the Pharmacy and Therapeutics Committee (PTC). The following guidelines are to be followed to set up DICs.

1. Professional and technical competence in the evaluation of literature will be a pre-requisite.

2. The DIC pharmacist should be familiar with electronics, basic computer literacy data processing methodology

3. The information with supporting documentation to permit independent, informed conclusions and decisions should be made available.

4. Written and verbal communication skills regarding pharmaco-therapeutic information is essential quality required from pharmacist.

4.2 Drug Information Resources

Pharmacists and pharmaceutical scientists assist patients in meeting their information needs with regard to drugs, therapies and diseases. Effectively communicating the wealth of information available to those needing is a major concern.

There are three resources available for drug information service

1. Primary sources

2. Secondary sources

3. Tertiary sources

Primary resources: The primary resource of the drug information is the scientific journals. The journal is the channel through which scientific research has been reported, evaluated and disseminated. These literatures provide up-to-date information on drugs.

Eg: American Journal of Health-Systems Pharmacy

Secondary sources: Compilations, commentaries and digests of the primary scientific literature are referred to as secondary literature. Drug monographs and treatises are also the secondary sources. Indexing and abstracting services are valuable tools for quick and selective screening of the primary literature for specific information, data, citation and articles.

Eg: Micromedix and Poisindex

Tertiary sources: It includes text books, compendia computer databases and review articles. Textbooks serve as a state-of-the-art summation for a particular area. Major draw backs associated with text books are insufficient information because of lack of space and informations are out of date.

Eg: Drug Design: Medicinal Chemistry [E.J. Ariens]

Compendium of Organic Medicinal Chemistry Drugs: [Raj. B. Durai raj and Magesh Sathaiah].

4.3 Evaluation of Literatures

Clinical pharmacist at DIC can provide complete and updated information regarding the drugs to health care professionals and patients. The clinical literatures give clinical pharmacist abreast of new developments to answer questions addressed by health professionals (physicians and nurses). Poorly analyzed literature makes them irrelevant for the use. So, critical evaluation of the available information is very much necessary.

The DIC pharmacist performs an impartial scholarly evaluation of new drugs and published literature. Hence, the DIC pharmacist should be professionally and technically competent in the evaluation, critical selection and utilization of drug literature. Critical evaluation of literature involves the following steps

1. The objective of the research should be determined first.

2. The profile of study population should be analyzed by assessing the following information.

    - Objective of the study
        - Is the goal of the study stated clearly?
        - Was the research limited to a single objective or were there multiple drugs / effects being tested?

    - Subjects of the study
        - Were the subjects used in the study is animals or human volunteers and healthy?
        - Number of subjects included in the study and their age, sex, race and other criteria.
        - Other disease details, if any, disease being treated.
        - Additional treatments given and their contraindications to the therapy.

3. The administration and details of treatment with the agent being studied like route, dose and frequency of administration in relation to factors affecting absorption.

4. The environment of the study and dates on which the trial began and ended.

    - Professionals who made the observations.
    - Whether the study was done on an inpatient or outpatient basis.
    - Description of the physical setting and length of the study.

5. The methods and design of the study

   The study design and the methods used to complete the study are very important in judging whether the study and the results are valid.

   - Methods of assessing the therapeutic effects and standardization protocol.

   - Control measures used to reduce variation that might influence the results.

   - Controls used to reduce bias.
     - Blind assessment: The professionals don't know who is a subject and who is a control.
     - Blind patients: The patients don't know whether they received the substance or a placebo.
     - Random allocation: Patients involved in the study have even chance of being group of subjects receiving the active drug or the group receiving controls.
     - Matching dummies: Comparison of a placebo / therapy to a recognized standard practice.

6. The result perspective to current knowledge and its significancy.

7. The complete list of authors, publications and references cited.

8. Evaluation of the literature analysis

   - Suitability of the subjects and validity of the measurement methods

   - Appropriateness of the data, design, dosage, duration and control

   - The comparability of treatment groups examined

   - If statistical tests were not done, were they unnecessary or overlooked?

   - Assessment of statistical methods

   Thus critical evaluation of each article is carried out and key article and journals are selected for storage at drug information centers.

4.4 Literature Databases

Print and electronic indices retains control over the phenomenal growth in the quantity of published information (includes books and journals). Earlier print medium helped in storage, retrieval and dissemination of information and are outdated the day they are published. Advances in computer technology have made most of the printed tools obsolete and many electronic indexes can be accessed from desktop computers. It facilitates quick identification of relevant information.

Scientific information retrieval and literature search, previously dominated by librarians, is now directly available to a widespread group of scientists through web search engines. These research groups in laboratories, universities and academic institutes were connected to the internet. It helps to search and obtain information, in performing analysis on research data. Some indexes even link to the full text articles themselves. The internet has number of resources (pharmaceutical databases) for information and become an important tool for biological scientists including pharmaceutical scientists.

Table 4.1 List of journals based on their discipline.

Pharmaceutical scientists	European Journal of Pharmacology
	Journal of Natural Products
	Pharmaceutical Research
	Indian Journal of Pharmacology
Clinical pharmacist	JAMA: Journal of American Medical Association
	New England Journal of Medicine
	American Journal of Health-Systems Pharmacy
	Annals of Pharmacotherapy
	Indian Journal of Pharmacology
Researches in pharmacy administration	Journal of Pharmaceutical Marketing and Management
	Pharmacoeconomics
Teachers of pharmacy	American Journal of Pharmaceutical education
	Journal of Pharmacy Teaching
	Indian Journal Pharmaceutical Education and Research
	The Indian Pharmacist

MEDLARS (MEDical Literature Analysis and Retrieval System) developed by National Library of Medicine (NLM) and MEDLINE made revolution in this field. The most widely used databases by pharmacists and pharmaceutical scientists are listed below

    1. MEDLINE

    2. EMBASE

3. International Pharmaceutical Abstract
4. Chemical abstracts
5. BIOSIS previews

MEDLINE and EMBASE are the large medical databases. Searching on-line databases appears to be easy–deceptively. But successful search requires a great deal of skill and prior experience.

MEDLINE: It is produced by US International Library of Medicine is the prominent bio medical database and it covers of *3500 highly* reputed journals. This database gives medical informations (clinical and therapeutic topics). PubMed and Internet Grateful Med (IGM) are the two search engines available are MEDLINE.

EMBASE: It is produced by Elsevier and covers *3500 journals.* EMBASE covers European literature in much more depth than does MEDLINE. This is stronger in drug information and in areas of biological science related to human medicine.

International Pharmaceutical Abstract (IPA): IPA is produced by the American Society of Health-System Pharmacists and covers publications including pharmacy trade magazines, state pharmacy journals and the meeting abstracts of pharmacy related associations. It provides a comprehensive collection of information on drug use and development. As a primary source of drug-related health literature, IPA provides pharmacists, poison information specialists, drug information centers, the pharmaceutical industry, health practitioners, pharmacologists, medical librarians, cosmetic companies, environmentalists, educators, toxicologists, and litigators with information from over 800 health journals throughout the world. Many pharmacy and pharmaceutical science topics are much better searched in IPA.

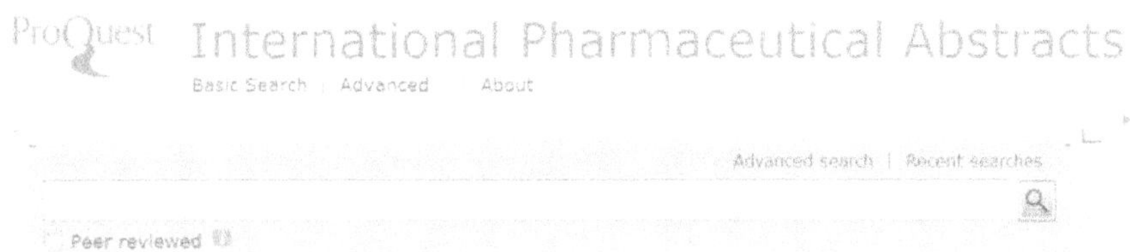

Chemical Abstracts: Chemical Abstract is the world's largest scientific database, produced by American Chemical Society's Chemical Abstracts Service in Columbus. It contains *72 million* abstracts from journals, patents, technical reports, books, conference proceedings and dissertations. It is the most important database for drug development.

BIOSIS Previews: This is online version of Biological Abstracts and the Bio Research index. It covers the literature of the life science, including pre-clinical toxicity and carcinogenicity studies.

Other databases

Iowa Drug Information Service	SEDBASE
NDA pipeline	Toxlit
Pharmaprojects.	Unlisted drugs
Scisearch	Drugs of the Future

4.5 PubMED

MEDLINE and PREMEDLINE are available freely through Internet Grateful Med (IGM) and PubMED. PubMED offers simple and advanced search options. Advanced search option enables search retrieval efficiency. Simple search can be carried out by entering keywords in a search window. PubMed enhance the search by combining key term and MeSH terms.

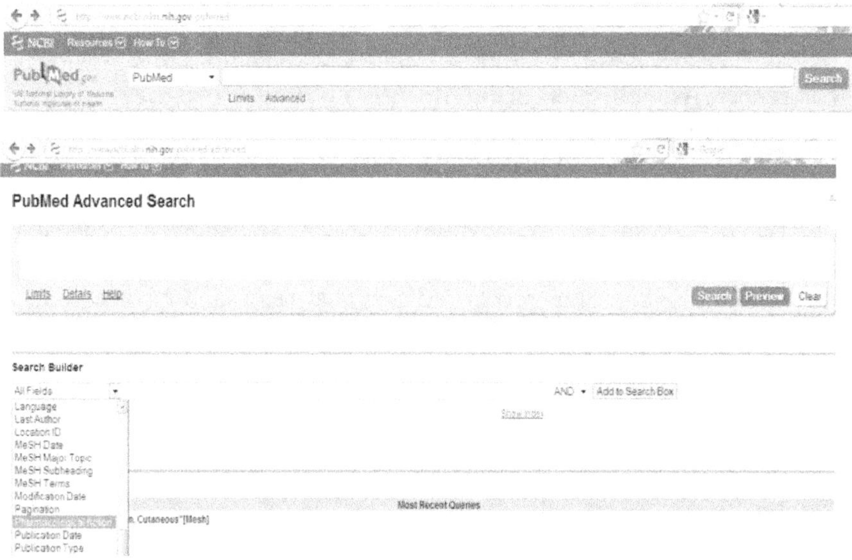

PubMed Features

1. It provides access to older references of INDEX MEDICUS back to 1951 and earlier.
2. It provides references to journals before they were indexed (Science, British Medical Journal and Annal of Surgery).

3. It provides spell checker, advanced search special tools such as ClinicalTrials.gov®, MedlinePlus®, and PubMed central.
4. It assists in finding search terms using Medical Subject heading (MeSH) browser.
5. Citations can be stored using My NCBI option and updates can be received through e- mail.
6. It provide link to full text articles and other subsets available in NLM.

Medical Subject Heading (MeSH) browser: MeSH is a controlled vocabulary used to index articles entered into the database. Subject experts at NLM read appropriate terminology to define those topics. The terms are then attached to the article as its index terminology and entered into MEDLINE along with article citation. Use of these terminologies in the search makes extraction of information more accurate and comprehensive. MeSH avoids the use of synonyms and acronyms. PubMed automatically link to MeSH terms and subheadings.

Searching through MEDLINE

1. Select MeSH option, enter the key term in search window

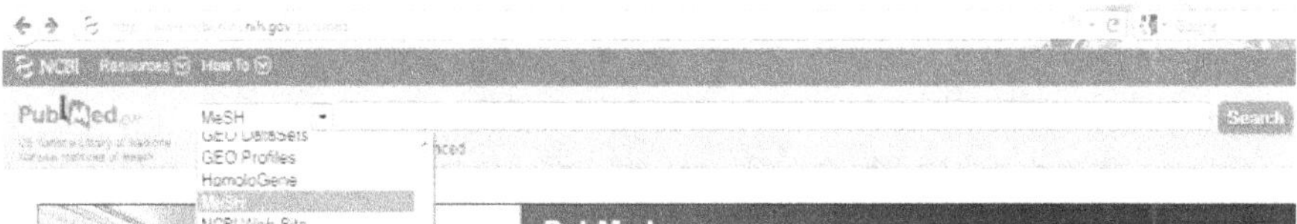

(a) MeSH browser tells us whether the key term entered is correct or not.
(b) Gives closely associated key terms.

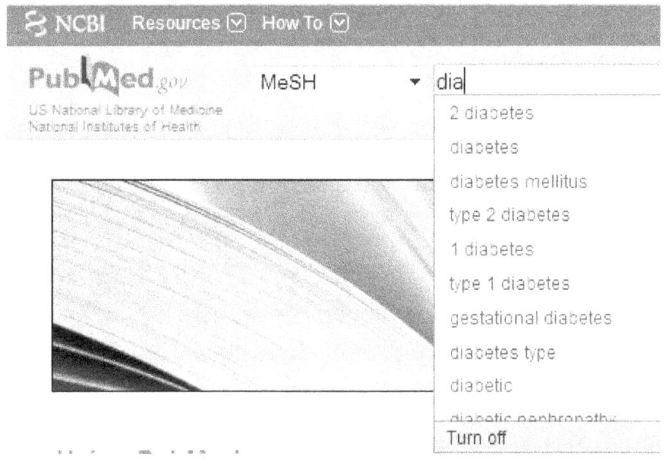

2. Select the correct key term from the list of result and add to search builder browser.

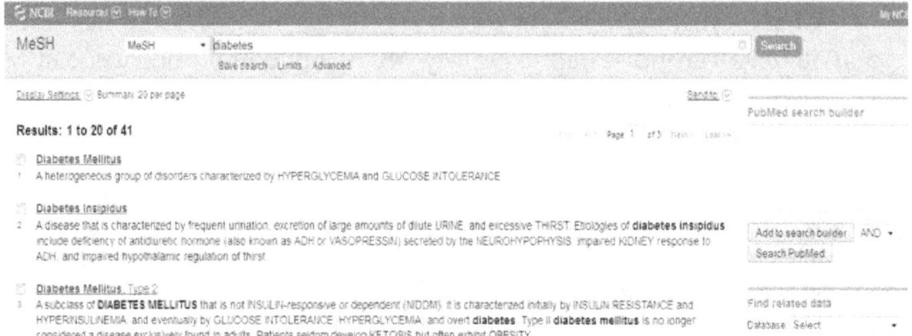

3. To many key terms can be entered using proper add button option.

4. AND, OR and NOT options can be used appropriately.

   (a) AND- Retrieve articles that are indexed under both topics.

   (b) OR- Retrieve articles that are indexed using either one or other topic.

   (c) NOT- Removes any articles that are indexed using that terminology.

5. Click on return to PubMED (executes search against MEDLINE).

6. Displays results

- Number of article in view can be changed by using Entrez date limit option).

- Number of free full-text articles and review can be viewed through filtered search.

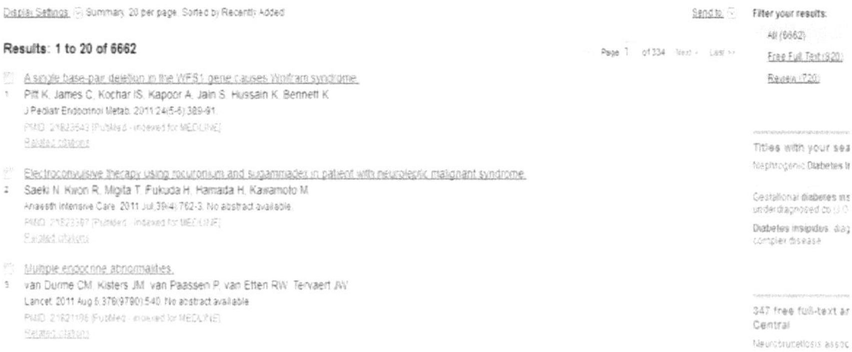

4.6 Information and Library Network (InfLibNet)

With globalization of education and competitive research the demand for the journals has increased over the years. Due to scarcity of funds, libraries have been forced to discontinue the scholarly journals, which have great impact to the users. In order to provide the current literature to academia, UGC-Infonet E-Journals Consortium has been set up by UGC to promote the use of electronic databases and full text access to journals by the Research and academic community.

It covers almost all areas of learning like Arts, Humanities, Social Sciences, Physical and Chemical Sciences, Life Sciences, Computer Sciences, Mathematics and Statistics etc. and other subject areas are to be added in near future. The programme is wholly funded by the UGC and monitored by **Information and Library Network (InfLibNet)** Centre, Ahmedabad. The INFLIBNET library plays a vital role in the collection development and dissemination of scientific and technical information. InfLibNet consists of 2000 documents on computer, communication, information and library science. The library is fully computerized by using Software for University Library (SOUL), which is integrated library management software.

It enables academia to access large number of scholarly journals from reputed publishers, aggregators and society publications. Under the consortium, about 4000 full text scholarly electronic journals from 25 publishers across the globe can be accessed. The consortium provides current as well as archival access to core and peer-reviewed journals in different disciplines.

Main Objectives of InfLibNet

1. To promote and establish communication facilities to improve capability in information transfer and access, which provide support to scholarship, learning, research and academic pursuit.

2. To provide and implement computerization of operations and services in the libraries and information centers of the country, following a uniform standard.

3. To evolve standards and uniform guidelines in techniques, methods, procedures, computer hard ware and software, services and promote their adoption in actual practice by all libraries, in order to facilitate pooling, sharing and exchange of centers towards optimal use of resources and facilities.

4. To provide reliable access to document collection of libraries by creating on-line catalogue of serials, theses / dissertations, books, monographs and non-book materials (manuscripts, audio visuals, computer data, multimedia, etc) in various libraries in india.

5. To provide access to bibliographic information sources with citations, abstracts, etc.

6. To facilitate scientists, engineers, social scientists, academics, faculties, researchers and students through electronic mail, file transfer, computer / audio / radio conferencing, etc.

7. To collobrate with institutions, libraries, information centers and other organizations in india and abroad in the field relevant to the objectives of the center.

Resources available through inflibnet:

http://unicat.inflibnet.ac.in/econ/freeurls.htm

      http://highwire.stanford.edu/lists/freeart/dtl

      http://www.doaj.org

      http://www.pubmed central.nih.gov

      http://www.biomedcentral.com/start.asp

      http://www.freemedicaljournals.com

      http://www.rsc.org/Publishing/CurrentAwareness/index.asp

      http://www.doaj.org

      http://www.bioline.org.br

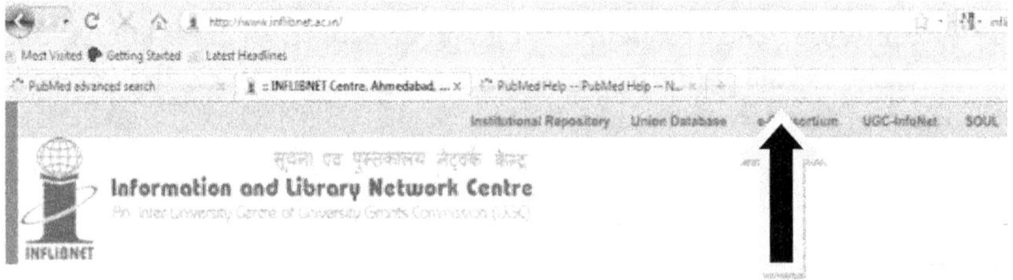

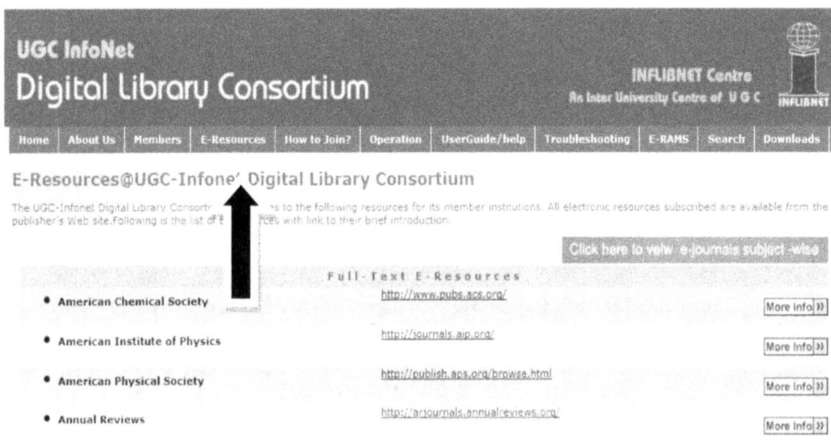

Information search through PubMed Central

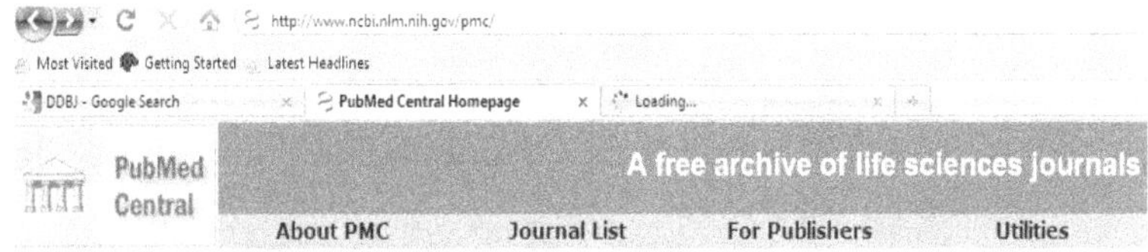

PubMed Central (PMC) is the U.S. National Institutes of Health (NIH) free digital archive of biomedical and life sciences journal literature.

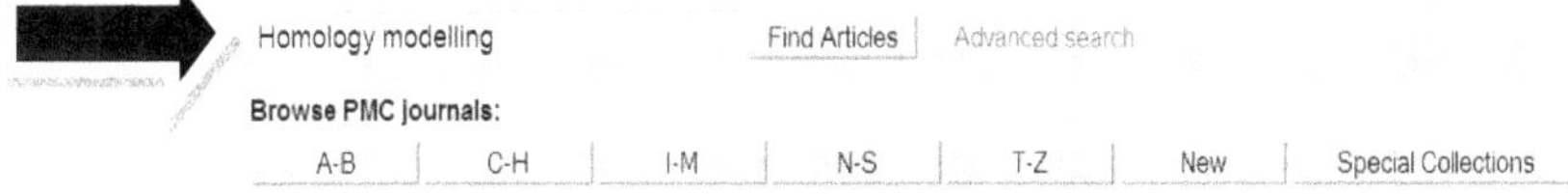

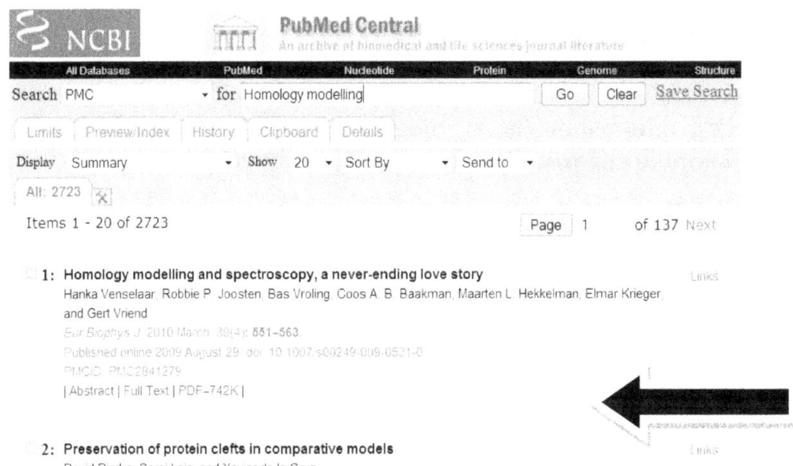

4.7 Written and Verbal Reports

The DICs through verbal, written or audio visual communications educate and counsel the patient and other health professionals. Written and verbal communication skills enable effective intra and inter-institutional dialogue regarding pharmaco-therapeutic information. It includes

1. Advising and educating patients for
    - Proper use of drugs, dosage form and route of administration
    - Identification, properties and storage conditions of drugs
    - Mechanism of action and pharmacokinetics
    - Directions, precautions and side effects
    - Therapeutic indications
2. Clarifying doubts regarding
    - Sexual problems, myths, contraceptives and family planning.
    - Socio-medical problems (drug addiction, drug abuse, alcoholism, smoking hazards)
    - Drug over dose, poisoning and drug toxicity.
3. Advise on self medication for minor complaints and on public health issues.

4.8 Drug Information Databases

Drug information databases are the best source of drug information and provide detailed information about the use and side effects of drugs.

PharmInfoNet   (http://www.pharminfo.com): Pharmainfo.net contains searches, information, news, blogs, profile pages, reviews, articles and videos for the pharmaceutical and healthcare professionals.

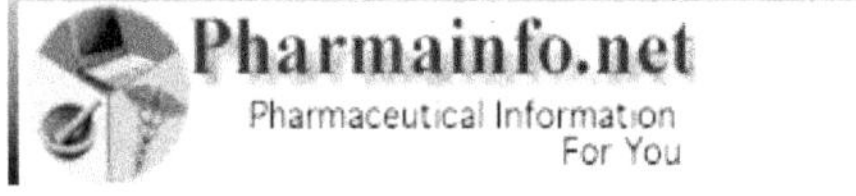

Pharmweb: http://www.pharmweb.net: Provides pharmaceutical and health related information.

MedlinePlus -MedlinePlus offers reliable, up-to-date health information and gives information about diseases, conditions, and wellness issues in more simplified language. Informations available in MedlinePlus are

- Health topics.

- Medical encyclopedia - an extensive collection of medical images as well as 4,000 articles about diseases, tests, symptoms, injuries and surgeries.

- Interactive health tutorials - narrated programs that use animated graphics to explain conditions and procedures in easy-to-read language.

- Drugs, supplements, and herbal information - prescription and over-the-counter medicines (OTC), herbs and supplements.

- Current health news – latest informations about medicine and health.

- Dictionary - spellings, definitions, and pronunciations of medical terms.

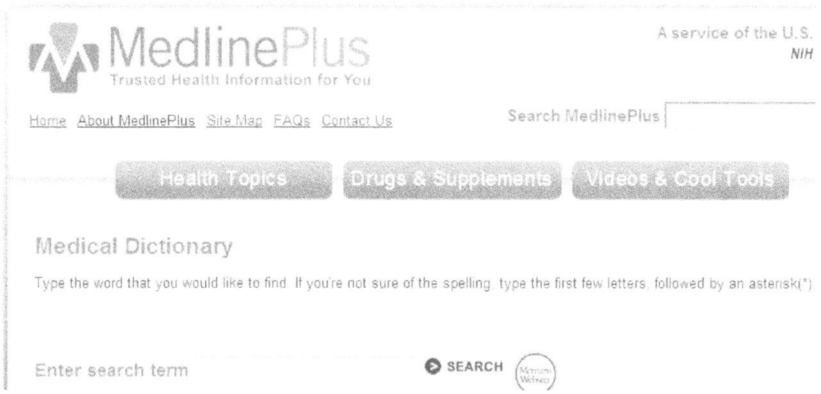

Drug information portal (http://www.nlm.nih.gov/learn-about-drugs.html)

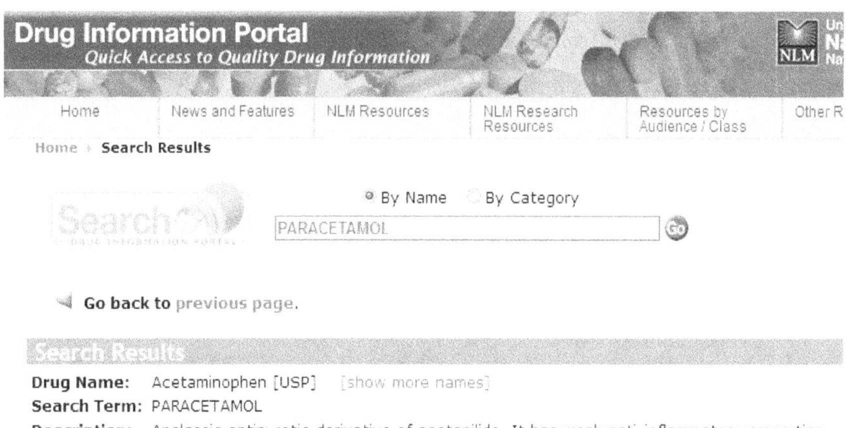

Drug @ FDA (http://www.accessdata.fda.gov/scripts/cder/drugsatfda/)

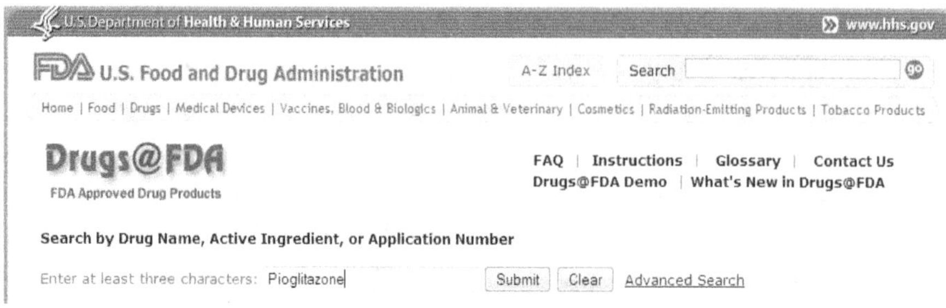

Search Results for 'Pioglitazone'

Products listed on this page may not be equivalent to one another.

Click on a drug name for more information:
Click on a column header to re-sort the table:

Drug Name	Active Ingredients
ACTOPLUS MET	METFORMIN HYDROCHLORIDE; PIOGLITAZONE HYDROCHLORIDE
ACTOPLUS MET XR	METFORMIN HYDROCHLORIDE; PIOGLITAZONE HYDROCHLORIDE
ACTOS	PIOGLITAZONE HYDROCHLORIDE
DUETACT	GLIMEPIRIDE; PIOGLITAZONE HYDROCHLORIDE
PIOGLITAZONE	PIOGLITAZONE HYDROCHLORIDE
PIOGLITAZONE HYDROCHLORIDE AND METFORMIN HYDROCHLORIDE	METFORMIN HYDROCHLORIDE; PIOGLITAZONE HYDROCHLORIDE

Iowa Drug Information Service (IDIS) database - IOWA

This database is a bibliographic indexing service for 200 premier medical and pharmaceutical journals. It supports the drug information role of pharmacists providing pharmaceutical care.

http://www.uiowa.edu/homepage/resources/listings/i/IA_drug_info_s erv.html

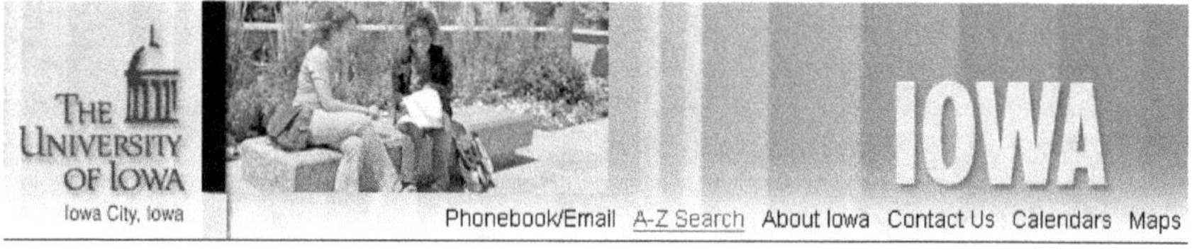

Iowa Drug Information Service (IDIS) - Resources for Iowans

The IDIS database provides an index to drug articles from biomedical literature via microfiche, compact disc, and computer access. For more information, call (319) 335-4800, e-mail idis@uiowa.edu, or visit the web site at www.uiowa.edu/~idis.

Drug Information System

It provides details about therapeutics, pharmacology, prescribing information and dosage regimen of drugs.

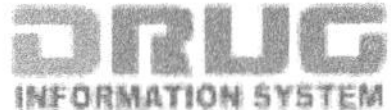

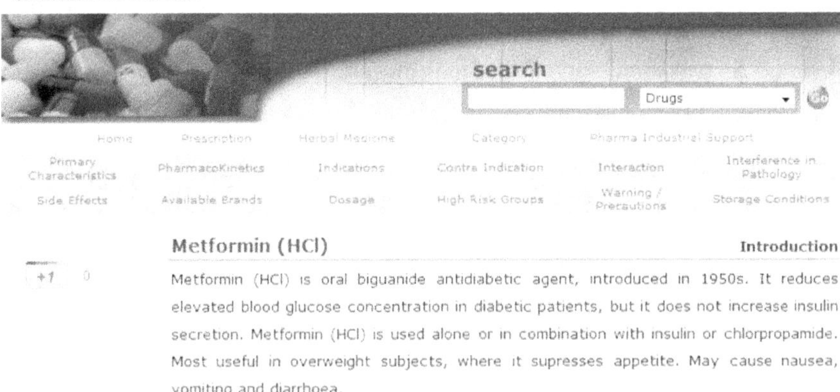

Toxicology Data Network (TOXNET)

TOXNET database includes toxicology, hazardous chemicals, environmental health and toxic releases. It gives extensive array of references to literature on biochemical, pharmacological, physiological, and toxicological effects of drugs and other chemicals.

http://toxnet.nlm.nih.gov/

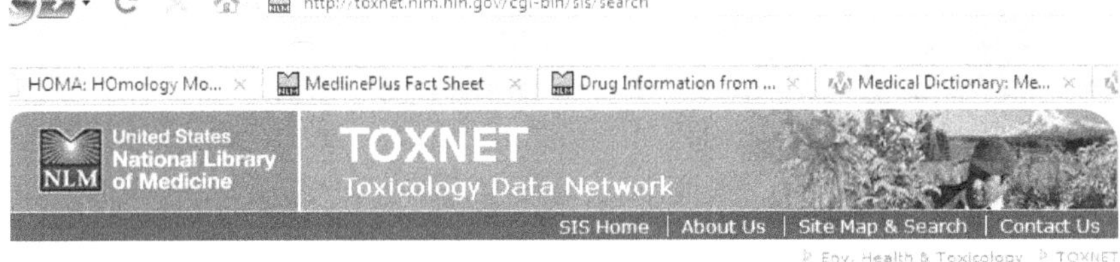

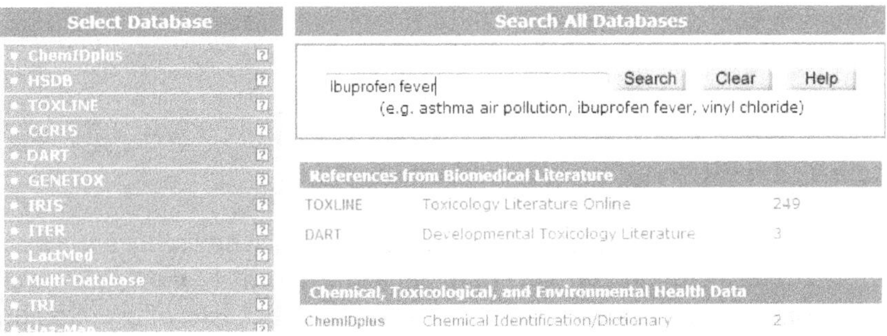

The international program of chemical society [http://www.who.int/ipcs/poisons/en/]

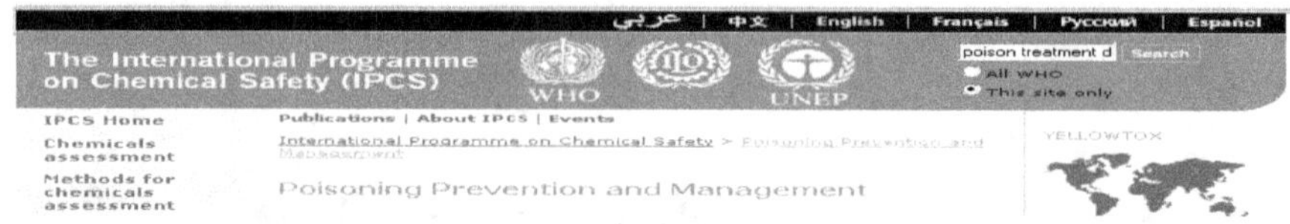

Asia pacific association of medical pharmacology

http://www.prn2.usm.my/apamt/pages/poison_arc.asp?cat=all

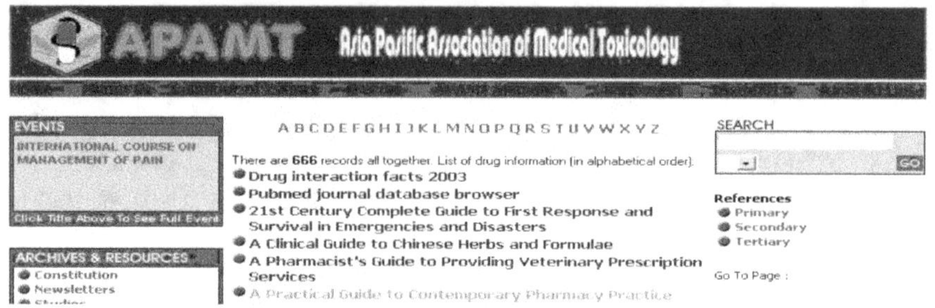

National Poison Data System (NPDS)

The National Poison Data System (NPDS) is the only comprehensive poisoning surveillance database in the United States. Maintained by the American Association of Poison Control Centers (AAPCC), contains detailed toxicological information on more than 18 million poison exposures reported to U.S. poison centers.

http://www.aapccpoisoncenters.com/npds/npds.html

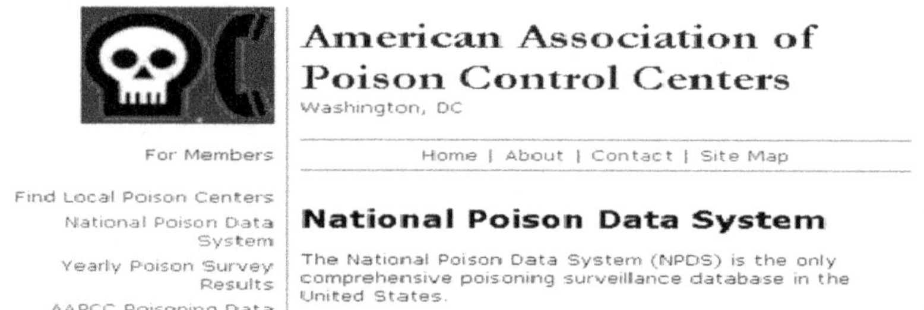

The Arizona Poison and Drug Information Center

It provides accessible poison and medication-related emergency treatment advice, referral assistance and comprehensive information on poisons and toxins, poison prevention and the safe and proper use of medications.

The immediate availability of the center's experts is especially crucial for rural communities that lack quick access to major medical facilities to healthcare professionals.

http://www.pharmacy.arizona.edu/outreach/poison/

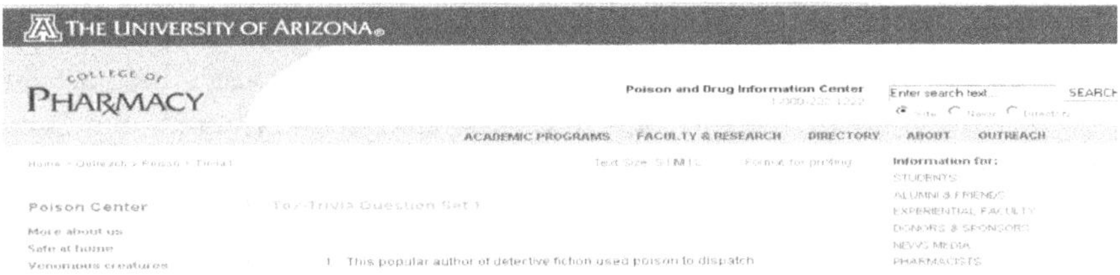

4.9 Databases used in Personalized Medicine

- **Drug candidate database:** A large number of chemical substance databases are available for drug research.

- **Digital database:** It includes official documents like pharmacopeia in CD-ROMs and web sites contains all the official drugs and their complete profile.

- **ADME knowledge base database:** ADME knowledge base database keeps all the informations related drug metabolizing enzymes, which help predicting the bioavailability and adverse effects of the drug.

- **Drug target database:** It includes the information on the primary targets and mode of action of the drugs. Signal transduction, perturbation in metabolic reactions and metabolic pathway are accumulated in this database. The affinity of the drug molecule to the macromolecule can be studied from this database.

- **Pathway database:** It covers the informations related to the transport pathway and of intracellular drug metabolism pathway.

- **DRUGDEX System:** It delivers unbiased drug information to physicians, pharmacists, and other health care professionals. This system provides independently reviewed data gathered from major drug centers and pharmacology services worldwide. These informations are prepared by MICROMEDEX editorial board and can be retrieved by generic name, manufacturer brand name, or indications. It contains details about drug dosage, pharmacokinetics, cautions, interactions, comparative drug efficacy, clinical applications, generic and brand names, indications and adverse side effects.

- **Drug Consults:** An excellent resource for information on herbal medications, medical and surgical materials, excipients, drugs of abuse, and health foods. Drug Consults are provided for investigational, international, FDA approved and over-the-counter preparations.

- **Product Index:** It documents wide-range of unbiased information related to drug therapy in the clinical setting. Product Indexes are provided for investigational, international, FDA approved, and over-the-counter preparations (OTC).

CHAPTER 5

PHARMACY AUTOMATION

Health information technology (HIT) is most promising tool for improving the overall quality, safety and efficiency of the health delivery system. HIT refers to the use of both computer hardware and software for storage, retrieval, sharing and use of health care information, data and knowledge for communication and decision making. HIT allows Health care providers to collect, store, retrieve and transfer information electronically.

5.1 Technologies

- **Electronic health record (EHR):** EHR previously known as the electronic medical records (EMR) reduces errors related to prescription drugs and preventive care.

- **Computerized provider order entry (CPOE):** CPOE also known as computerized physician order entry (CPOE) is a process of electronic entry of medical practitioner instructions for the treatment of patients. These orders are communicated over a computer network to the departments (pharmacy, laboratory, or radiology). CPOE decreases delay in order completion, reduces errors related to handwriting or transcription and simplifies inventory and posting of charges.

  EHR and CPOE provide access to legible patient information with legible physician order.

- **Clinical decision support system (CDSS):** CDSS provides physicians and nurses with real-time diagnostic and treatment recommendations. It is interactive decision support system software designed to assist health professionals with decision making tasks.

57

- **Picture Archeiving and Communication System (PACS):** PACS captures and integrates diagnostic and radiological images from various devices (X-ray, MRI), stores and disseminates them to a medical record. A PACS consists imaging modalities [X-rays, computed tomography (CT) and magnetic resonance imaging (MRI)], workstations for interpreting and reviewing images, and archives for the storage and retrieval of images and reports.

- **Bar Coding:** An optical scanner is used to electronically capture information encoded on drugs, devices, lab and radiological reports. Barcode system prevents errors in drug dispensing.

- **Radio Frequency Identification (RFID):** RFID uses radio-frequency electromagnetic fields to transfer data from a tag attached to an object, for the purposes of automatic identification and tracking. This technology tracks patients throughout the patient hospital, and links lab and medication tracking through a wireless communications system.

- **Automated Dispensing Machines (ADMs):** ADMs is a computerized drug storage device allows medications to be stored and dispensed. They also are called unit-based cabinets (UBCs), automated dispensing devices (ADDs) and automated distribution cabinets (ADCs).

- **Electronic Material Management (EMM):** Health care organizations use EMM to track and manage inventory of medical supplies, pharmaceuticals and other materials

- **Interoperability:** Interoperable HIT will improve individual patient care through early detection of infectious disease outbreaks and improved tracking of chronic disease management.

5.2 Applications

The applications of HIT for hospitals, physicians are mentioned below

- **HIT in hospitals**
  - (a) Administrative and financial department
    - Billing and cost accounting system.
    - Patient registration system.
    - Electrical material management.
  - (b) Clinical department
    - Computerized provider order entry for drugs.

- Lab test procedures, electronic health record and result reporting.
- Prescription and electronic monitoring of patients in intensive care units.

(c) Infrastructure maintenance

- Voice recognition system for transcription.
- Physician orders and medical records.
- Bar-coding technology for drugs, medical devices and inventory control.
- Information security system.

- **HIT for Physicians**

(a) Administrative and financial department

(b) Clinical

- Receiving lab results and other clinical information online
- Electronic prescribing
- Clinical decision system support
- Electronic health record
- E-mail communication with patients

(c) Infrastructure maintenance

(d) e-Prescribing: It is computer to computer transfer of prescription data from physician to pharmacies. It includes medication history and new prescriptions.

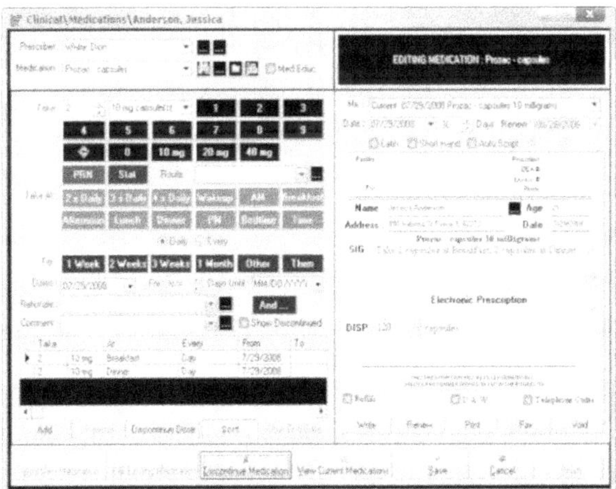

Fig. 5.1 Image showing the view of e-prescription.

5.3 Merits

The rate of growth for prescription volume is projected to be 10 times the rate of new available pharmacists. Pharmacy automation

1. Pharmacy automation reduces liability associated with prescription dispensing errors and increases patient care.

2. Pharmacy automation improves patient counseling, reduces mental and physical tension and saves pharmacists and technician time.

3. Pharmacy automation reduces the shortage of services rendered by pharmacists and improves pharmacy administration efficiency.

4. Pharmacy automation reduces labor costs and escalates prescription volume.

5.4 Barcodes

Barcodes are information carrying graphical patterns designed for easy and reliable automatic retrieval. A bar code is an optical machine-readable representation of data, provides detailed up-to-date information quickly with more confidence. Barcodes helps in keeping track of a large number of items in a store. Barcodes are widely used in shop floor control applications software. Retail chain membership cards use bar codes to uniquely identify a consumer.

5.4.1 Types of Barcodes

One dimensional (1D) barcodes or symbologies: Bar codes represent data in the widths (lines) and the spacings of parallel lines. These graphical patterns vary in a single dimension (e.g. horizontal) and are constant in the other (vertical) dimension. One-dimensional barcodes are employed in low information content applications like product index registry (e.g. automatic price tagging and inventory management) and serial number registry (e.g. test-tube tagging in automated medical tests).

Two-dimensional barcodes: Two-dimensional (2D) barcodes are graphical patterns composed usually of dots also known as 2D matrix codes or symbologies. They are rendered using two-toned dots (e.g. black dots on a white background), and occupies rectangular area. In order to convey more information on the same surface area, the constancy in the vertical dimension has to be abandoned for more intricate patterns. 2D Barcodes come in patterns of squares, dots, hexagons and geometric patterns within images.

5.4.2 Barcodes in Pharmacy

The National Drug Control (NDC) number encoded in the bar code is automatically recorded when the symbol is scanned. The scanner is interfaced to a database or other software application that checks the NDC against the prescription order to validate that the correct medication and dosage were dispensed.

The FDA investigated bar code medication administration processes (storing and dispensing medication from the hospital pharmacy) and concluded that they would reduce medication errors by 50 % and potential adverse drug events. Barcodes identifies the item by manufacturer / distributor, product code (product strength, dosage form, formulation), and package type. Lot codes and expiration dates encoded on labels trigger appropriate alerts.

Barcode systems automatically record the date and time of all transactions. Prior to dispensing medication, the nurse scans the bar codes on their own ID badge, the patient wristband, and the medication-specific unit-dose label. The patient-specific barcode is usually a unique serial number that corresponds to a database record that contains the formulation and patient identification details.

2D barcode prescription system (2DBPS): Improves pharmacists activities. Patient delivers paper prescription with 2D barcode issued by clinic to pharmacy. Pharmacist scans in the 2D barcode, validates and dispenses the drug. Prescription data is stored in the 2DBPS database for other activities.

Managing inventory in hospitals

Maintaining accurate inventory is a very complex procedure and Hospitals utilizes barcodes and controls inventory supply of consumable items (medication and supplies), x-rays, lab results, diagnostic tools., etc. Barcodes are also used in for the maintenance of patient medical record folders and accout files. Barcodes helps in locating the right materials and making them available in right place.

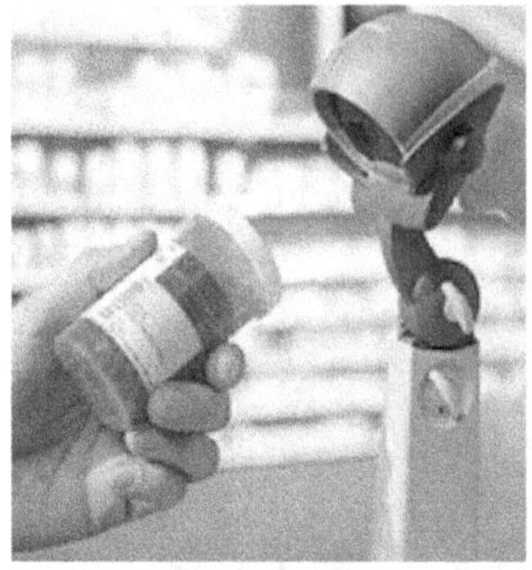
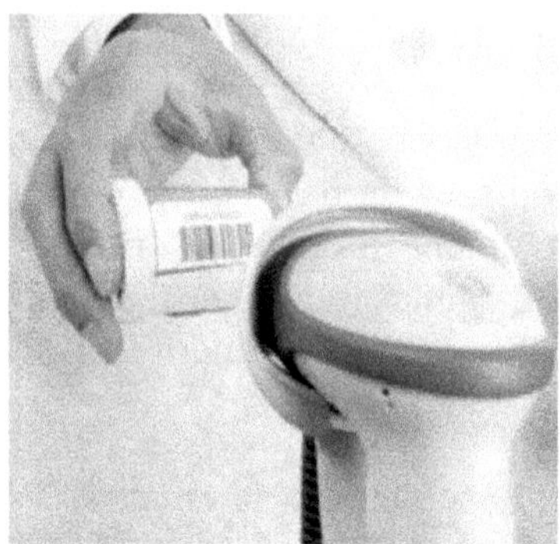
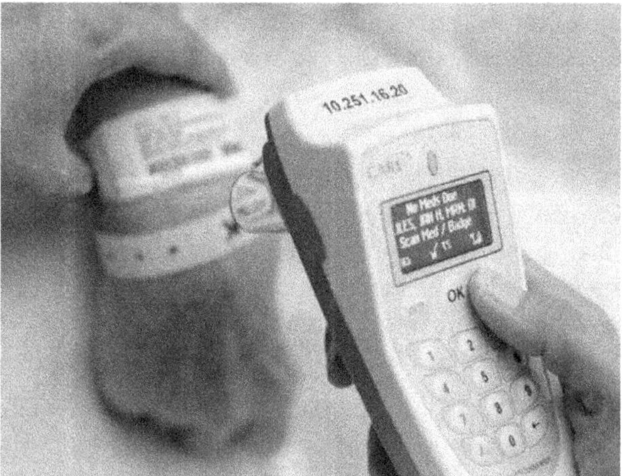

Fig. 5.2 Pictures shows the scanning of barcodes present in the medicine container and wrist band of patient.

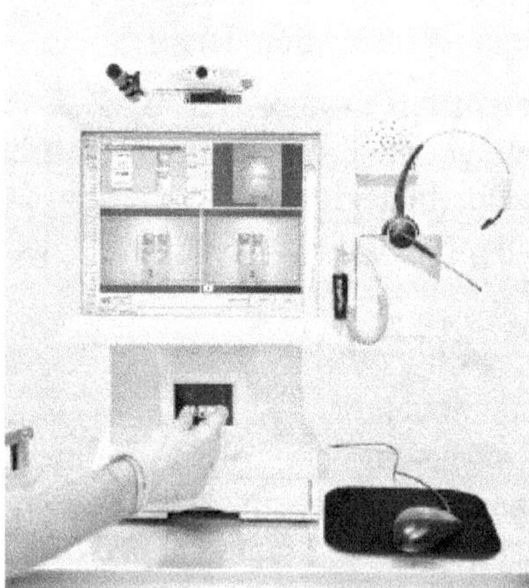

Fig. 5.3 Picture shows the checking of medicine for correctness of medication.

Pharmacists can set a strong foundation for patient safety initiatives by developing a comprehensive program to ensure the implementation of automated medication administration systems. Integrated thermal printers produce medication and bar code labels and supports equipment that doesn't offer bar coding capabilities.

5.5 Advantages of Barcodes

- **Improved operational efficiency:** Barcodes permits faster and accurate recording of data and quick tracking of them.

- **Reduced errors:** Barcodes are more accurate and permits 1 error per 36 trillion characters.

- **Automated recording:** Barcodes allows automated replenishment of inventory process.

5.6 Automated Dispensing Devices

Automated dispensing devices improves the efficiency of prescription processing and allow pharmacists to focus on providing patients with education on their medication and working with prescribers on improving the selection and use of medications. Automated dispensing systems are drug storage cabinets that electronically dispense medications in a controlled fashion and track medication use. Internal electronic devices track nurses accessing the system, track the patients for whom medications are administered. These devices reduces rates of medication errors, increased efficiency for pharmacy and nursing staff, ready availability of medications and improved pharmacy inventory and billing functions.

McLaughlin dispensing system: It includes a bedside dispenser, a programmable magnetic card and a pharmacy computer. It is a locked system that is loaded with the medications prescribed for a patient. A light above the patient's door illuminates at the appropriate dosing time, the bedside dispenser drawer unlocks automatically to allow a dose to be removed and administered.

Baxter ATC-212 dispensing system: It uses a microcomputer to pack unit-dose tablets and capsules and are stored in calibrated canisters that are designed specifically for each medication. Canisters are assigned a numbered location, which is thought to reduce mix-up errors upon dispensing. When an order is sent to the microcomputer, a tablet is dispensed from a particular canister. The drug is ejected into a strip-packing device where it is labeled and hermetically sealed.

Pyxis Medstation (Medstation Rx): This is an automated dispensing devices kept on the nursing unit and pharmacists can keep these units loaded with medication. Physicians orders entered in the pharmacy computer will be transferred to Medstation, where patient profiles are displayed. Each nurse is provided with a password that must be used to access the Medstation.

Controlled Substance dispensing/tracking System: It increases the accuracy and accountability of controlled substance transactions through the use of system access security controls, bar codes, and integration with the Pyxis Medstation.

Centralized robotic dispensing device: It can store up to 15,800 unit dose packaged medications with bar code identification on the labeling. The system has the ability to pack and store medications from bulk supplies, unload the medications into 24 h patient medication bins and place back into storage medications (that are returned following patient discharge).

ScriptPro SP200 robotic prescription dispensing system: This delivers filled and labeled vials to the pharmacist for final approval. The system utilizes bar code technology throughout the various filling and checking steps for accuracy and quality control.

BPOC Bedside Device: It contains Wireless Laptop computer with a touch screen and bar code scanner.

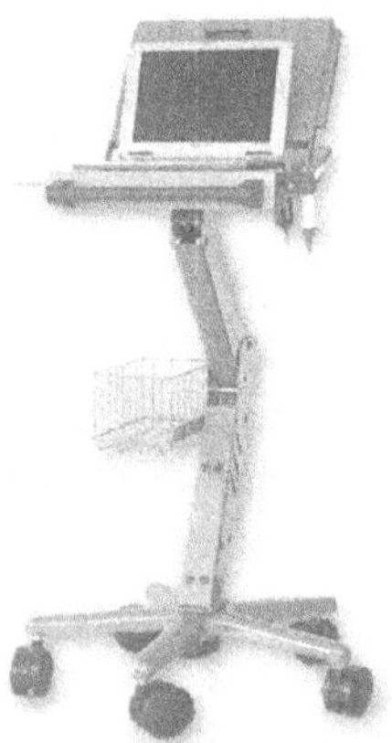

Fig. 5.4 BPOC bedside device.

DRUG RESEARCH

The discovery, development and design of new drugs / medicines are multifaceted and enormously difficult process. Concepts of organic chemistry, pharmacology, microbiology, biochemistry and molecular biology shaped drug discovery process. The advent of genomic sciences, DNA sequencing, combinatorial chemistry, cell-based assays and high throughput screening (HTS) has led to a new concept of drug discovery. Drug search can be conveniently grouped into following streams

Drug discovery: Drug discovery process involves the identification of compounds with activity against a specified target.

Drug development: Drug development process involves optimization of lead molecules and generation of analogs. Its main aim is to improve pharmacokinetic (ADME) properties, increase potency and to decrease toxicity associated with parent molecule. It also includes formulation development.

Drug design: Designing molecules with more complementarity for the active sites of the receptor protein is called as drug design. It involves in the identification of target, ligand and its 3D structural studies.

<h1>CHAPTER 6</h1>

DRUG DISCOVERY

Natural sources are of good origin for the discovery of many existing drugs and still useful in drug discovery process. Drugs obtained from natural sources are grouped below.

1. Extracts of plant sources: Morphine, pilocarpine, vincristine.
2. Extracts of animal sources: Shark liver oil, honey.
3. Products of microorganisms: Penicillins, macrolides, aminoglycosides.

Traditionally drug discovery process has relied on experimental trial and error screening and is based on

- In depth investigations of active constituents in herbs and plants (quinine).
- Accidental effects observed during biochemical investigations (penicillin).
- Massive screening (mefloquine).
- Exploitation of biochemical functions (pyremethamine).
- Observed side effects (minoxidil).

Modern drug discovery process involves identification and optimization of the molecules for clinical applications. Typical drug discovery process includes the following procedures:

- Lead identification
- Lead optimization / geometry optimization
- Pharmacokinetic studies
- Bio-assay
- Clinical studies

6.1 Lead Identification

Lead identification plays a very important role in the drug discovery process. The lead structure will be modified to get next generation of compounds.

6.1.1 Chance Observation – Serendipity

'Serendipity' in drug discovery implies the finding of one observation during the other research program. Most of the discoveries in chemotherapy are result of a false hypothesis or due to chance observation. Penicillin is discovered by Alxender Fleming (1928), when *Staphylococcus aureus* culture was stored in unusual conditions. During the preparation of benzheptoxdiazines, benzodiazepines analog of chlordiazepoxide is formed in an unexpected reaction, and it is lead for the generation of tranquilizer agents.

Penicillin   Chlordiazepoxide

Observation of flies attracted to the sugar-rich urine of experimental dogs with pancreas removed led to the discovery that the pancreas is related to blood sugar regulation and diabetes. Molecules designed for one disease sometimes fails to produce expected effect, but it produces effect in some other target. Azidothymidine (anti-HIV agent) developed for cancer therapy and sildenafil (drug used in erectile dysfunction) was developed for heart ailments are the examples of this kind.

Sildenafil

6.1.2 Lead Identification Methods

The below mentioned methods are employed in the lead identification process.

- Random screening
- Non-random screening
- Drug metabolism studies
- Clinical observations
- Identification from Marketed drugs
- Natural ligands

Random Screening: The biological activity testing of compounds (natural/synthetic) without considering their structure is known as random screening. Random screening method of lead identification is also known as non-selective/blind/mass/broad screening/dedicated random screening. Anti-hypercholesterolemic agents lovastatin (mevinolin) and pravastatin are discovered by random screening. Currently high throughput screening (HTS), a very rapid and sensitive robotic *in vitro* screens are used universally.

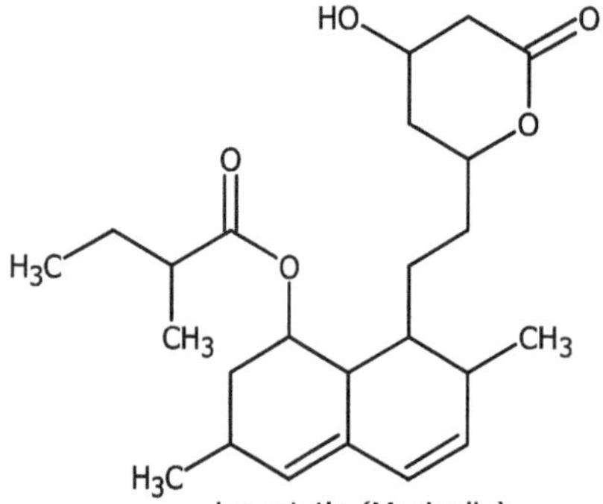

Lovastatin (Mevinolin)

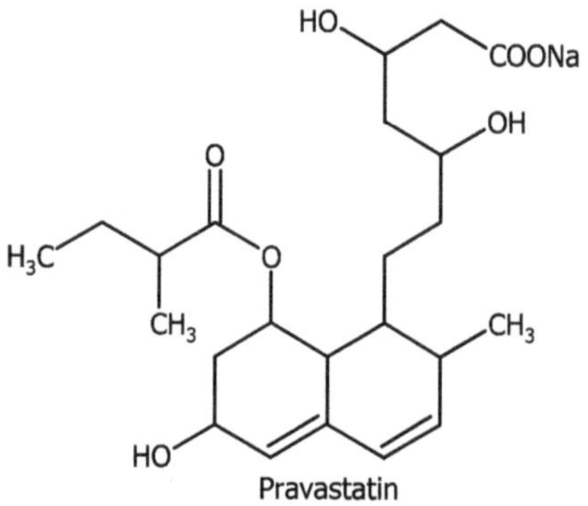

Pravastatin

Non-random screening: Only compounds with similar structures will be screened for their biological activity. This method is also known as rationally directed random screening, targeted and focussed screening.

Drug metabolism studies: Biochemical degradation products (metabolites) of drugs are tested for their biological activity potential to know whether the activity is due to drug or its metabolite. If metabolite is found to be active then that product alone can be administered and those compounds become lead for next generation molecules. The toxicity (abnormal heart rhythm) of anti-histamine terfenadine is not associated with its metabolite fexofenadine, this made fexofenadine itself to enter into market.

Terfenadine   -CH$_3$
Fexofenadine -COOH

Clinical observation: Drugs with multiple pharmacological activities are exploited as lead for their secondary pharmacological activity. Antihistamine dimenhydrinate is used in the treatment of motion sickness and anti-hypertensive minoxidil is having hair revital property.

Dimenhydrinate

Minoxidil

Marketed drugs: Targets for marketed drugs are mostly known and it becomes lead for next generation drugs. The main drawback is patent for commercialization.

Natural ligands: Designing drug from natural ligand involves rationalization, and known as rational drug design. Rational drug design is becoming major route for drug discovery. Norgestrel, long and strong acting progestational agent is developed from weak and short acting natural ligand progesterone. Similarly 17-α-ethynylestradiol is designed from 17-β-estradiol.

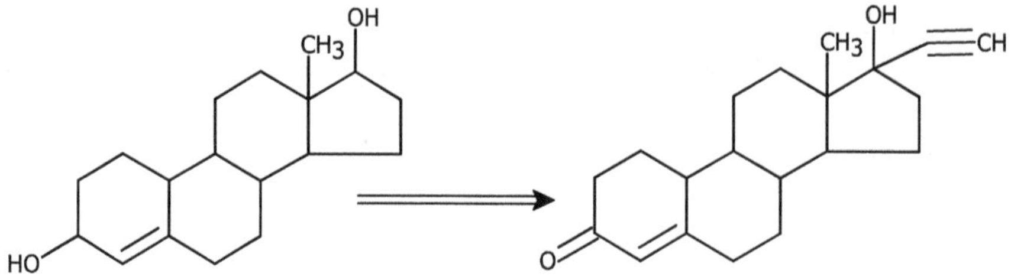

Progesterone   Norgestrel

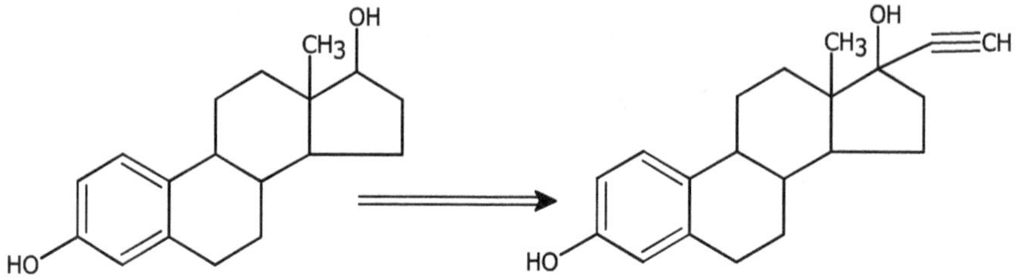

Estradiol   Ethinyl estradiol

6.2 Lead Optimization

Drug development process involves improvement of pharmacokinetic (ADME) properties to increase potency and to decrease toxicity associated with parent molecule. In the past, lead finding activities were mainly directed towards affinity and selectivity rather than molecular properties and metabolic liabilities. During the past few years, there has been an increasing awareness of the need for developing drug-like properties of a molecule. These are the balance of bio-physicochemical requirements for the molecule to reach its site of action. Lead optimization process involves collection and analysis of structural activity relationship (SAR) data and serves for this purpose. Once the lead compound is identified it must be systematically altered to maximize the therapeutic index and minimize the side effects.

The major goals of lead optimization process are:
1. To amplify desired activity of the lead molecule
2. To improve the bioavailability of lead molecule
3. To optimize potency and to improve specificity
4. To eliminate or reduce the toxicity associated with lead molecule
5. Modification of agonist to antagonist

The two major steps involved in the lead modification are:
- Identification of pharmacophore
- Lead modification approaches

6.2.1 Identification of Pharmacophore

Investigation of numerous lead compounds to identify the pharmacophore and auxophore (parts of the structure) which are responsible for biological response as well as unwanted side effects. A functional group(s) / nucleus present in a molecule that interfere with a receptor and produce the biological activity are known as pharmacophore. The other atoms / groups present in the structure are called as auxophore, it may be essential for the integrity of the molecule and may interfere with the pharmacophore in binding pattern. Removal of group(s) or introduction of group(s) will result in the conformational change and alters the biological activity. A decrease in potency on removal of a group will suggest that it is pharmacophoric part and an increase/decrease in potency refers it as an auxophoric group.

6.2.2 Lead Modification Approaches

- Functional group modification
- Structural activity relationship (SAR)
- Molecular modification

Functional group modification: The antibacterial agent, carbutamide was found to have anti-diabetic activity as a side effect. To remove the antibacterial activity and improve anti-diabetic potential various modifications are done. Replacement of amino group of carbutamide with methyl group (tolbutamide), retains the anti-diabetic effect. Further change of methyl group with chloro group and shortening of liphophilic alkyl side chain gave chlorpropamide, with extended half life and 6 fold increase in activity.

	R	R^1
Carbutamide	NH_2	C_4H_9
Tolbutamide	CH_3	C_3H_7
Chlorpropamide	Cl	C_3H_7

Structure activity relationship: Drugs can be classified into structurally specific drugs and structurally non-specific drugs. Activity and potency of structurally specific drugs are very sensitive to even small change in chemical structure. (eg; Skeletal muscle relaxants of quaternary ammonium salts).

N-Methyl nicotine   N-Methyl morphine

Molecules with diverse structures shows similar biological activity are known as structurally non-specific drugs. (Eg; Gaseous anaesthetics)

Halothane   Isoflurane   Enflurane

The size and shape of the molecule is most significant with respect to biological activity. Incorporation of any group to unsubstituted position in the lead or replacing existing group may results in:

(a) Analogues with a different size and shape.

(b) Introduction of chiral center (impose conformational restrictions).

These modifications introduce the change in pharmacokinetic and pharmacodynamic properties of the newer analogues.

Rigidity/flexibility of molecule: Dissection of rings or the rigidification of flexible molecule is the most common lead modification approach. Molecules with several rotatable bonds may adopt different conformations, which influences the biological activity. Different conformations can be frozen by joining certain atoms / groups (cyclization). This bioactive conformation may increases (agonist) or decreases (antagonist) the biological activity of molecule. Anti-ulcer drug thioburimamide when converted to oxoburimamide shows no activity because of the rigidity it gains by intramolecular hydrogen bond interaction.

Thioburimamide

Oxoburimamide
(extented conformation)

Oxoburimamide
(Cyclized conformation

Privileged structures: Elements of known bioactive molecule are used as the core for generating libraries.

Molecular Modification

Homologation: Homologation is a process of increasing the chain length of molecule by a constant unit and show either increase or decrease in biological activity. In many cases, lengthening of carbon chain increases its bio-activity as it increases the lipophilicity (important for penetration). But lengthening beyond certain level decreases its activity, because of no optimal balance between lipophilicity and hydrophilicity. (eg: antibacterial effects of alcohols)

Chain branching: Chain branching lowers the potency of a compound because the branched alkyl chain is lipophilic than the corresponding straight alkyl chain (lower Log P). Chain branching interferes with receptor binding of chlorpromazine (antipsychotic) and promethazine (antihistamine).

Chlorpromazine

Promethazine

Ring chain transformation: Transformation of alkyl substituents into cyclic analogue, often does not affect its potency.

The conversion of acyclic alkyl groups in chlorpheniramine in to cyclic group gives triprolidine, both are active anti-histaminergic agents.

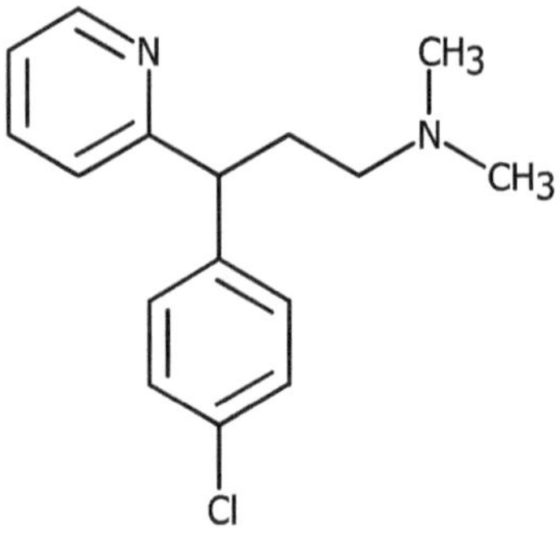

CH3
N
CH3

Chlorpheniramine

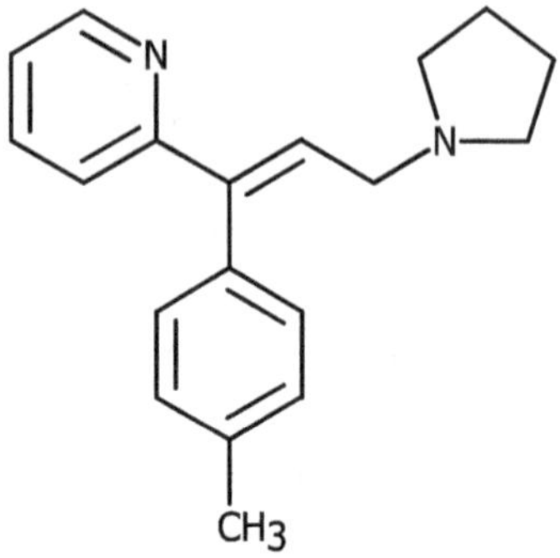

Triprolidine

Bio-isosterism: Bioisosterism is a strategy of medicinal chemistry for the rational drug design of drugs applied to a lead compound as a special process of molecular modification.

6.3 Bio-Isosterism

Two molecules or molecular fragments containing identical number and arrangement of electrons are termed as isosteres and the existence of such phenomenon is termed as isosterism.

Eg: CO and N_2 (**CO = 6 + 8 = 14 and N_2 = 7 + 7 = 14**)

These isosteres will have similar physicochemical properties in most instances. Replacement of atom or group of atoms in a molecule by another group with similar electronic and steric properties is an important lead optimization process. It induces modifications in size, shape, electronic distribution, chemical reactivity, liphophilicity and hydrogen bonding capacity of molecules.

Isosteric modification led to a fruitful yield of new and improved drug. The widespread application of the concept of isosterism to modify biological activity has given rise to the term bio-isosterism, an important tool in rational drug design.

- Friedman defined bio-isosteres as "compounds similar that of isosteres and having similar bioactivity".
- Thornber explained bio-isosteres as, "subunits / groups / molecules possessing similar physicochemical as well as bioactive properties".

- Langmuir postulated that substances possessing atoms or groups with the same number of valence electrons as isosteres and phenomenon as isosterism.

Grimm's hydride displacement law: Grimm postulated hydride displacement law as, "an atom belonging to groups 4A, 5A, 6A, 7A on the periodic table change their properties by adding a hydride and become isoelectronic pseudoatoms".

Grimm's hydride displacement law					
6	7	8	9	10	11
C	N	O	F	Ne	Na
	CH	NH	OH	FH	-
		CH_2	NH_2	OH_2	FH_2^+
			CH_3	NH_3	OH_3^+
				CH_4	NH_4^+

Erlenmeyer further broadened Grimm's classification and redefined isosteres as "atoms, ions and molecules in which the peripheral layers of electrons can be considered identical. He proposed that elements in the same column of the periodic table are isosteric and his concept of isoelectric ring later became ring isosterism.

Number of peripheral electrons				
4	5	6	7	8
N^+	P	S	Cl	ClH
P^+	As	Se	Br	BrH
S^+	Sb	Te	I	IH

Alfred Burger (1970) modified this definition as "compounds or groups that possess near-equal molecular shape and volumes, approximately the same distribution of electrons and which exhibit similar physical properties".

Burger classified bioiososteres in two groups.

1. Classic bio-isosteres
2. Non-classic bio-isosteres

Any bioisosteric replacement should be rigorously preceded by careful analysis of the following parameters

(a) Size and volume and electronic distribution of the atoms

(b) Degree of hybridization, polarizability, bonding angles, inductive effect and mesomeric effects of the atoms

(c) Degree of lipid and aqueous solubility (Log P and pKa)

(d) Conformational factors

6.3.1 Classic Bio-Isosteres

- Mono valent atoms /groups
    - Fluorine vs hydrogen replacement
    - Amino-hydroxyl interchanges
    - Thiol-hydroxyl interchanges
    - Fluorine, hydroxyl, amino and methyl group interchanges (Grimm's concept)
    - Chloro, bromo, thiol and hydroxyl group interchanges (Erlenmeyer's concept)
- Di valent atoms /groups
- Tri valent atoms /groups
- Tetra valent atoms /groups
- Ring equivalents

Classic bio-isosteres			
Monovalent	**Divalent**	**Trivalent**	**Tetravalent**
OH, -NH$_2$, -CH$_3$, -OCH$_3$	- CH$_2$ -	=CH-	=C=
- F, -Cl, -Br, -I	- O -	=N-	=Si=
-SH, -SR	-S-	=CH-	=N$^+$=
-PH$_2$, -Si$_3$,	-Se-	=As-	=P$^+$=
	-Te-	=Sb-	=As$^+$=
			=Sb$^+$=

Modification of Mono Valent Atoms / Groups

- Fluorine vs hydrogen replacement: Steric nature of hydrogen and fluorine are similar, but their difference in the electronegativity is responsible for their different pharmacological properties. Introduction of fluoro atom to 5th position of uracil in place of hydrogen alters the biochemical pathway of thymidylate synthase. 5-Fluorouracil is closely similar to uracil and becomes good substrate for thymidylate synthase and thus produces antagonistic activity. The antagonistic effect is due to the inductive effect of fluorine atom, which is responsible for covalent binding to thymidylate synthase.

Uracil

5-Flurouracil

- Amino-hydroxyl interchanges: The hydroxyl group present in the folic acid is replaced with amino group (retains tautomeric nature of hydroxyl group) to get aminopterin. Tautomeric nature and hydrogen bonding capability of amino group facilitates the bonding with dihydrofolate reductase. Thus aminopterin inhibits the binding of folic acid to the enzyme, which is essential for the cell growth function and expresses antibacterial activity.

X = OH (Folic acid)

X = NH$_2$ (Aminopterin)

The similar steric size, spatial arrangement and the ability of these functional groups to act as either hydrogen bond donors / acceptors is utilized here.

- Thiol-hydroxyl interchanges: Hydrogen bond donating or accepting nature of both thiol and hydroxyl groups are utilized in this approach. In 6-thioguanine, an anticancer drug oxygen atom present in the guanine is replaced with thio group. This change in the groups contributes to different pharmacological activity.

X = O (Guanine)

X = S (6 -Thioguanine)

- Fluorine, hydroxyl, amino and methyl group interchanges (Grimm's concept): Monovalent substitution of fluorine, hydroxyl and amino in place of hydrogen. Replacement of -CH$_3$ group of SC-58125 with bio-isostere -NH$_2$ group gave anti-inflammatory drug celecoxib. First pass metabolism of SC-58125 due to the vulnerable soft metabolic site of -CH$_3$ group is overcome by this modification.

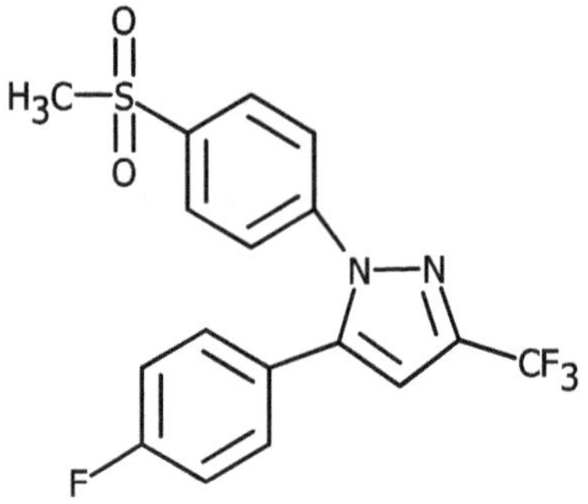

SC-58125 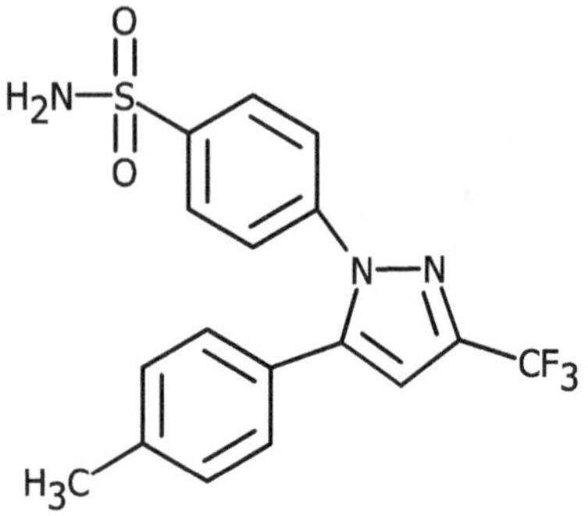   Celecoxib

- Chloro, bromo, thiol and hydroxyl group interchanges (Erlenmeyer's concept): Thioamide and thiomethyl groups of tolrestat (aldose reductase inhibitor) is substituted with amide and methoxy group to generate oxotolrestat.

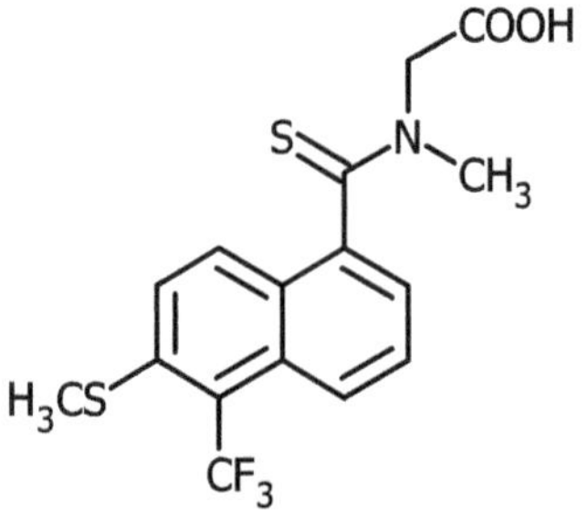

Tolrestat 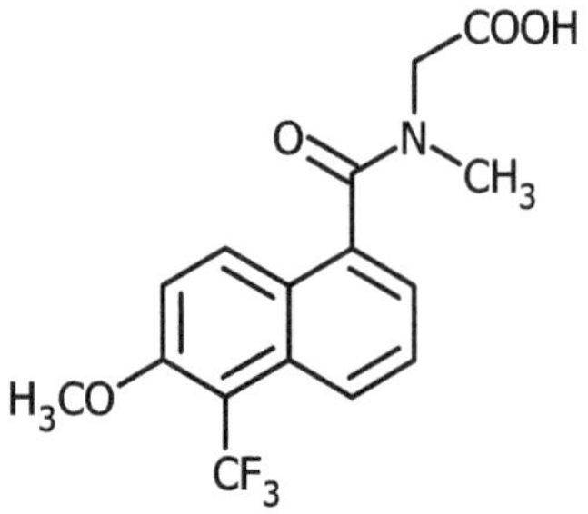   Oxotolrestat

Modification of Divalent Atoms / Groups

Divalent isosteres can be classified into two subtypes

1. Bio-isostere replacement involving double bonds: C=C, C=N, C=O and C=S.

2. Bio-isostere replacement involving two single bonds: C-C-C, C-NH-C, C-O-C and C-S-C.

- Bio-isostere replacement involving double bonds: In anti-diabetic drug tolrestat, the replacement of -C=S with -C=O gives oxotolrestat which retains the aldose reductase inhibitory activity.

- Bio-isostere replacement involving two single bonds: Attachment of these bio-isosteres to two different substituent's makes chemical and polar substituent's less pronounced. The bond angle or the conformation associated with the use of these divalent bio-isosteres may be an important factor associated with retention of biological activity. (eg: antihistamines)

Modification of Trivalent Atoms/Groups

Bio-isosteric replacement of –CH= with –N= is an example of trivalent modification approach. In cholesterol, replacement of two CH groups in side chain with N gives 20, 25 - diazacholesterol which is more potent inhibitor of cholesterol biosynthesis. The greater electronegativity of nitrogen is responsible for the inhibitory activity.

Cholesterol

20,25-Diazacholesterol

Modification of Tetravalent Atoms / Groups

Replacement of quaternary nitrogen with tertiary carbon is classical example of this type. Structure activity studies of acylcarmitine analogues, a carnitine acyl transferase inhibitors includes replacement of the hydroxyl group of carnitine with amino and as well as quarternary nitrogen with carbon to get trimethyl ammonium group.

Acylcarmitine analogues

Ring Equivalents

Similar physicochemical properties observed for benzene and thiophen is basis for the ring equivalents. Replacement of pyrazole heterocyclic ring of celecoxib with isoxazole and pyridine gave valdecoxib and etoricoxib respectively.

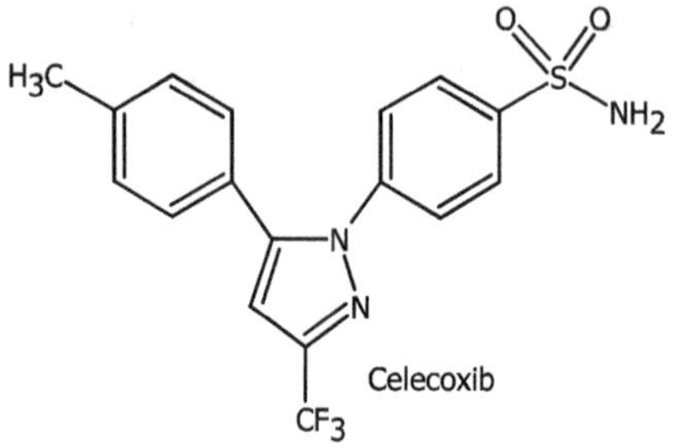

Celecoxib

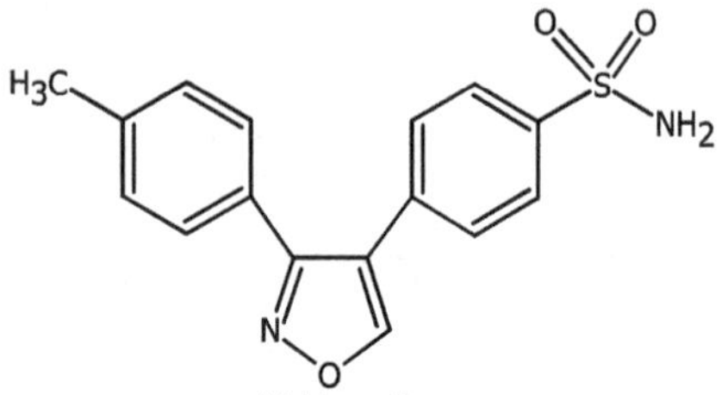

Valdecoxib

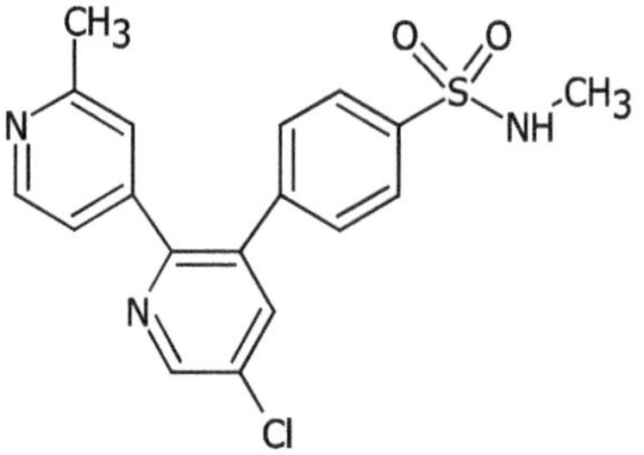

Etoricoxib

In antihistamine mepyramine, pyridyl group is introduced in place of phenyl group in antergan gave more potent antihistamine.

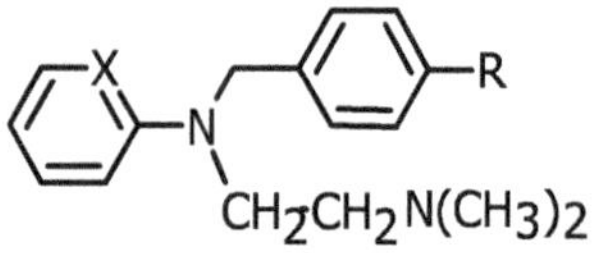

	X	R
Antergan	CH	H
Mepyramine	N	OCH_3

The trivalent substitution of –CH= with –N= is commonly used in modern drug design. In antibacterial agent norfloxacin, this substitution gives enoxacin having same clinical effect.

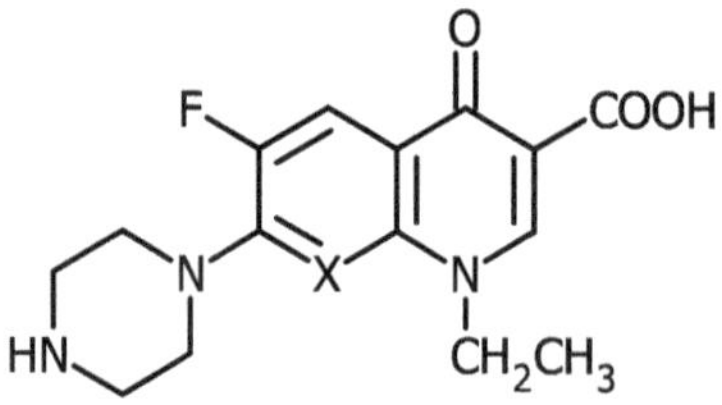

	X
Norfloxacin	-CH-
Enoxacin	-N-

6.3.2 Non-Classical Bio-Isosterism

- Cyclic vs non-cyclic: Local anaesthetic agents lidocaine and mepivacaine is the best example of this type. Both open chain lidocaine and closed ring structure in mepivacaine retain their biological activity.

Lidocaine   Mepivacaine

- Functional groups: Diverse functional groups are known for their bio-isosteric relationship with the carboxylic group. Losartan, angiotensin-II antagonist is developed from lead EXP 7711, where carboxylic group is exchanged with tetrazole group.

EXP 7711   Losartan

- Retroisomerism: It involves the inversion of functional group present in the lead compound. Retroisosteric relationship is present in new selective COX-2 inhibitor leads. In which methyl-sulphonylamine and methylsulphonamide functions is observed. This confers metabolic susceptibility and distinct pKa values. The higher activity of compound is due to the interaction of groups with Arg513 and Ser353 residues present in COX-2, methylsulphonamide group favours this interaction.

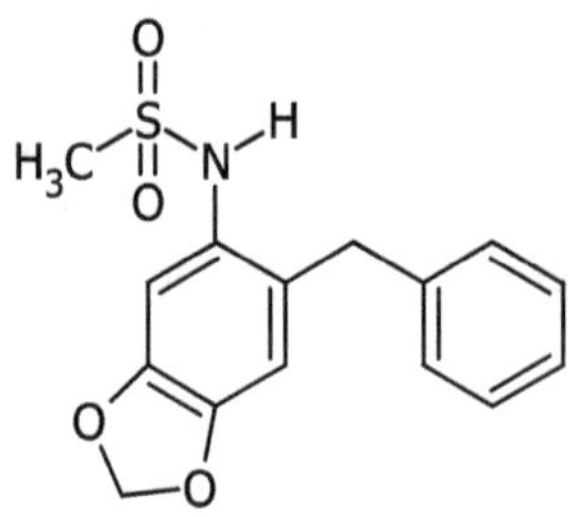

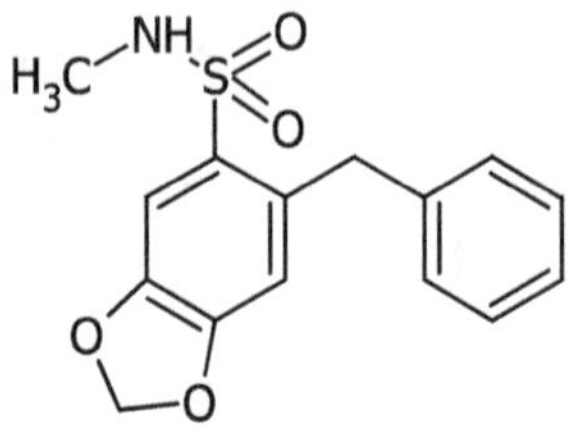

6.3.3 Applications of Bio-Isosterism

1. Structure: Geometry (size, shape and hydrogen bonding) of the structure can be modified to get more complementary structure for the receptor binding.

2. Receptor interactions: Change in the geometry facilitates the specific drug receptor interactions

3. Pharmacokinetic properties: Bio-isosteric modification can be used to alter the absorption, distribution and excretion pattern of the compound.

4. Metabolism: Bio-isosteric modification assists in the rapid / slow elimination of molecule depending upon the necessity.

CHAPTER 7

DRUG DEVELOPMENT

Pharmacokinetic events are highly dependent on permeation and protein recognition. Permeation depends mainly on size, shape, lipophilicity, hydrogen bonding capacity and vander waals radii. In protein recognition, hydrophobicity and hydrogen bonding capacity play major role. Medicinal chemist's utilises metabolic profile (bio-transformation) of the molecules in drug design and lead optimization strategies to reduce the cost and time. It also helps to explore the pharmacokinetic and / toxicological properties. The main utilities of bio-transformation concepts are listed below

- Understanding the biochemical aspects of drugs
- Prediction of metabolism
- Designing of prodrug and soft drug

7.1 Significance of Bio-Transformation

Bio-transformation has much influence on drug development process, helps understanding the following major bio-chemical reactions

1. Formation of active metabolite from drug
2. Formation of active metabolite from prodrug
3. Formation of inactive metabolite
4. Formation of reactive and toxic metabolite
5. Complex kinetics in metabolic pathway (inhibition of metabolic pathway by metabolite)
6. Vast change in the physiochemical properties than drug

Almost all therapeutic agents show some undesirable bio-physicochemical properties. Integrating metabolic considerations into drug design and lead optimization strategies overcome pharmacokinetic and pharmacodynamic defects. For these reason medicinal chemists give more attention to chemistry of metabolic reactions and quantitative structure metabolism relationship. Minimizing or eliminating these undesirable properties while retaining therapeutic efficacy can be achieved by

1. Biological approach: Alters the route of administration if patient experience any difficulty with existing mode.
2. Physical approach: It modifies the design of the dosage form to controlled drug delivery form.
3. Chemical approach: Enhances drug selectivity and minimizes the toxicity

7.2 Chemical Approach in Drug Development

Chemical approach uses three different strategies for optimization of drugs to effect design and development of new drugs with desirable features.

- Design of hard drugs
- Design of soft drugs
- Design of prodrugs

7.3 Hard Drugs

Biologically active and non-metabolizable compounds are known as hard drugs. It resists bodily biotransformation, thus no toxic metabolites are generated. Eg: Biphosphonates.

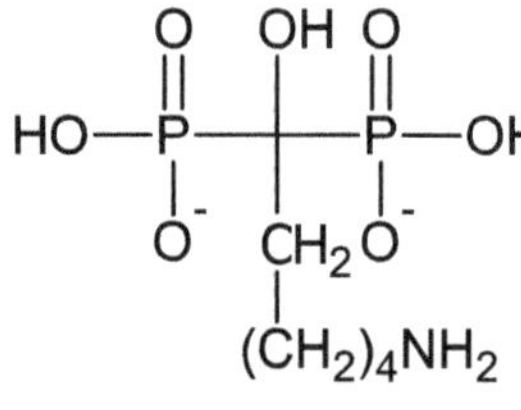

$$HO-\underset{\underset{O^-}{\overset{O}{\|}}}{P}-\underset{\underset{(CH_2)_4NH_2}{\overset{OH}{|}}}{\underset{CH_2}{|}}-\underset{\underset{O^-}{\overset{O}{\|}}}{P}-OH$$

Neridronate

7.4 Soft Drugs

Soft drug design helps in design of safer drugs with an increased therapeutic index by integrating metabolic considerations. Soft drugs are active isoelectric-isoelectronic analogues of a lead compound. They are deactivated in a predictable and controllable way after exerting their therapeutic effect by rapid metabolism.

The goal of soft drug design is not to avoid metabolism, rather to control and direct metabolism that yields inactive species. Higher doses of less potent but much less toxic soft compounds are often preferred over lower doses of more potent and toxic compounds. Inclusion of metabolically sensitive site on the molecule makes possible the design and prediction of its major metabolic pathway and avoids the formation of undesired toxic, active or high energy intermediates.

7.4.1 Types of Soft Drugs

- Soft analogs
- Active metabolite based soft drugs
- Inactive metabolite based soft drugs
- Pro-soft drugs
- Activated soft compounds
- Natural soft drugs

Soft analogues: Close structural analogues of known active drugs that have a specific, metabolically sensitive moiety built into their structure to allow a facile, one step and controllable deactivation and detoxification after achieving their therapeutic activity. Eg: Conversion of cetyl pyridinium chloride in to isosteric soft analog and decamethonium bromide in to succinyl choline.

$$N^+\!-\!CH_2\!\cdot\!CH_2\!\cdot\!CH_2\!-\!(CH_2)_{12}\!-\!CH_3$$
Cetyl pyridinium chloride

$$N^+\!-\!CH_2\!-\!O\!-\!\overset{O}{\overset{\|}{C}}\!-\!(CH_2)_{12}\!\cdot\!CH_3$$
Isosteric soft analog

$$H_2C\!-\!CH_2\!-\!CH_2\!-\!CH_2\!-\!CH_2\!-\!N(CH_3)_3Cl^-$$
$$H_2C\!-\!CH_2\!-\!CH_2\!-\!CH_2\!-\!CH_2\!-\!N(CH_3)_3Cl^-$$

Decamethonium bromide

$$H_2C\!-\!O\!-\!\overset{O}{\overset{\|}{C}}\!-\!CH_2\!\cdot\!CH_2\!-\!N(CH_3)_3Cl^-$$
$$H_2C\!-\!O\!-\!\underset{O}{\overset{\|}{C}}\!-\!CH_2\!\cdot\!CH_2\!-\!N(CH_3)_3Cl^-$$

Succinyl choline chloride

Active metabolite based soft drugs: Many metabolites of drugs (by oxidative conversions) retains significant activity of the parent drug. Bufuralol, a potent non-selective β-antagonist undergoes stepwise oxidative metabolism to form corresponding hydroxyl and keto intermediates. These metabolites are active and have different half live than bufuralol. The active metabolite ketone retains most of the activity and is deactivated by further oxidation.

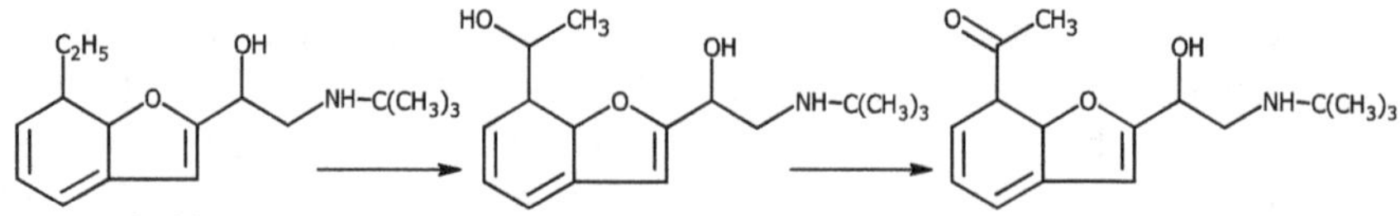

Bufuralol

Inactive metabolite based soft drugs: Active compounds designed with a known inactive metabolite of an existing drug as their starting molecule. It involves the chemical conversion of the metabolite into an isosteric / isoelectric analog of the original drug to allow the metabolic conversion to occur in a controllable manner after achieving their therapeutic activity.

Inactive metabolite based soft drug approach involves three stages
1. Activation stage: chemical modification of known inactive metabolite of a drug
2. Predictable metabolism: New soft analogue upon metabolism yields inactive metabolite without producing toxic intermediate
3. Controllable metabolism: Molecular modification of molecules controls transport, binding properties and rate of metabolism

Pro-soft drugs: Inactive prodrugs of a soft drug of any of the above classes, including endogenous soft molecules are known as pro-soft drugs. These are converted enzymatically into the active soft drug and deactivated. Prodrugs are ideally inactive by design and are converted into an active drug by a predictable mechanism. Soft drugs are active and are designed to achieve controllable metabolic deactivation. Hence it is possible to design a "pro-soft drug" but designing "soft prodrug" is not possible.

Activated soft compounds: Activated soft compounds are designed by introducing non-toxic, inactive pharmacophoric group into the drug structure in order to activate it to exhibit a certain pharmacological activity. Eg: Soft chloramines.

Soft chloramines release positive chlorine (Cl^+) before or after penetrating the microbial cell walls. They have much lower chlorine potential and are much less corrosive than conventional chloramines.

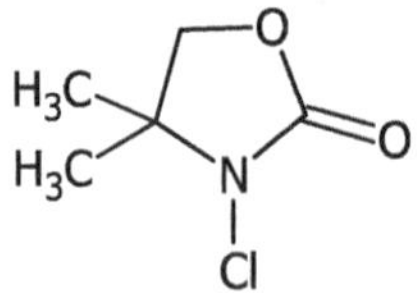

Soft chloramines

Natural soft drugs: Several endogenous substances are considered as natural soft drugs because of their predictable metabolism. Eg: Epinephrine, Dopamine, GABA, Oestradiol, Hydrocartisone etc.

Adrenalone diester through combined reduction-hydrolysis (biotransformation) delivers epinephrine in to eye.

Adrenalone ester   Epinephrine

7.4.2 Applications of Soft Drugs

1. Soft drugs produce increased therapeutic index.
2. Soft drugs undergo predictable metabolism and forms non-toxic metabolites.
3. Improves pharmacokinetic insufficinencies and site specificity
4. Applied in developing selective and safer ocular drug delivery systems
5. Applicable in local delivery of steroids to eye and brain
6. Allergic responses and cataracts observed in long term glucocorticoid therapy have been removed by this strategy
7. Inactive metabolite based approach is most useful in designing selective soft drugs. Esmolol (β-blocker) and remifentanil (opioid analgesic) were developed through this strategy.
8. Selectivity based metabolism can be achieved exploiting differential enzyme distribution in vertebrates. Site directed β-blockers (betaxoxime) is designed to be activated in the eye and avoids undesirable side effects (optic neuropathy and decreased level of HDL).

7.5 Prodrugs

Prodrug design is useful in optimization of clinical application of drug (lead modification approach) and corrects a flaw in a drug candidate. Prodrug is chemically modified inert drug precursor, which upon biotransformation liberates the pharmacologically active parent compound. The conversion of prodrug to drug occurs before / during / after absorption and at specific site.

Active drug $\xrightarrow{\text{Chemical derivatization}}$ Prodrug $\xrightarrow{\text{Biochemical conversion}}$ Active drug

In vivo conversion of prontosil to sulphanilamide generated the idea about prodrug concept.

Prontosil

Biochemical conversion

Sulphanilamide

7.5.1 Types of Prodrugs

- Carrier linked prodrugs
  - Bipartate prodrugs
  - Tripartate prodrugs
  - Mutual prodrugs
- Bioprecursor prodrugs

7.5.2 Carrier Linked Prodrugs

A carrier linked prodrug contains an active drug linked to a carrier group which can be removed enzymatically (ester hydrolysis to carboxylic acid). The bond to the carrier group must be labile enough to allow the active drug to be released efficiently *in vivo*. The carrier group should be nontoxic and biologically inactive when detached from the drug.

Carrier linked prodrugs can be sub divided into bipartate, tripartate and mutual prodrugs.

Bipartate prodrug: A bipartate prodrug is a prodrug in which active drug is attached to the carrier. In chloramphenicol palmitate, palmitate is carrier will get released in *in vivo* enzymatic hydrolysis.

Chloramphenicol palmitate → Chloramphenicol

Tripartate prodrugs: The prodrug linkage in bipartate prodrugs is too labile or stable and renders it ineffective. A tripartate (a self-immolative) prodrug overcomes this problem. In a tripartate prodrug the carrier is not connected directly to the drug, but rather to a linker that in turn attached to the drug. Eg: bacampicillin and pivampicilllin (prodrugs of ampicillin).

Ampicillin

	R	**R**^{1}
Bacampicillin	$-CH_3$	$- OC_2H_5$
Pivampicillin	$-H$	$- C(CH_3)_3$

Mutual prodrugs: A mutual prodrug is bipartate / tripartate prodrug in which the carrier is synergistic drug to the drug to which it is linked. The combination of amoxicillin and the β-lactamase inactivator potassium clavulanate is used for oral treatment of infections is an classical example of this kind.

Amoxycillin

Potassium clavulanate

7.5.3 Bioprecursor Prodrugs

A bioprecursor prodrug is a compound that is metabolized into drug. Unlike the carrier linked prodrug, a bioprecursor prodrug contains a different structure that cannot be converted into active drug by a simple cleavage of a group. Bio-precursor prodrugs mostly utilize oxidative or reductive activation reactions.

Levodopa is a prodrug for the neurotransmitter dopamine. High polar nature of dopamine restricts its transport through blood-brain barrier. Levodopa (even more polar) uses amino acid transporter to cross blood-brain barrier and a decarboxylase enzyme present in brain tissue removes the acid group and generates dopamine.

Levodopa   Dopamine

An anti-ulcer drug omeprazole is a bio-precursor, which upon smiles rearrangement converts in to an active form. The active form of omeprazole through covalent interaction with proton pump produces inhibition of acid secretion.

Omeprazole

7.5.4 Applications of Prodrugs

Prodrugs to alter aqueous solubility: Chloramphenicol, an antibiotic has bitter taste and can be converted into more hydrophobic palmitate ester (due to long chain fatty acid group), which is tasteless. It doesn't dissolve easily on the tongue (tasteless) and is quickly hydrolyzed once swallowed.

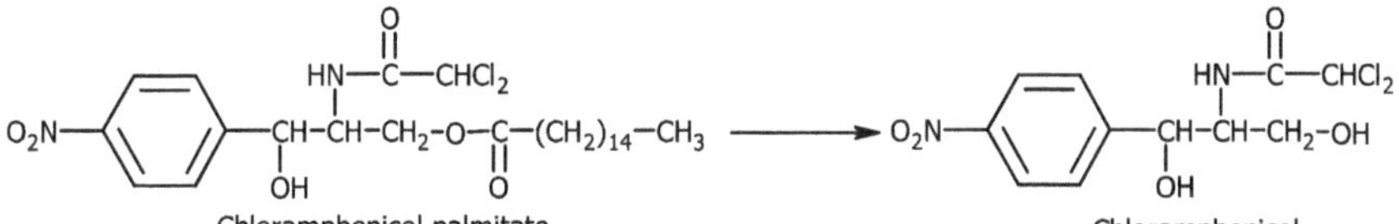

Chloramphenicol palmitate

Chloramphenicol

Prodrugs for improved absorption and distribution: Epinephrine absorption through cornea is difficult because of its more hydrophilicity. Dipivaloylepinephrine (dipivefrin), a prodrug form of epinephrine used for anti-glaucoma therapy, is able to penetrate the cornea better than epinephrine. Two protected hydroxyl groups present in the epinephrine is protected in dipivefrin, which increases liphophilicity and in turn penetration. The cornea and aqueous humor have significant esterase activity, once absorbed an esterase releases the drug.

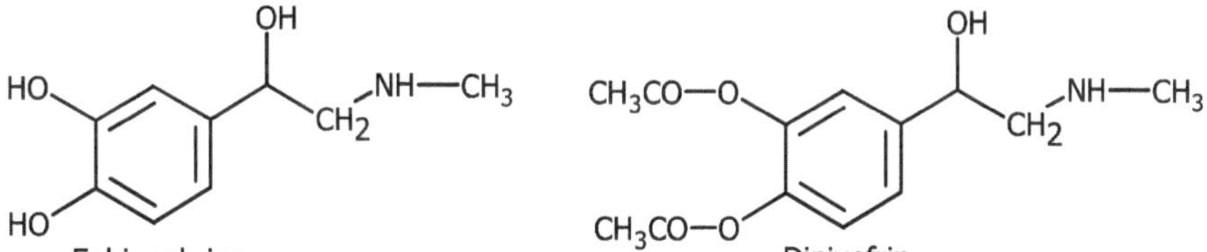

Ephinephrine

Dipivefrin

Prodrugs for site specificity: Site specific drug delivery requires activation of prodrug by enzyme found predominantly at the desired site of action. Tumor cells contain a higher concentration of phosphatases and amidases than normal cells. Diethylstilbestrol phosphate was designed for site specificity delivery of diethylstilbestrol to prostatic carcinoma tissue. Phosphatases present in tumour cells hydrolyse diethylstilbestrol phosphate into diethylstilbestrol.

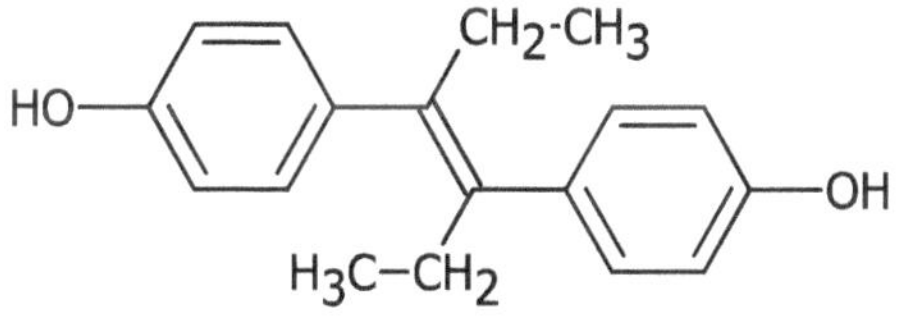

Diethyl stilbesterol

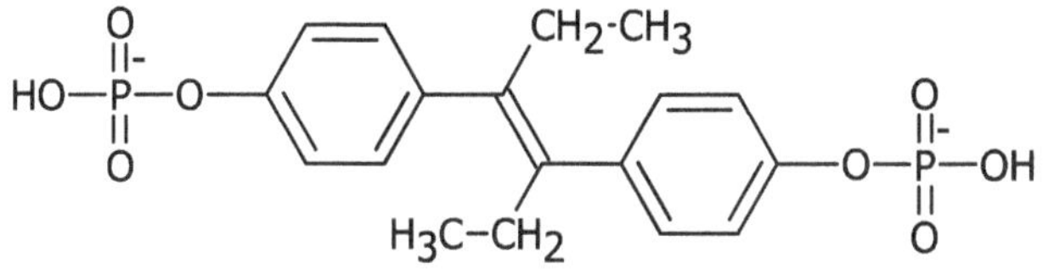

Diethyl stilbesterol diphosphate

Prodrugs for stability: Antihypertensive drug propranolol shows much lower bioavailability because of first pass elimination in oral adminstration. The major metabolites are propranolol O-glucuronide, p-hydroxypropranolol and its O-glucuronide. The hemisuccinate ester of propanolol was prepared to block glucuronide formation.

Propronolol

Prodrugs for slow and prolonged release: Antipsychotic fluphenazine has a short duration of activity due to its polar carboxylic group. Prodrug form of fluphenazine, fluphenazine enanthate and fluphenazine decanoate have longer duration of action (for about a month). On metabolic hydrolysis drug gets converted into active form.

	R
Fluphenazine	-H
Fluphenazine ethanthate	-CO (CH$_2$)$_5$ CH$_3$
Fluphenazine decanoate	-CO (CH$_2$)8 CH$_3$

Prodrugs to minimize the toxicity: The gastric irritation and ulceroginicity associated with aspirin is due to the accumulation of the salicylic acid in the gastric mucosal cells. Esterification of aspirin greatly suppresses gastric ulcerogenic activity.

Aspirin

Prodrugs to eliminate formulation problems: High toxicity associated with disinfectant formaldehyde limits its direct use as medicine. Formaldehyde with ammonia produces a stable methenamine. In acidic pH of urine, methenamine hydrolyses to formaldehyde and ammonium ions and is used as a urinary tract antiseptic.

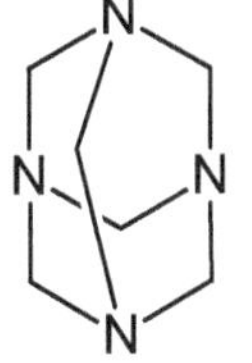

Methenamine

7.6 Targeted Prodrug Design

Prodrugs can be designed to target specific enzymes or carriers by considering enzyme-substrate specificity or carrier-substrate specificity in order to overcome various undesirable drug properties. Targeted prodrug design is classified into two types:

1. Targeting specific enzymes
2. Targeting specific membrane transporters

Targeting specific enzymes: The enzyme-targeted prodrug approach can be used to improve the oral drug absorption and site-specific drug delivery. In the case of improving oral drug absorption, gastrointestinal enzymes are the main targets for prodrug design. The use of a nutrient moiety as a derivatizing group permits more specific targeting for gastrointestinal enzymes to improve oral drug absorption. Glycosidase activity of the colonic micro flora offers an opportunity to design a colon-specific drug delivery system. Glycoside derivates are hydrophilic and poorly absorbed from the small intestine, but once they reach the colon they can be effectively cleaved by bacterial glycosidases to release the free drug.

Targeting specific membrane transporters: The targeted prodrug approach uses membrane transporters to facilitate the transport of polar nutrients such as amino acids and peptides. Prodrugs can be designed to resemble the intestinal nutrients structurally and to be absorbed by specific carrier proteins. p-nitrophenyl-β-D-glucopyranoside was found to be actively absorbed by glucose transporters and its permeation was comparable with that of D-glucose.

Site-specificity delivery can be obtained from tissue-specific activation of a prodrug, which is a result of metabolism by an enzyme that is either unique for the tissue or present in the tissue at a higher concentration compared with other tissues.

7.6.1 Enzyme-Activity Prodrug Therapy

Enzyme-activity prodrug therapy involves the following two step approach

1. Targeting drug-activating enzyme in tumors is first step and
2. Systemic administration of nontoxic prodrug (substrate of exogenous enzyme expressed in tumors).

The net gain is that a systemically administered prodrug can be converted to high local concentration of an active anticancer drug in tumors.

To be clinically successful both enzymes and prodrugs should meet certain requirements.

- Prodrug-activating enzyme should be either of non-human origin or a human protein that is expressed only at low concentration in normal tissues.

- The prodrug should be a good substrate for the expressed enzyme in tumors and not activated by endogenous enzyme in non-tumor tissues.

- The prodrug must be able to cross the tumor cell membrane for intracellular activation.

- The activated drug should be highly diffusible or actively taken up by adjacent non-expressing tumor cells to show 'bystander killing effect' (the ability of a drug to kill neighbouring non-expressing cells).

- The half-life of active drug should be long enough to induce bystander killing effect, but short enough to avoid drug leaking out of the tumor cell.

- Cytotoxicity difference between prodrug and active drug should be as high as possible.

7.6.2 Enzyme Prodrug Strategies

Enzyme prodrug strategy can be divided into two major classes.

1. Delivery of active enzymes onto tumor tissues
    - Antibody Directed Enzyme Prodrug Therapy (ADEPT)
2. Delivery of genes that encode prodrug activating enzymes into tumor tissues
    - Gene Directed Enzyme Prodrug Therapy (GDEPT)
    - Genetic Prodrug Activated Therapy (GPAT)
    - Virus Directed Enzyme Prodrug Therapy (VDEPT)

Antibody Directed Enzyme Prodrug Therapy (ADEPT): An antibody raised against a particular tumor cell line is conjugated with the enzyme that is needed to activate an antitumor prodrug. Antibody-enzyme conjugate accumulates on the tumor cell and the excess conjugate not bound to the tumor cell will be cleared from blood and normal tissues. The antibody enzyme conjugated present on the tumor surface catalyzes the conversion of the prodrug to the active drug.

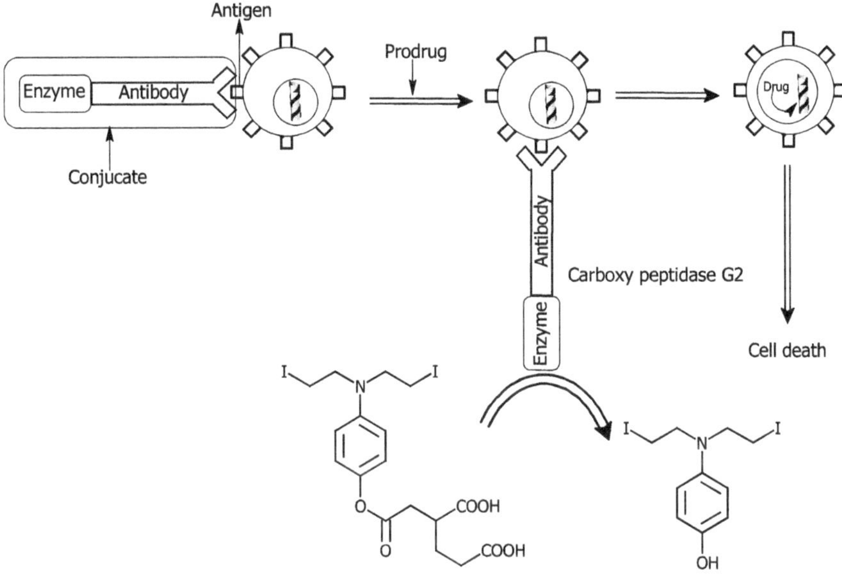

Fig. 7.1 Antibody directed enzyme prodrug therapy.

Gene Directed Enzyme Prodrug Therapy (GDEPT): GDEPT also called as suicide gene therapy and involves two steps. In first step a gene encoding the prodrug-activating enzyme is delivered through liposomes. The prodrug is then administered which is activated to drug by the enzyme expressed by the gene delivered previously.

Genetic Prodrug Activation Therapy (GPAT): GPAT is a variation of GDEPT, which uses known transcriptional differences between normal and tumor cells to drive the selective expression of a drug-metabolizing enzyme to convert a nontoxic prodrug into a toxic moiety.

Virus Directed Enzyme Prodrug Therapy (VDEPT): VDEPT relies on the use of viral vectors for efficient delivery of "suicide gene" encoding an enzyme, which converts non-toxic prodrug to cytotoxic agent. The VDEPT system requires a gene expressing a non-endogeneous enzyme, which is able to activate the prodrug. The gene must be expressed in a sufficient number of target cells at high levels compared to normal cells and the total catalytic activity achieved, its distribution must be sufficient for therapeutic benefit.

Table 7.1 Differences between a hard drug and a soft drug.

Hard drugs	Soft drugs
• Non-metabolizing compounds characterized by high lipid solubility and accumulation in adipose tissues and organelles.	• Biologically active, therapeutically useful compounds with predictable and controllable metabolism.
• Poor substrates for metabolizing enzymes.	• Active substrates for metabolizing enzymes.
• Hard to metabolize.	• Easy to metabolize.
• Metabolically sensitive parts are sterically hindered or the hydrogen atoms are substituted with halogens to block oxidation.	• Metabolically sensitive parts are not sterically hindered.
• Gives toxic or active products after metabolism.	• Gives non toxic or inactive products after metabolism.

Table 7.2 Difference between prodrug and soft drug.

Prodrug	Soft drug
• Prodrugs are derivatives of bioactive molecules which are inactive and converted *in vivo* to the active form.	• Soft drugs are bioactive molecules which are active and converted *in vivo* to the inactive form.

7.7 Bio Assay

Bio assays measures the potency of the new or chemically undefined substance on living matter. This also evaluates the side effect profile (toxicity) of the test molecule and determines the specificity of the substance to receptors. Bioassays can be divided in to the following categories

- *In Silico* screen: Screening through computer algorithms (virtual screening)
- *In Vitro* screen: Screening on sub-cellular organelles including cell based assays

  Ex Vivo Screen: Tissue based assay

- *In Vivo* Screen: Animal based assay includes preclinical and human clinical trials.

***In silico assay*:** It involves the screening of database representative sets (compounds) to identify hit molecules (which are likely to produce biological potential) prior to the experimental synthesis of molecules. It enable the selection of limited subset molecules to identify the novel chemical entities having selectivity for target molecule (receptor). This includes 2D and 3D similarity searching, ligand and target based pharmacophore mapping and molecular docking.

***In Vivo* assay:** In this assay both test and standard compounds are administered to animals to derive dose-response relationship and explore their potency. Animals will be selected on the basis of species, strain, gender and weight.

***Ex Vivo* assay:** Cells or tissues from human or animal donors can be (cultured in the laboratory) used to assess the test compound potential. This type of assay requires similar process management as that of in vivo assay to minimize variability.

***In Vitro* assay:** It includes experimental biology studies, which are conducted in isolated components of an organism. These experiments are most commonly known as test tube experiments.

7.8 Clinical Studies

Study of drug effectiveness in human system is called as clinical trials. Its study involves battery of tests to generate safety and efficacy data of for the drugs, diagnostics, devices and therapy protocols. It is described in four temporal phases (phase I-IV), recently phase 0 trial also introduced in to the procedure.

Phase 0: It involves micro-dosing of the several drugs. It provides essential human pharmacokinetic and pharmacodymanic data earlier in drug development process. Hence this more sophisticated method supports in the design and clinical development of agents.

Phase I: It involves the administration of the investigational drugs to the healthy volunteers to determine the dose tolerance and nature of adverse reactions. This study also involve in the pharmacokinetic assessment and drug-drug interaction analysis.

Phase II: This involves the study of effect of investigational drugs unhealthy volunteers (patients) of homogenous population. The efficacy and safety of the drugs for the particular therapeutic indication will be evaluated.

Phase III: These studies provide the adequate basis for the approval of drug launch in to market. It explores the dose-response relationship in wider populations, different stages of disease and drug use with other combinations.

Phase IV: It involves the assessment of additional drug-drug interaction dose-response, safety studies and use of drug in approved indication. It monitors the use of drugs in very large populations and identifies additional use of drugs.

New technologies are developed in order to increase the success rate and to help reducing the cost of drug discovery process. In present days the following newer drug discovery technologies are being used

- siRNA approach
- Ultra high throughput screening (ultra HTS)
- Combinatorial chemistry
- Genomics, proteomics and toxicogenomics approaches
- Bio-physical techniques (NMR spectroscopy and X ray crystallography)
- Structure based drug design

<h1>CHAPTER 8</h1>

DRUG DESIGN

Designing molecules with more complementarity for the active sites of the receptor protein is called as drug design. It involves mainly the identification of target, ligand and their 3D structural studies.

- Drug design is an integrated developing discipline which involves the study of effects of biologically active compounds on the basis of molecular interactions in terms of molecular structures or its physico-chemical properties.

- Drug design involves either total innovation of lead or an optimization of already available lead.

- The current trend in the drug design is to develop new clinically effective agents through the structural modification of a lead nucleus.

8.1 Rational Drug Design (RDD)

Advancement in the understanding of physiological mechanism, identification of target protein, identification of natural ligand and use of biophysical techniques (X ray crystallography and NMR spectroscopy) in 3D structural determination of target proteins and ligands gave path for "rational drug design".

Drug discovery is also guided by scientific understanding of chemical structures, pharmacological actions and mechanism of disease. Rational drug design utilises knowledge on physiological and chemical properties of target and its interactions with molecules to design newer ligands. Development of cimetidine (H_2-blocker) from histamine, a natural ligand is the good example for rational drug design.

These traditional methods provided most existing drugs but the entire process is laborious and expensive. In order to further the drug discovery, a rational drug design (RDD) approach is emerged. Rational drug design is based on the principle that biological properties of the molecules are related their structural features. It includes physicochemical properties, Log P, hydrogen bonding and 3D structures (geometry) of both ligand and receptor protein.

8.2 Types of Rational Drug Design

- 1st generation rational drug design
- 2nd generation rational drug design

1st **generation rational drug design:** It involves prediction of bio-physical properties of the molecules using theoretical equations. Liphophilicity (Log P), steric substituent constant (Es), electronic effects (σ) and molar refractivity (MR) are the important drug-likeness parameters are useful in predicting the biological activity of the molecule. This strategy concentrates on two dimensional aspects (2D) of the molecules and hence known as 2D-quantitative structure activity relationship (2D-QSAR).

2nd **generation rational drug design:** This strategy considers molecular properties of three dimensional (3D) structures of molecules and supports their visualization (2D-QSAR concentrates on 2D-structural properties). Hence this procedure is called as 3D- quantitative structure activity relationship (3D-QSAR).

8.3 Second Generation Rational Drug Design Strategies

1. Direct design: It involves the designing of molecules based on the 3D features of a receptor binding sites
2. Indirect design: It involves the designing of molecules based on the comparative analysis of known active and inactive molecules (pharmacophoric concept)
3. Database search: It involves the designing of molecules based on the pharmacophoric concept and search against 3D databases.
4. 3D automated drug design: New lead compounds are generated on the basis of a active binding site of the protein.
5. Molecular mimicry: It involves design of mimics of selected reference ligands.

8.4 Rational Drug Design Techniques

Various techniques used in rational drug design are:

1. Quantitative Structure Activity Relationship (QSAR)

2. Virtual screening
   (a) Cheminformatics
   (b) Molecular modelling
3. Protein crystallography
4. NMR spectroscopy
5. Homology / comparative modelling
6. Molecular graphics

Quantitative Structure Activity Relationship (QSAR): Steric effect is an important physicochemical parameter of quantitative structure activity relationship, used in both lead discovery and lead modification process. Mutual approach of ligand and receptor is depends on the steric and electronic effects excerted by the molecules, which ultimately decide the molecular interaction.

Virtual screening: Virtual screening uses computer-based methods to discover new ligands on the basis of biological structures. Virtual screening has emerged as an adaptive response to the massive throughput synthesis and screening paradigm.

Cheminformatics: Cheminformatics is an integral part of the drug discovery process, from lead identification through lead development. 2D similarities and substructure searching can be done through cheminformatics. The basic principle behind this is compounds with common structural features will have similar biological activity.

Molecular modeling: Docking is a molecular modeling method, which predicts the preferred orientation of one molecule (target) to a second molecule (ligand) when bound to each other. Docking is frequently used to predict the binding orientation of small molecule drug candidate to their targets. Virtual screening based docking is an emerging technology in rational lead discovery based on receptor structure.

Protein crystallography: Purified proteins (targets) will be subjected for crystallization and it yields 3D structure with great accuracy. Structures of the target protein complexed with drugs can be determined by X-ray crystallography. Complexed structure reveals major/minor conformational changes of the protein and is useful in the designing of newer molecules.

NMR spectroscopy: A survey by GSK (2006) indicates that only about 50 % of all screening techniques produces quality leads that are worthy of further evaluation. Upon binding to the receptor, the apparent molecular weight and hydrodynamic radius of a small ligand change dramatically.

This is due to the conformational changes of ligand upon binding to the target and ligand. A dedicated "editing experiments" by NMR spectroscopy provide a powerful tool for the structure determination of a protein-ligand complex. It explains the exact intermolecular interactions and thus helps in the identification of best fit molecule.

Homology modeling / comparative modeling: It is a methodology helps in predicting protein / target structures based on the general observations that proteins with similar sequences have similar structures. When crystal structures of proteins are not available, homology modeling is the alternative method to predict the 3D structure of the target. A combination of homology modeling and docking is effective virtual screening tool in ligand identification and ligand optimization.

Molecular graphics: Molecular modeling techniques with the aid of various theoretical calculations suggest useful drug molecules. Promising molecules need to be synthesised and tested for its efficacy.

QUANTITATIVE STRUCTURE ACTIVITY RELATIONSHIP (QSAR)

Quantitative structure activity relationship uses parameters assigned to the various functional groups and modifies the structure of a compound. These parameters (also known as descriptors) are a measure of the potential contribution of its group to a particular property of the parent drug. In a typical procedure a series of related compounds are examined and the relevant parameters of their substituent groups compared with the biological activities of the compounds. 2D-QSAR establishes mathematical relationships in the form of an equation between biological activity and measurable bio-physicochemical properties. The structure of the most promising derivatives are predicted which helps in molecular modifications.

The important breakthrough of 2D-QSAR

- **Richet rule:** Richet observed that narcotic actions of group of compounds are inversely proportional to their water solubility.

- **Overton and Meyor theory:** This theory explains that the tad pole narcoses of group of structurally non-specific compounds are due to their liphophilicity.

- **Ferguson principle:** Ferguson related the biological activity to their thermodynamic property.

The pharmacokinetic and pharmacodynamic property of the molecule is depends upon the solubility (Log P), electronic (σ) and steric features (E_s) of the molecule.

$$\text{Log (BA)} = a \text{ Log P} + b\sigma + c \text{ Es}$$

9.1 QSAR Descriptors

- **Solubility parameters**
    - Water solubility
    - Partition coefficient [Log P]
    - Hansch substituent constant [π]
    - Fragmentation constant [f]
    - Chromatographic R_m value [R_m]
- **Electronic parameters**
    - Hammett substituent constant [σ]
    - Inductive substituent constant [σ_1]
    - Taft substituent constant [σ^*]
    - Swain-Lupton constant
- **Steric parameters**
    - Taft-steric substituent constant
    - Charton steric constant
    - Molar refractivity
    - Molecular connectivity
    - Sterimol parameter
    - Parachor

9.2 Solubility Parameters

9.2.1 Predicting Water Solubility

Empirical approach: Lemke developed constants based on carbon solubilising potential of organic functional groups. If the solubilising potential of the functional groups exceeds the total number of carbon atoms present in the molecule (excluding the carbon atom in functional group) then the molecule is considered to be water soluble. Functional groups that can interact either through intramolecular hydrogen bonds / ion-ion interaction will decrease the solubilising potential of each group. Since most drug molecules are polyfunctional, polyfunctional values are considered instead of monofunctional values.

Functional group	Monofunctional molecule	Polyfunctional molecule
-OH (alcoholic)	5-6	3-4
-OH (phenolic)	6-7	3-4
-O- (ether)	4-5	2

Table *Contd...*

Functional group	Monofunctional molecule	Polyfunctional molecule
-CHO (aldehyde)	4-5	2
-CO- (ketone)	5-6	2
$-NH_2$ (amine)	6-7	3
-COOH (carboxyl)	5-6	3
-COO- (esteric)	6	3
-NH-CO- (amide)	6	2-3
$-NH_2-CO-NH_2$, $-CO_3$, -CO-NH-	6	2

Calculation of solubility of ibuprofen

CH_3

CH_3

H_3C COOH

Ibuprofen

Ibuprofen contains	1 aromatic amine	- can solubilise 3 carbons
	1 tertiary alkylamine	- can solubilise 3 carbons
	1 ester group	- can solubilise 3 carbons

Total number of carbon atoms in the molecule is   = 21

Solubilizing potential of the functional groups are   = 9

Since, solubilizing potential of the functional groups is less than the total number of carbon, ibuprofen is water insoluble, but the hydrochloride salt is soluble in water.

Analytical approach: Calculating approximate logP of a molecule gives details about their solubility. Hydrophobic substituents constant is usually referred as ClogP and are given in the table.

Fragment	π value	
-C (aliphatic)	+ 0.5	
-Phenyl	+ 2.0	
-Cl	+ 0.5	
$-NO_3$	+ 0.2	
-IMHB	+ 0.65	
-S	0.0	
-COO		-0.7

Table *Contd...*

Fragment	π value
-CO-NH-, -CO-N-	-0.7
-OH, -O-	-1.0
$-NH_2$, -NH, -N	-1.0
NO_2 aliphatic	-0.85
NO_2 aromatic	-0.28

Calculation of solubility of ibuprofen

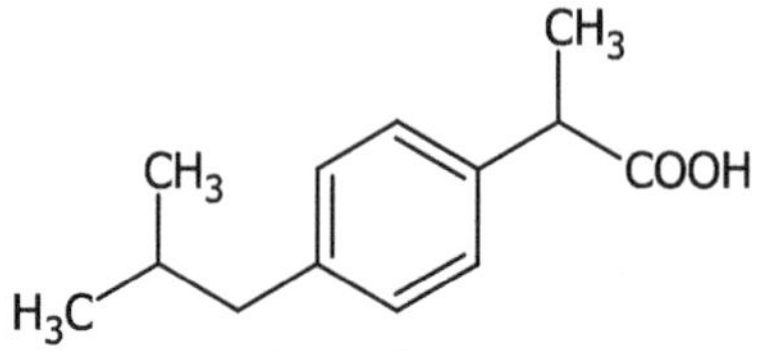

Carbon (6×0.5) $= 3$

Phenyl (1×2.0) $= 2$

COOH (1×-0.7) $= -0.7$

$\overline{}$

$\quad\quad\quad\quad\quad\quad + 4.3$

$\overline{}$

Log P (expt) $=$

ClogP $= + 3.68$

9.2.2 Partition Coefficient

In order to reach its site of action drugs must possess interactive properties with both lipoidal biomembrane and aqueous bio-phase. The first step in drug transport is a slow diffusion of drug through membrane. This process is very slow and highly dependent on the molecular structure of the drug. Liphophilicity is a measure of drug solubility in biological lipid membranes. Lipophilicity can be measured by distribution of the drug between an aqueous and non-aqueous phase. Hansch designed a model, consists of n-octanol as a non-aqueous phase (which simulates a lipid membrane) and aqueous buffer (which simulates the bio-phase) to determine the lipophilicity. Hansch described this measure of the solubility in n-octanol-water system as partition coefficient (Log P).

$$\text{Log } P = \frac{\text{Compound}_{org}}{\text{Compound}_{aq}} \, (1 - \alpha)$$

α = Degree of dissociation of compound in water

Partition coefficient is a free energy related parameter which expresses the relative free energy change occurring on movement of compound from one phase to another. n-octanol has a long saturated alkyl chain, a hydroxyl group for hydrogen bonding and it dissolves water to the extend of 1.7 M (saturation). This combination of lipophilic chains, hydrophilic groups and water molecules makes n-octanol very similar to those of natural membranes and macromolecules. Colander model for the drug transport to its site of action and the relative potency of the drug is expressed as

$$\text{Log} (1/C) = K_1 \, \text{Log} \, P + K_2$$

Larger Log P enhances more drug interaction with lipoidal membrane.

1. As Log P approaches infinity (Log $P = \infty$) (lipophilicity predominates) micelles will form and drug remains in lipoidal membrane.

2. It will be localized in the lipophilic phase with which it comes into contact first.

3. As Log P approaches zero (Log $P = 0$) (more water soluble) molecule will be localized in the aqueous phase because of its inability to cross lipid membrane.

The optimum Log P refers to the balance between aqueous and lipid solubility (so that drug transport in both site 1 and site 2 are to maximum extent) and results in good biological activity response.

Estimation of Log P

Shake flask method: Shaking the separatory flask containing varying volumes of n-octanol and water with added drug gently ensures the complete distribution of the compound between two phases. Determination of concentration of the compound in each phase can be done by normal titrimetry, gas chromatography and HPLC techniques. The partition coefficient of a compound can be derived from the equation

$$\text{Log} \, P = (\text{Compound})_{\text{org}} / (\text{Compound})_{\text{aq}}$$

The reverse phase HPLC (RP-HPLC) method is applicable for compounds with wide range of lipophilicity and results produced are accurate. RP-HPLC method is also used to determine the Log D value.

Choice of organic phase: More accurate results may be obtained if the organic phase is matched to the area of biological activity being studied.

1. n-octanol usually gives most consistant results for drugs absorbed in the gastro intestinal tract.

2. Less polar solvents (eg: olive oil) frequently give more consistant correlations for drugs crossing the blood-brain barrier.

3. More polar solvents (eg: chloroform) gives consistant values for buccal absorption.

Some of the commercially available software packages to predict Log P are listed below

Day light	-	ClogP
ACD	-	logP
CTIS	-	AUTOLOG
Scivision	-	Sci logP
Bio-Rad	-	Predict It Log P and log D,

9.2.3 Hansch Substituent Constant
(Lipophilicity / Hydrophobic Substituent Constant)

Drug biological activity is influenced by lipophilicity, electronic and steric properties of the substituents at specified position. The environment of a substituent also got significant influence on its bio-chemical property. Hansch and co-workers derived substituent constant (π) for the contribution of individual atoms and groups to the partition coefficient. These substituent constants are additive and constitutive in nature.

$$\pi = \log (P_X / P_H) = \log P_x - \log P_H$$

Log P_x = Partition coefficient for the molecule with substituent X

Log P_H = Partition coefficient for the molecule with substituent H

A positive π value indicates that a substituent has higher lipophilicity.

A negative π value indicates that a substituent has lower lipophilicity.

Additive property: Multiple substituents exert an influence equal to the sum of the individual substituents.

Constitutive property: Effect of substituent may differ depending on the molecule to which it is attached or on its environment.

Groups	Aliphatic	Aromatic		
		o	**m**	**P**
OH	-1.16 (1°)	-0.41	-0.49	-0.61
	-1.39 (2°)			
	-1.43 (3°)			
Cl	0.39	0.71	0.76	0.70
F	-0.17	-	0.22	0.15
I	1.00	0.93	1.18	1.43
Br	0.60	0.84	0.96	1.19
COOH	-0.67	-1.26	-	-
COCH₃	-0.71	-1.26	-	-
CH₃	0.52	0.84	0.51	0.56
OCH₃	0.47	-0.98	-	-
NH₂	-1.19	-1.40	-1.29	-1.30
NO₂	0.85	-	0.11	0.22
CN	-0.84	-1.47	-	-
CONH₂	-1.71	-2.28	-	-

[As a rule Log P or π is lowered by 0.2 unit per branch,
since branching in an alkyl chain lowers the lipid solubility].

Calculation of Log P

- **For diethyl stilbesterol**

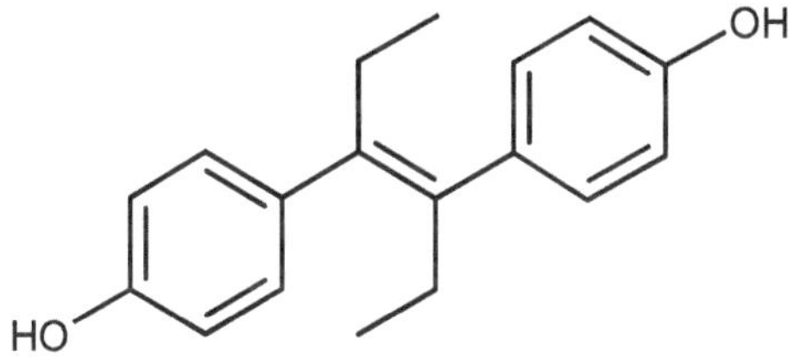

$$\text{Log P} = 2\,\pi\,CH_3 + 2\,\pi\,CH_2 + \pi\,CH = CH + 2\,\text{Log P}_{PhOH} - 0.4$$
(2 branch)

$$\text{Log P} = (2 \times 0.52) + (2 \times 0.52) + 0.72 + (2 \times 1.46) - 0.4$$

$$\text{Log P} = 5.32 \text{ (predicted)}$$

Log P = 5.07 (experimental)

The constant for CH=CH is calculated by adopting the following concept.

In conjucated systems, π values are fairly constant

π value for -CH=CH-CH=CH- is 1.38 ± 0.046

So, $\pi_{CH=CH} = 1/2\,\pi_{(CH=CH-CH=CH)} = 1/1.38 = 0.72$

The constant for CH=CH–CH=CH is calculated through following strategy.

Log P of naphthalene – log P of benzene

$$\text{Log P} \quad - \quad \text{Log P}$$

$$= 3.45 - 2.13 \quad = 1.32$$

Log P of indole – log P of pyrazole

$$\text{Log P} \quad - \quad \text{Log P}$$

$$= 2.14 - 0.75 \quad = 1.39$$

Log P of quinoline – log P of pyridine

$$\text{Log P} \quad - \quad \text{Log P}$$

$$= 2.03 - 0.65 \quad = 1.38$$

Log P of anthracene – log P of quinoline

$$\text{Log P} \quad - \quad \text{Log P}$$

$$= 3.40 - 2.03 \quad = 1.37$$

- **For diphenhydramine**

$$CHO-CH_2-CH_2-N\begin{cases} CH_3 \\ CH_3 \end{cases}$$

$$\text{Log P} \quad = \quad 2\,\pi_{Ph} + \pi\,CH + \pi\,oCH_2 + \pi\,CH_2 + \pi\,N(CH_3)_2 - 0.2$$

$$\text{Log P} \quad = \quad 2 \times 2.13 + 0.5 - 0.73 + 0.5 - 0.95 - 0.2$$

$$\text{Log P} \quad = \quad 3.38 \text{ (predicted)}$$

$$\text{Log P} \quad = \quad 5.07 \text{ (experimental)}$$

$$\text{Log P for benzene} \quad = \quad 2.13$$

$$\pi\,CH \quad = \quad \pi\,CH_3 = 0.5$$

π oCH$_2$ value is obtained by subtracting 1.5 (2 π CH$_3$ + π CH$_2$) from 0.77 (Log P of CH$_3$CH$_2$ OCH$_2$ CH$_3$)

$$\pi\, oCH_2 \;=\; Log\, CH_3CH_2\, OCH_2\, CH_3 - 2\,\pi\, CH_3 + \pi\, CH_2$$
$$=\; 0.77 - (2 \times 0.5) + 0.5$$
$$=\; -\,0.73$$

π N(CH$_3$)   value is obtained by subtracting 3.63 (π Ph (CH$_2$)$_3$) from 2.68 (Log P of CH$_3$CH$_2$ OCH$_2$ CH$_3$)

$$\pi\, N(CH_3)_2 \;=\; Log\, P\, Ph\,(CH_2)_3\, N(CH_3)_2 - \pi\, Ph\,(CH_2)_3$$
$$=\; 2.68 - 2.13 + 3 \times 0.5$$
$$=\; -\,0.73$$

1 branch $=\; 0.2 \times 1 = 0.2$

9.2.4 Fragmentation Constant

The values for CH$_3$ and CH$_2$ are same in Hansch method, hence it is considered inadequate method. An alternative approach for calculating Log P is by using fragmentation constant is established.

$$Log\, P = \Sigma\, af$$

a = number of times the group occurs

f = hydrophobic fragmentation constant

Groups	(f)Values
$-\!\overset{\textstyle\mid}{\underset{\textstyle\mid}{C}}\!-$	0.20
-COOH	−1.11
-H	0.23
-OH	−1.64
-NH$_2$	−1.54
-O	−1.82

For hydrocarbon chains 0.12 (n-1) is substracted, where n = number of bonds between carbons and between carbon and hetero atoms (except hydrogen).

Calculation for n-propanol (CH$_3$CH$_2$ CH$_2$OH)

$$= (3 \times C) + (7 \times H) - (3 \times CH) - (1 \times OH)$$
$$= (3 \times 0.2) + (7 \times 0.23) - (2 \times 0.12) - (1 \times -1.64)$$
$$= 0.6 + 1.61 - 0.24 - (1.64)$$
$$= 2.21 - 1.84$$
$$= 0.33$$

But, Hansch method gives

$$= 3 \times 0.52 + (1 \times -1.16)$$

$$= 1.56 - 1.16$$

$$= 0.40$$

9.2.5 Chromatographic R_m Value

R_f value of chromatography is related to partition coefficient and can be used as a measure of liphophilicity. Partition coefficient becomes difficult to determine experimentally, if the solubility of the solute is considered greater in one phase then in the other. R_m value from reverse phase paper and thin layer chromatography (RP-TLC) can be used as an alternative to calculate Log P value.

$$R_m = \log (1/R_f + 1)$$

$$\text{Log P} = R_m + \text{constant}$$

Chromatogram can be run on thin layer [impregnated with liquid paraffin / silicone oil / ethyl oleate / n-octanol] using acetone-water as moving phase. Extrapolation of R_f values to zero acetone concentration gives R_m value. This value can be used as a substitute for partition coefficient in QSAR investigation.

9.3 Electronic Parameters

The distribution of electrons in its structure determines the type of bond the drug forms with its target and ultimately it results in biological activity. Electronic parameters quantify these qualities by giving a value, which is a measure of electron donating or electron withdrawing power. The electronic parameter σ depends on the electronic properties of the substituents on the ring, hence it is known as substituent constant. Most important electronic parameters are

- Ionization
- Hammett substituent constant
- Inductive substituent constant
- Taft substituent constant
- Swain-Lupton constant

9.3.1 Ionization

Ionization will have a profound effect not only on its interaction with a receptor but also on its lipophilicity. Most drugs are weak acids or weak bases and their degree of ionization can be determined by the dissociation constant (pka) of the drug and pH of the environment influences their lipid / water solubility. The electrostatic forces interacting between the ion and cell-wall serve to repel or bind the ion, thus decreasing cell penetration.

The non-ionized molecules possess the higher lipid-solubility and pass most membrane barriers more rapidly than ionized molecule. Equilibrium is established between the ionized and non-ionized form of a molecule when the pH of the medium equals to pKa of the molecule. An electron withdrawing/donating group attached to the molecules alters pka of the molecule. Electron withdrawing groups will lower the pka (acidic) and electron donating groups increases the pka (basic). This is considered as an important lead modification approach and used in the design of H_2 blockers (cimetidine). All 5,5-disubstituted barbituric acid derivatives are CNS depressants, whereas barbituric acid and its 5-mono substituted derivatives are inactive.

The pKa values for acids and bases can also be calculated from σ substituent constant by using the following formula

$$pka = 4.20 - 1.00 \, \Sigma\sigma$$

Calculation of pka for propranolol

$$pka = 4.21 - 1.00 \, (\Sigma\sigma) \qquad = 3.2 \, (0.71 + 0.12)$$
$$= 3.2 + 0.93 \qquad\qquad = 2.976$$

9.3.2 Hammett Substituent Constant

Hammett proposed that the electronic effects (both inductive and resonance effects) of a set of substituent's should be similar for different organic reactions. The electron withdrawing group attached to the aromatic benzoic acid would increase the acid strength of the carboxyl group and it increases with electron withdrawing power. Substituent constants (σ) are assigned to groups according to their influence on the acid strength of benzoic acid.

$$\sigma_x = \log (k_x / k_o) = \log k_x - \log k_o$$

k_o = dissociation constant for benzoic acid

k_x = dissociation constant for substituted benzoic acid

Electron withdrawing groups in X pulls electron density from -COOH group to the ring and makes it more acidic (increases the dissociation constant). Electron donating groups in X decreases the acidic strength of COOH. More conveniently, Hammett substituent constant (σ) can be expressed as

$$\sigma_x = pka^o - pka^x$$

pka^o = acid strength of benzoic acid = 4.19

pka^x = acid strength of substituted benzoic acid = 4.36

So, the change in acid strength brought about by the methyl group is

$- 0.17$ (4.19- 4.36).

The value of σ_x for a specific substituent containing both inductive and mesomeric contributions so it varies with the position of substituent. Hence, Hammett substituent constants are a measure of both inductive and mesoemeric effects. σ value for substituent at meta position is (σ_m) different from that in para position (σ_p). The meta (σ_m) substituent constant result from inductive effect, but not para substituent constant (σ_p) corresponds to the net inductive and resonance effect. Therefore σ_m and σ_p for the substituent are not same.

Ortho substituent constant (σ_o) can't be calculated because of possible steric interactions and polar effects. In body fluids ortho groups compete for the water molecules, forms an ordered structure around receptor. It reduces the expected Log P and π values. This effect is known as ortho effect, and can be calculated by

$$\pi \, \Delta \, ortho = \pi \, o\text{-substituent} - \pi \, p\text{-substituent}$$

But, the linear free energy relationship (LFER) is observed for meta and para substituent constant.

9.3.3 Inductive Substituent Constant (σ_1)

The para substituent constant (σ_p) has a greater resonance component hence the inductive contribution alone can be calculated.

$$(\sigma_1) = \tfrac{1}{2}\,(3\,\sigma_p + \sigma_m)$$

σ_1 = Inductive substituent constant

σ_p = Inductive substituent constant (pala)

σ_m = Inductive substituent constant (meta)

It mainly describes the polar effects of substituents on aliphatic system.

9.3.4 Taft Substituent Constant (σ^*)

It is the measure of polar effects of substituent in aliphatic compounds, when group doesn't form part of a conjugated system. They are based on the hydrolysis of esters and are calculated by

$$(\sigma^*) = 1/\,2.48\,[\,\log\,(k\,/\,k_o)_B -- \log\,(k\,/\,k_o)_A\,]$$

$(k\,/\,k_o)_B$ = rate constants for base hydrolysis

$(k\,/\,k_o)_A$ = rate constants for acid hydrolysis

In Taft substituent constants methyl group, rather than hydrogen (used in other constants) is considered as standard group. It uses propanoic acid as a reference point and it is given zero value. Taft and inductive substituents are related by the equation

$$\sigma^* = 2.51\,\sigma_1$$

9.3.5 Swain-Lupton Constant

It represents the contributions due to the inductive field (F), mesomeric and resonance components of Hammett constant. Swain-lupton constant quantifies the inductive and mesomeric effects of the substituent. Swain-Lupton constant is also known as Field-Inductive constant (F), suggests that the polar effects was the components in both hammett electronic constants σ_m and σ_p.

$$F = b0 + b1.\ \sigma_m + b2.\ \sigma_p$$

Groups	Hammetts		Inductive	Tafft	Swain-Lupton	
	σ_m	σ_p	σ_I	σ^*	F	R
H	0.00	0.00	0.00	0.49	0.00	0.00
CH_3	-0.07	-0.17	-0.05	0.00	-0.04	-0.13
C_2H_5	-0.07	-0.15	-0.05	-0.10	-0.05	-0.10
C_6H_5	0.06	-0.01	0.10	0.60	0.08	-0.08
OH	0.12	-0.37	0.25	-	0.29	-0.64
Cl	0.37	0.23	0.47	-	0.41	-0.15
Br	0.39	0.27	0.45	-	-	-
I	0.35	0.30	0.39	-	-	-
NO_2	0.71	0.78	-	-	-	-
OCH_3	0.12	-0.27	0.25	-	-	-

9.4 Role of Inductive and Resonance Effects in Biological Activity

In general fluorine substitution, excerts diminished electron withdrawal effect at distal sites and donates a lone pair of electrons by resonance. This effect is commonly referred as mesomeric effect. The opposing resonance and field effects will nearly cancel.

Fluorine is the smallest substituent available for the replacement of hydrogen in organic compounds. Hydrogen will be abstracted from enzyme substrates as an H^+ ion, where as fluorine doesnot readily yield the corresponding F^+. Substitution of fluorine into aromatic ring lowers the propensity of the aryl π electrons to interact with neighbouring cationic groups. The strength of the interaction is reduced progressively as the number of fluorine substituent's increases. The aryl group participates in a π-π stacking interaction with aromatic side groups, this types of interaction is perturbated much less by fluorine substituents. In enzyme inhibitors, fluorine is substituted for hydrogen. Flourine is strongly electronegative and possess prominent inductive effect. Inductive effect of fluorine reduces their enzymatic inactivities.

5-Fluoro uracil - thymidine synthetase inhibitor: Thymidine synthetase is inactivated by the deoxyribonucletide metabolite of 5-fluoro uracil. A thiol group of thymidylate synthetase attack the 6th position of the uracil moiety and 5th position of carbon react as carbocation with methyl tetrahydrofolate. Regeneration of enzyme required removal of hydrogen at position 5.

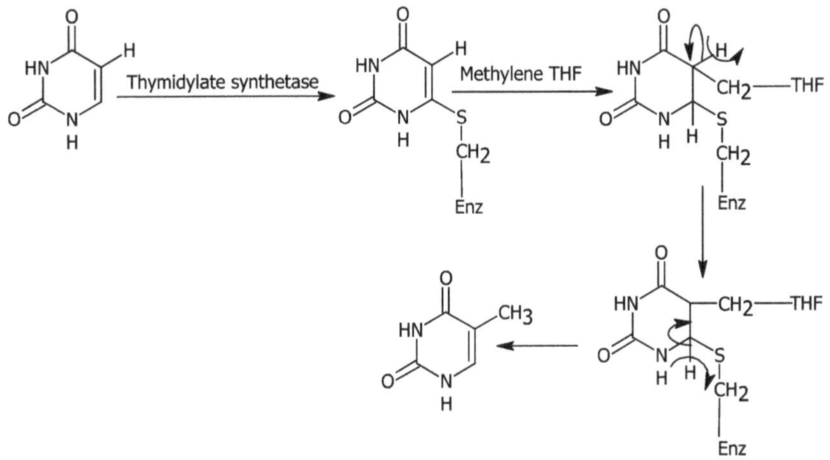

Fig. 9.1 Denova synthesis of thymidine.

But this pathway is blocked by fluorinated inactivators; 5-fluorouracil inactivates *s*-adenosyl methionine (SAM) and 5-flouocysteine inactivates cytosine methylase of DNA and RNA due to their inductive effect of fluorine, which results in its covalent binding to thymidylate synthetase.

Lignocaine - local anaesthetic agent: Procaine, a local anaesthetic agent containing carboxylic group is quickly hydrolysed, but amide group containing lignocaine reduces the hydrolysis. The presence of 2 methyl groups (in 2nd and 5th position) on the aromatic ring in lignocaine helps shield the carbonyl group from attack by nucleophile or enzymes and prolongs the activity.

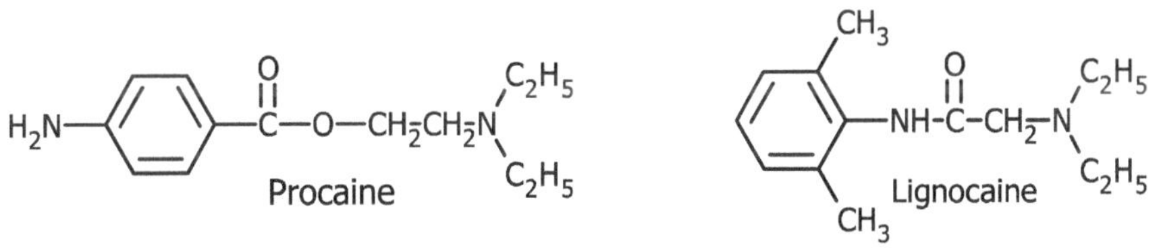

The local anaesthetic activity of procaine is however greater than that of procainamide, because the dipolar character of the carbonyl group in procaine is more pronounced. In procainamide the amine group resonance is offset by the amide resonance so that the magnitude of the C = O dipole is decreased.

Electron donating groups in *para* or *ortho* positions increases local anaesthetic potency. Proparacaine, propoxyparacaine and tetracaine increases electron density of the ring by both inductive and resonance effect and has enhanced local anaesthetic potency. Resonance effect gives rise to zwitterionic from and electrons are localised on carbonyl carbon this makes binding with sodium channel.

9.5 Steric Parameters

Interaction of a drug with its receptor involves complementarity between these two molecules and can be explained by steric effect. It explains the relationship between the shape and size of the drug, and also the dimension of the target and drugs. Different steric features of the drugs are responsible for the difference in drug-receptor bonding and also cause change in biological activity response. Various parameters used to describe the steric features are

- Taft-steric substituent constant
- Charton steric constant
- Molar refractivity
- Molecular connectivity
- Sterimol parameter
- Parachor

9.5.1 Taft-Steric Substituent Constant (E_S)

Taft steric substituent constant is the more important QSAR descriptor. It is the measure of the bulkiness of the group and its effect on the closeness of contact between the drug and the receptor site.

$$E_s = \text{Log } K \times COOCH_3 - \text{Log } K\ CH_3COOCH_3$$
$$E_S = \log (K / K_0)$$

where K_o = Rate of acid hydrolysis for substituted parent ester

K = Rate of acid hydrolysis for substituted ester

Normally standardized to methyl group, E_S = CH_3 = 0. Hencock claimed that this reaction is under the influence of hyperconjucation so developed corrected E.

$$E_s^c = E_s + 0.306(n-3)$$

where n = No. of alpha hydrogen atoms

9.5.2 Charton Steric Constant

Charton demonstrated the strong relation between Es and van der walls radii.

$$v_x = r_x - r_H = r_x - 1.20$$

v_x = Upsilon parameter

r_x = van der walls radii of substituent

r_H = van der walls radii of hydrogen

9.5.3 Molar Refractivity (MR)

Molar refractivity (MR) is the molar volume corrected by the refractive index. It represents the size and polarizability of the molecule. MR is the measure of steric factors and bulkiness of the molecule and molar refractivity shows a strong correlation with ligand binding. Both Log P and molar refractivity increase with alkyl chain length, so Log P and molar refractivity show a strong correlation. Polar functional groups increase molar refractivity, but decrease Log P. Molar refractivity is a measure of non-lipophillic interactions Log P is a measure of lipophillic interactions. MR can be explained by the Lorentz-Lorentz equation:

$$MR = \frac{(n^2 - 1)}{n^2 + 1}\left[\frac{MW}{d}\right]$$

where n = Index of refraction, MW = molecular weight, d = density

9.5.4 Molecular Connectivity ($^m x$)

It describes the manner in which the atoms are connected in the molecule.

$$^0x = \Sigma\,(\delta_i)^{-1/2}$$

δ_i = Number assigned to each non-hydrogen atom

m = denotes order of parameter.

9.5.5 Sterimol Parameter

Molecular refractivity will not explain the 3D shape of the molecule. Sterimol parameter describes the size and shape of substituents in a congeneric series.

9.5.6 Parachor

Parachor is a secondary derived function depends upon surface tension, density and molecular weight of the molecule.

$$P \;=\; \gamma^{1/4}\, M / (D\text{-}d)$$

where, M = Molecular weight; γ = Surface tension; D = Density

When the vapour density is negligibly small

$$P' \;=\; V\, m\, \gamma^{1/4}$$

$$Vm \;=\; \text{Molecular volume}$$

9.6 QSAR Methods

1. Free energy methods
   (a) Ferguson effect
   (b) Hansch analysis
   (c) Free wilson analysis
   (d) Martin and Kubinyi analysis

2. Statistical methods
   (a) Discriminant analysis
   (b) Prinicipal component analysis
   (c) Factor analysis
   (d) Clustor analysis
   (e) Combined multivariate analysis

9.6.1 Ferguson Effect

The concentration of the drugs within the receptor cell is critical for its activity, [*i.e* relative saturation of drug in cell and surrounding body fluid (thermodynamic activity) determines its effect].

$$\text{Biological effect} \;=\; C_e / C_s$$

where, C_e = Effective concentration; C_s = Solubility

9.6.2 Hantsch Analysis

Hantsch postulated two states for drug for drug action. This linear free energy related approach is also known as extra thermodynamic method.

- Random walk of the molecule: Travel from site of administration to site of action, passes through membranes, related to Log P [f(P)]

- Attachment to the receptor site: Attachment of drugs to its target mainly depends upon its shape, expressed as k_x.

Liphophilicity and electronic factors are responsible for the biological activity, hence

$$\text{Biological activity} = R_b = f\,(P)\,K_x\;\;C$$

9.6.3 Free-Wilson Analysis

Structure activity based method optimizes substituents in molecular frame work. Introduction of particular group at any position of the molecule changes the relative potency. This is method of choice when mechanism of action and physico-chemical properties of drugs are unknown. The method is based upon an additive mathematical model in which a particular substituent in a particular molecular pattern is assumed to make an additive and constant contribution to biological activity. Introduction of particular substituent at a particular molecular position always lead to a quantitatively similar effect on biological potency

$$BA \;\; = \; \epsilon\, a_i\, X_i + \mu$$

where a_i = Contribution of substituent

X_i = ith substituent

μ = Average activity

Advantages

- Physicochemical constants are not required.
- Any type of quantitative data can be analysed.

Limitations

- Large number of molecules with varying substituent's combinations is required for the analysis.
- Intra molecular interactions cann't be explained.

9.7 QSAR Applications

1. QSAR serves as an integral part of drug design, discovery and development

2. Optimum hydrophobicity for the CNS permeation can be established through Log P values

3. QSAR predicts the bioavailability of the molecules through different approaches

4. Hammet equation reveals the influence of electron releasing and withdrawing groups [electronic an resonance effects] in the biological activity

5. Hansch equation provides information on drug-receptor interactions (electronic, steric and hydrophobic)

6. Free-Wilson models approximates the chemical features responsible for observed biological activity

CHAPTER 10

VIRTUAL SCREENING

Drug-likeness is a qualitative concept used in drug design. It is estimated from the molecular structure before the substance is even synthesized and tested. It can be deduced as a delicate balance among molecular properties affecting pharmaco-dynamics and pharmacokinetics of molecules which ultimately affects their absorption, distribution, metabolism, and excretion in human body like a drug. Molecular properties include molecular weight, electronic distribution, hydrophobicity, hydrogen bond donors/acceptors, solubility, viscosity, and other related properties. Selection of suitable molecular descriptors for predicting the drug-likeness of a molecule is of prime importance for the screening of drug-like molecules.

10.1 Drug-Likeness

Lipinski "rule of five" (RO5) helps in predicting drug-likeness. According to RO5 the molecules having molecular weight > 500, Log P > 5, hydrogen bond donors (HBD) > 5 and hydrogen bond acceptors (HBA) > 10 have poor absorption or permeation. Pharmacodynamic aspect of molecules is not given any consideration by RO5 which deal with drug action. CLog P values greater than 3 or significantly more likely to be toxic.

Polar surface area is directly correlated with the sum of HBD and HBA. Total polar surface area (TPSA) and number of rotatable bonds are related to the pharmacodynamic aspects of drug action. Molecular flexibility is of primary importance in chemistry since it influences the chemical and biological properties of compounds as well as their interactions with other molecules. Rotatable bond is a very good descriptor of oral bioavailability of drugs.

TPSA has been shown to be a very good descriptor characterizing drug absorption, including intestinal absorption, bioavailability and blood-brain barrier penetration. TPSA decides the passive transport of compounds across biological membranes. TPSA value of < 140 Å^2 is acceptable for many drugs, whereas for penetration into blood brain barrier it should be > 60 Å^2.

10.2 Cheminformatics

Use of chemical databases in drug design is known as cheminformatics, it encompasses the design, creation, organisation, storage, management, retrieval, analysis, dissemination, visualisation and use of chemical information. Cheminformatics is defined as "mixing of information resources to transform data into information, and information into knowledge, intending for better rapid decisions in the arena of drug lead identification and optimisation." Cheminformatics uses computer and information techniques to solve the problems in the field of chemistry, these *in silco* techniques has wide range of applications in rational drug design process. Cheminformatics refers to the systems and scientific methods used to store, retrieve, and analyze the immense amount of molecular data that are generated in modern drug-discovery efforts.

Chemical databases contain encoded chemical structures along with molecular and atomic data. Most chemical databases store 2D and 3D structural models in different domain (2D and 3D domain) and can be searched separately.

Chemical databases are of two types

1. Analytical / experimental database: It contains libraries of reference materials with defined techniques.
2. Computed models: It contains structure derived from quantum mechanical methods or molecular mechanics.

Modern drug discovery requires systems that have the ability to access and manipulate large quantities of data quickly and easily. Cheminformatics has become an integral part of the drug-discovery process, from lead identification through development. For the effective implementation of chemoinformatics different firms and organisations follow various approaches which includes compound registration (Database Creation), library enumeration, navigating virtual libraries, access to primary and secondary scientific literature, QSAR (quantitative structure/activity relationships), physicochemical property calculations and integrated chemical structure based property databases. These approaches require tools not only for the analysis of experimental data, but also for the generation of calculated properties of molecules.

In general, the data present in cheminformatics database fall into four categories:

1. **Structural:** The molecular structure data are the most unique aspect that differentiates cheminformatics from other database applications. Molecular structure refers to the 1-, 2-, or 3-D representations of molecules.

2. **Numerical:** Numerical data includes biological activity, pKa, log$P$, or analytical results.

3. **Annotation / text:** Annotation includes information such as experimental notes that are associated with a structure or data point. The protocols are categorized by the type of task: for example, substructure / similarity searches, database access and property calculators.

4. **Graphical:** Any structure or data point may have associated graphical information such as spectra or plots.

Considering the vast number of molecules in most corporate databases (not to mention external sources) and the large quantity of data associated with these molecules, the need for sophisticated information systems is clear. Modern drug discovery requires systems that have the ability to access and manipulate large quantities of data quickly and easily. However, information archival and retrieval is not enough. It is also necessary to have tools that can effectively analyze and organize these data in order to make it useful for effective decision making.

10.2.1 Applications

- Cheminformatics predicst the drug-likeness (virtual screening) of molecule prior to synthesis.
- Cheminformatics aids screening in a number of different ways, including
  - Library design
  - Similarity searching and clustering
  - Pharmacophore modeling
  - Design of experiments (DOE)

Library design: Pharmaceutically relevant small molecules can be retrieved using ISIS-MDL molecular descriptors.

The selections of compounds are made using a variety of methods, such as

1. Dissimilarity selection
2. "Optiverse" library selection
3. Jarvis–Park clustering
4. Cell-based methods

All these methods attempt to choose a set of compounds that represent the molecular diversity of the available compounds as efficiently as possible.

Similarity searching and clustering: Similarity searching involves the identification of all molecules in a database that are loosely related to the query structure. Similarity searching has been widely used in the discovery of compounds with similar biological activity but different chemical structure (or at least different enough to allow patenting of the new structure); this has been termed "leapfrogging" or "scaffold hopping".

2D structure searching: 2D structure searching involves the identification of user defined molecules in a chemical database. Sub structure search identifies chemical structures with equal / larger in size. It involves normal, sub similarity and super similarity. In 2D substructure following query features can be set.

- Atom lists [C, N, O]
- Bond types [single / Aromatic]
- Chain bond [acyclic]
- Hydrogen count
- Substituent count
- Ring specifications

3D structure searching: A set of atom types with set of distance constraints, orientation of side chain, height of the group about the plane of ring (geometric concepts) are important criteria in 3D database search. Mentioning of functional nature of groups (hydrophilic, hydrophobic) also facilitates the search.

The relative positions of atoms in 3D coordinate spaces known as pharmacophore are given importance. Rigid and flexible 3D searching are the two types of 3D structure searching.

Pharmacophore Modeling: Pharmacophore modeling has been used in library design once common pharmacophores from known actives have been identified. Initially designed for smaller datasets, pharmacophore modeling is being increasingly applied to HTS data. The advantage of this methodology offers to the researcher is that it suggests common structural themes even from a diverse set of active compounds. This can then help rationalize the observed activity and much more quickly suggest directions in which the actives can be modified to optimize activity (*i.e.,* helping in the hit to lead optimization stage of discovery).

Design of experiments: DOE has been successfully applied only in cases where limited libraries of related compounds (e.g., peptides) were being evaluated. The reason for this is intuitively obvious, as one of the assumptions of DOE is that variability in the descriptors is continuous and related to activity over a smooth response surface, so that trends and patterns can be readily identified. With HTS data both of these assumptions are generally not true, as molecules can display discontinuous responses to changing features, and the SAR of even related compounds does not map to a smooth continuous response surface.

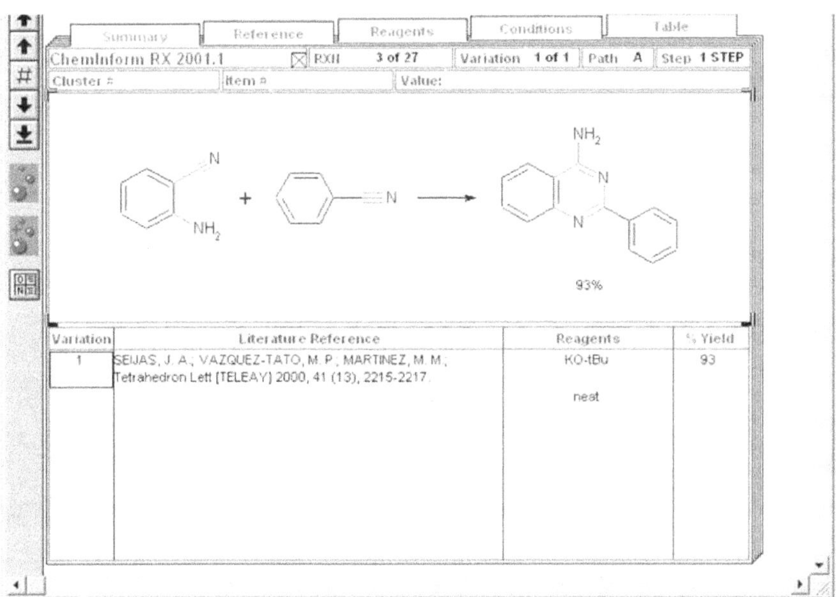

Variation	Literature Reference	Reagents	% Yield
1	SEIJAS, J. A.; VAZQUEZ-TATO, M. P.; MARTINEZ, M. M.; Tetrahedron Lett [TELEAY] 2000, 41 (13), 2215-2217.	KO-tBu neat	93

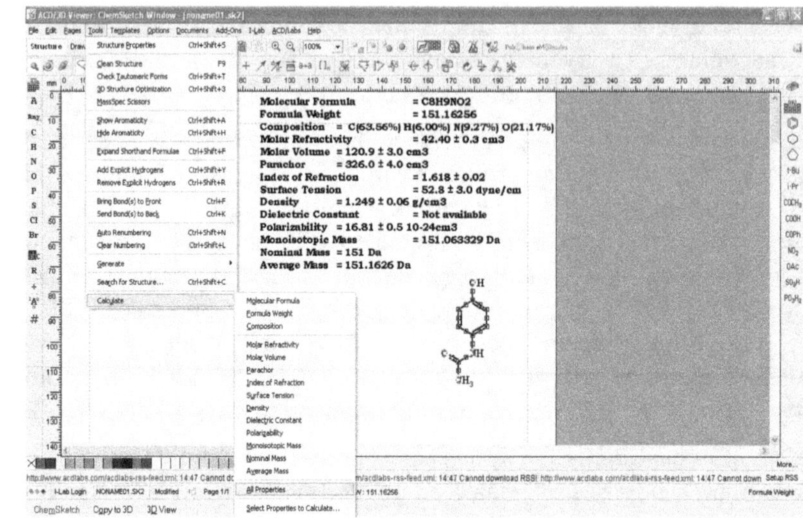

10.3 Drug-Likeness Analysis

The rule of five is now widely used to filter out compounds likely to have poor pharmacokinetic properties early on in drug discovery. Also, other factors such as substructures with known toxic, mutagenic or teratogenic properties affect the usefulness of a designed molecule. Drug-likeness can be estimated for any molecule, and does not evaluate the actual specific effect that the drug achieves (biological activity). Some of the online tools available for drug-likeness analysis are

- Molinspiration
- Molsoft
- Chemicalize.org
- Vcc lab

Molinspiration

1. Open www.molinspiration.com
2. Select 'Calculation of molecular properties and bioactivity'
3. Draw the structure in the draw applet
4. Select the appropriate options

    (a) Calculate properties: To know the drug like properties

    (b) Predict bioactivity: To know their possible binding affinity to the receptor

    (c) Galaxy 3D generator: To view 3D structure

Select substituent ▾

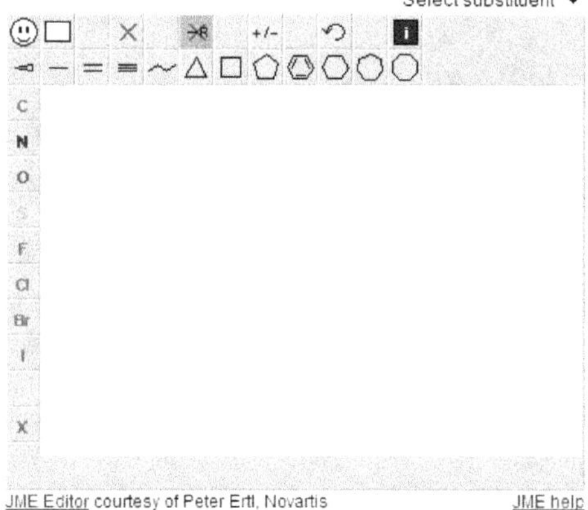

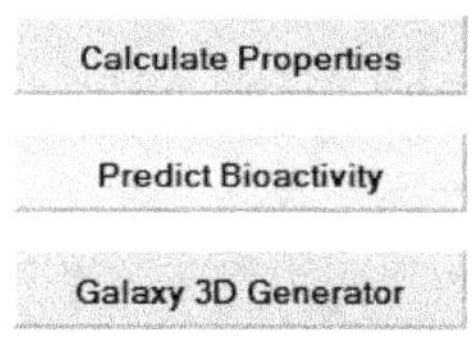

Molinspiration home

Molinspiration products and services

Molinspiration services FAQ

Molinspiration RESTful web services

Terms of service

© Molinspiration Cheminformatics 2011

JME Editor courtesy of Peter Ertl, Novartis   JME help

Select substituent ▾

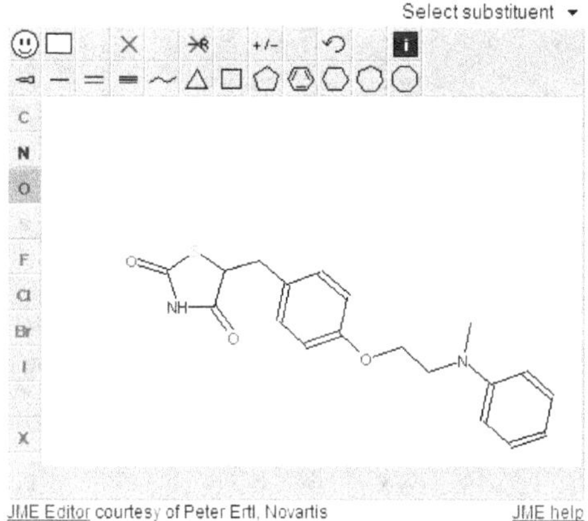

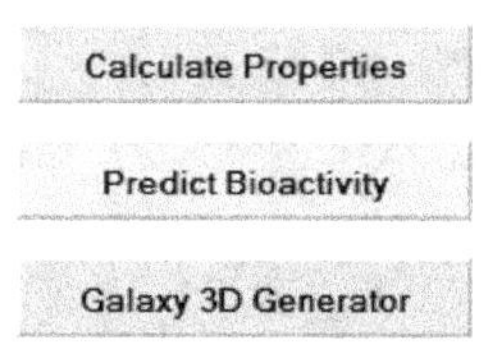

Molinspiration home

Molinspiration products and services

Molinspiration services FAQ

Molinspiration RESTful web services

Terms of service

© Molinspiration Cheminformatics 2011

JME Editor courtesy of Peter Ertl, Novartis   JME help

miSMILES CN(CCOc2ccc(CC1SC(=O)NC1=O)cc2)c3ccccc3

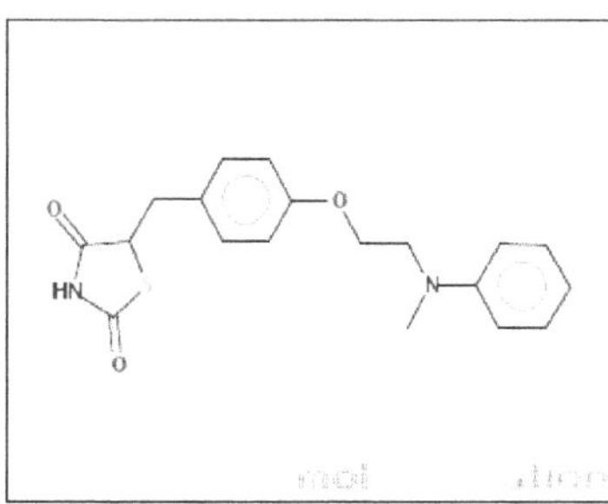

Molinspiration property engine v2011.04

miLogP	3.246
TPSA	58.641
natoms	25.0
MW	356.447
nON	5
nOHNH	1
nviolations	0
nrotb	7
volume	318.671

Get data as text (for copy / paste).

Get 3D geometry BETA

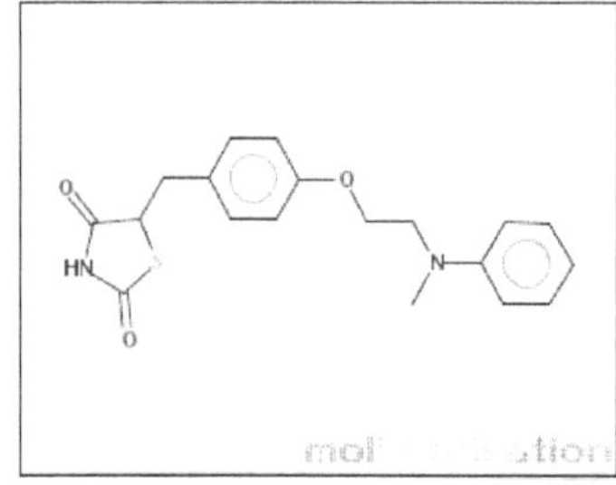

miSMILES CN(CCOc2ccc(CC1SC(=O)NC1=O)cc2)c3ccccc3

Molinspiration bioactivity score v2011.06 NEW

GPCR ligand	0.04
Ion channel modulator	-0.75
Kinase inhibitor	-0.81
Nuclear receptor ligamd	0.38
Protease inhibitor	-0.27
Enzyme inhibitor	-0.20

Get data as text (for copy / paste).

Get 3D geometry BETA

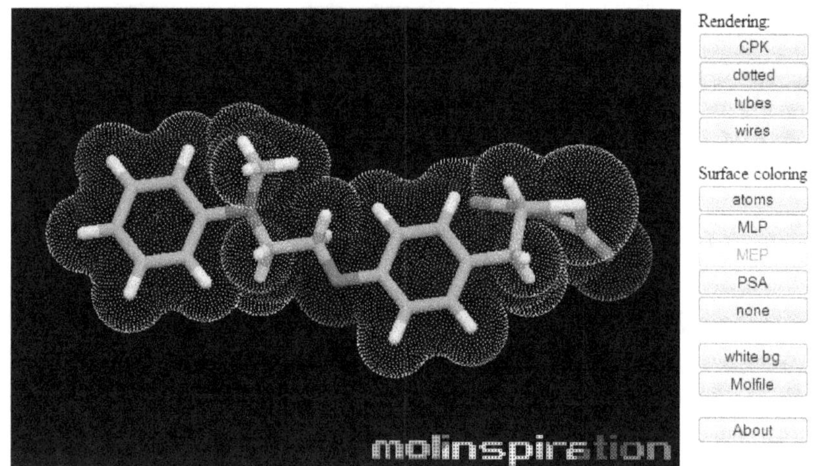

<h1>CHAPTER 11</h1>

TARGET IDENTIFICATION

The essential step in rational drug design (RDD) is the identification of target linked to specific disease and development of a drug with a specific affinity to the target. A key molecule involved in a particular metabolic pathway (specific to disease) is known as target. Drug targets have following characteristics

1. Possess special binding sites for small molecules (endogenous and exogenous)

2. Biomolecular structure undergo conformational change, when binds to small molecules (reversible)

3. Conformational change induces cellular regulation

4. Produces therapeutic effect on pathological conditions (diseases) upon binding to drugs

Physiology based drug discovery and target-based drug discovery are two different fields in the discovery and development of drugs. The principle behind physiology based drug discovery is disease phenotype. Target-based drug discovery begins with the identification of the function of a potential therapeutic drug target and understanding its role in the disease process. Target identification and validation reduces the failure rate and increases the efficiency of drug discovery process.

Target identification is to find the best interaction mode between the potential target candidates and small molecule probes. Identifying small molecules that bind to target proteins may help elucidate information on their role in the biological process. Target identification is the process of identifying new targets (protein or DNA/RNA) whose modulation might inhibit or reverse disease progression. The main goal of target identification is to discover the specific targets that are modulated by particular chemical molecules.

Advancement in molecular biology (genomics and proteomics) is the main driver of the target based drug discovery. Conventional pharmaceutical approach   finds drugs for targets, whereas genomics (chemical biology) finds targets for known drugs. The newly revealed potential target pool shows promising prospect for drug development. Molecular biology research suggest that there are 5,000 – 10, 000 established and potential drug targets in human.

11.1   Target Identification Technologies

There are three distinct and complementary approaches are available for discovering the protein target of a small molecule.

1. Direct biochemical approach: Biochemical affinity purification finds target proteins for small molecules. This method provides information about molecular mechanisms of efficacy or toxicity relevant to human disease. Small molecule optimization can be carried out by this approach, when 3D structure of target is known.

2. Genetic interaction methods: Genetic manipulations can also be used to identify protein targets.

3. Computational inference methods: Pattern recognition generates hypotheses to compare small molecule effects to known reference molecules (genetic perturbations).

11.2 Cutting Edge Technologies in Target Identification

11.2.1 Activity based Probe Design

The small molecules used in chemical proteomics are called activity based probes (ABPs). Generally they consists of three basic elements and are

1. Reactive functional groups: These groups present in ABPs covalently attaches to the active site of an enzyme. The ABPs use electrophilic groups of irreversible enzyme inhibitors to form a covalent bond with a nucleophilic group of the enzyme active site.

   - Affinity based labelling probe: they contains photolabile groups that can be converted into a highly reactive intermediate after irradiation with UV light.

   - Masked electrophile: Masked electrophile gets activated upon enzyme cleavage.

2. Tags: Tags are used for the identification and purification of modified enzymes. Tags facilitate the detection of probe-labelled targets after gel elelctrophoresis.

   - Radioactive ABPs: Display high sensitivity
   - Fluorophoric tags: Valuable alternative to imaging systems. It can be utilized for *in vivo* imaging of protese activity.
   - Biotinylated ABPs: Facilitates both visualization and purification of targets and have been used for characterization of labelled proteins by in-gel digestion and tandem mass spectroscopy analysis.

3. Linkers: Linkers connects functional group and tag. They provide selective binding interactions and prevent steric congestion. Linkers influences the specificity of the ABP. Polypeptides are often used as linkers due to their ease of preparation and compatibility with solid phase chemistry.

Diseases such as cancer, rheumatoid arthritis and osteoporosis are associated with elevated levels of protease activity. ABPs aid in the monitoring and profiling of protease activities throughout disease stages.

11.2.2 Microarrays

Micro array technology identifies novel transcriptional cascades, biological processes and disease markers. Microarrays assess gene and protein expression and validates at the targets at the tissue and cell levels (tissue and cell micro arrays).

1. Nucleic acid microarray: Data generated from genome sequencing projects in several organisms has provided the opportunity to build comprehensive maps of transcriptional regulation. Array based gene expression analysis has enabled parallel monitoring of cellular transcription at the level of the genome. Nucleic acid microarrays had a significant impact on understanding of normal and abnormal cell biochemistry.

2. Protein microarray: Protein and peptide microarrays have an impact on drug discovery. It examines enzyme-substrate, DNA-protein and protein-protein interactions.

3. Tissue and cell based micro arrays

The two important DNA microarray techniques are

- **Gene expression profiling:** DNA microarrays in the disease altered gene expression (up / down regulated) leads to changes in the structure or function of cells.

- **Gene knockout screening**: This technology is based on the transgenic 'gene knock out' (transgeneic animals). Inactivation of genes for cyclooxygenase (COX) lowers inflammatory reactions, which reflects in the clinical efficacy of drug acting on it.

11.2.3 Serial Analysis of Gene Expression (SAGE)

Polymerase chain reaction (PCR) based serial analysis of gene expression (SAGE) detects all transcriptional RNAs. This technology is more sensitive than micro arrays.

11.2.4 Antisense Technology

Antisense technology is a powerful method of rational drug design useful in discovering more specific treatments for diseases. It is recognised to be efficient tools for the identification of gene expression in a sequence-specific way. The antisence technology uses oligonuleotides and is known as antisense oligonucleotides (AS-ODs).

Antisence oligonuleotides (AS-ODs) are short (7-30 nucleotide) sequences of nucleic acid designed to bind to a specific region of a target mRNA. AS-ODs bind to the target mRNA and inhibits mRNA translation, these effects are acute and reversible.

11.2.5 Small Interfering RNA

Small interfering RNA (siRNA) activates sequence specific RNA-induced silencing complex (RISC). Activated RISC destroys functional mRNA of cell.

11.2.6 Zinc Finger Proteins

Zing finger proteins (ZFPs) have remarkable versatility for recognising different sequences of DNA and variation in the amino acid sequence. ZFP transcription factors (ZFP-TFs) can be applied to potential new drug target validation.

11.3 Computational Approaches in *In Silico* Target Fishing

In silico target fishing is an emerging technology that enables the prediction of biological targets of compounds on the basis of chemical structures.

Computational approaches useful in the prediction of target from chemical structures are

1. Chemical similarity searching
2. Data mining learning
3. Bioactivity spectra
4. Docking to protein databases

11.3.1 Chemical Similarity Searching

It involves comparison of compound structure to a database of compounds with known targets. Any chemical descriptor can be used in this connection. In more recent years, web-based search engines have become available for finding chemically similar bioactive structures. Web-based chemical similarity searching databases available are:

- PubChem: http://pubchem.ncbi.nlm.nih.gov/
- Chembank: http://chembank.broad.harvard.edu/
- Relibase: http://relibase.rutgers.edu/ http://relibase.ccdc.cam.ac.uk/

Similarity searching for target fishing can be performed with 3D chemical descriptors. The 2D descriptors are powerful for similarity searching in annotated databases. But, 3D descriptors are more appropriate, when the orphan compound has low 2D similarity to all database molecules.

11.3.2 Data Mining Learning

Data mining is an ideal approach for target prediction and it involves automated extraction of patterns and associations from large databases. Target prediction can be achieved by comparing orphan compound features with correlated features in each target class. First, associations between target names and chemical substructures can be extracted automatically across target class sets with inductive machine learning. Chemical features correlated with specific target binding are then stored in the form of multiple target models. Drug databases useful for target fishing are

- Comprehensive Medicinal Chemistry

  http://www.mdl.com/products/knowledge/ medicinal_chem/index.jsp

- Ashgate drugs

  http://www.cambridgesoft.com/ database/details/?db=2

- World Drug Index

  http://scientific.thomson.com/products/wdi/

In silico prediction of activity spectra for substances (PASS) by training models on the chemical features of activity classes is newer technological outcome. PASS predictions are incorporated into the NCI database browser and recent successes were reported using the PASS technology to guide medicinal chemistry, including in the design of novel cognition enhancers.

11.3.3 Bioactivity Spectra

The activities of a compound across a protein panel, cell line panel, HTS screening panel or DNA microarray is termed as "bioactivity spectra". The biospectra of a compound is related to chemical structure and therefore can be used for predicting compound's activities. Bioactivity spectra have also shown great promise with respect to mining pharmacology data and predicting adverse drug reactions (ADRs). ADRs can be predicted on the basis of its profile similarity to others compounds with known ADRs.

11.3.4 Docking to Protein Databases

Performing ligand-target docking to a wide panel of proteins using their 3D structures is an alternative approach for target identification.

11.4 Target Validation

Target validation is the process of finding the importance of target in the specific disease. Lack clinical efficacy in phase II clinical trial is the important reason for the termination of one-third of the molecules from the drug development program. This is mainly due to the improper target validation. New drug target validation provides insight into the pathogenesis of target related diseases. The next step after measuring the biological activity of the molecules for their biological response (inhibitory, stimulatory and antagonistic activity), is target evaluation.

Target validation establishes sensitive, reproducible and robust high throughput screening (HTS) method for studying the biological potential of molecules. Target validation process demonstrates the relevance of target through knock-out (loss of function) and knock-in (gain of function) in animal models (transgenic animals). Target validation process involves the following steps

1.   Discovering a biomolecule of interest (target discovery)

2.   Evaluation of new targets

3.   Design of bioassay and high throughput screen

4. Hits identification and evaluation: Small molecules obtained from HTS provide useful tools for the validation of new targets.

11.5 Target Validation Approaches

Target validation involves studies in molecular level model, disease-related cell-based models and in intact animals.

- Molecular level assay: Screening of a specific enzyme inhibitor usually involves mixing the enzyme and samples together to detect a decrease in the substrate or to determine an increase in the product in this enzyme catalytic process.

- Cellular level Assay: Validation at cell level provides confirmation of cell-free results.

- Animal model: Animal models validate the target at whole level. Therapeutic effect observed for the hits through animal model confirms their promising effect. Disease models of transgenic animals present

11.6 Bioinformatics in Target Discovery

The functional and positional information's of targets derived from bioinformatics supports the target identification and validation process. The bioinformatics tools have enabled *in silico* cloning of target candidates.

11.7 Single Nucleotide Polymorphs (SNPs)

SNPs are the key factors in personalised medicine and system biology to investigate relationship between sequence variation and physiological function *in silico*.

11.8 Binding Database

Binding database is a web accessible database contains measured binding affinities for known ligands. It focuses mainly on the interactions of drug-targets with small, drug-like molecules. It contains 910, 836 binding data for 6, 263 protein targets and 378, 980 small molecules. Binding database contains "Find my compounds targets" option for the identification of targets for the ligands. It allows one to draw the ligand or upload ligand in suitable format (*.sdf) to identify its possible targets.

Find my Compound's Targets

This page allows you to enter one or more Compounds and quickly see a list of Targets th

Draw one compound, or upload a file of compounds, and click the GO button to see a list

- Similarity: 0.85   (≥ 0.85)
- Substructure
- Exact

Affinity Filter(nM):   ≤ IC50 ▾ ≤   (Optional)

GO

If the chemical draw program does not appear below this text, you may need to download and install Java (free)

File Edit View Insert Atom Bond Structure Calculations Tools Help

Browse for and upload your compound file. Acceptable formats are detailed here. Example

Choose File No file chosen

11.9 Potential Drug Target Database (PDTD)

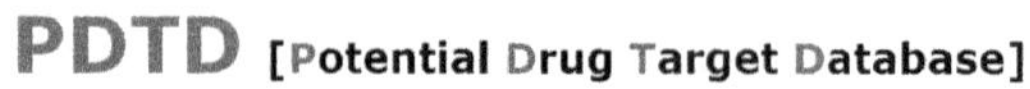
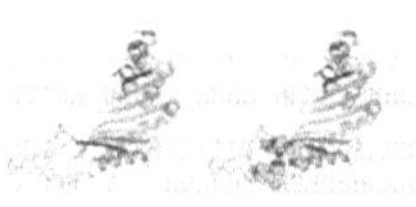

PDTD is a web-accessible protein database for *in silico* target identification. The database covers diverse information (protein and active site structures) of potential drug targets in both pdb and mol2 format. Each target is categorised by nosology and biochemical function. Each target is given PDB ID, target name, target category, related disease, structure and active site. PDTD provides link to Protein Data Bank (PDB), Uniprot, Therapeutic Target Database (TTD), Drug Bank, Thomson Pharma, Kegg and Enzyme structure database.

11.10 PharmMapper Server

PharmMapper server is a freely accessed web server designed to identify potential target candidates for the given small molecules using pharmacophore mapping approach. Pharmacophore is the spatial arrangement of features essential for a molecule to interact with a specific target receptor in a specific binding mode. PharmMapper hosts a large, pharmacophore database (namely PharmTargetDB) annotated from all the targets information in Target bank, BindingDB, DrugBank and potential drug target database. PharmMapper automatically finds the best mapping poses of the query molecule against all the pharmacophore models in PharmTargetDB.

PharmMapper may serve as a valuable tool for identifying targets for a novel synthetic compound, a newly isolated natural product, and a compound with known biological activity or an existing drug whose mechanism of action is unknown.

11.10.1 Experimental Procedure for Target Identification through PharmMapper Server

1. Open htttp://59.78.96.61/pharmmapper/

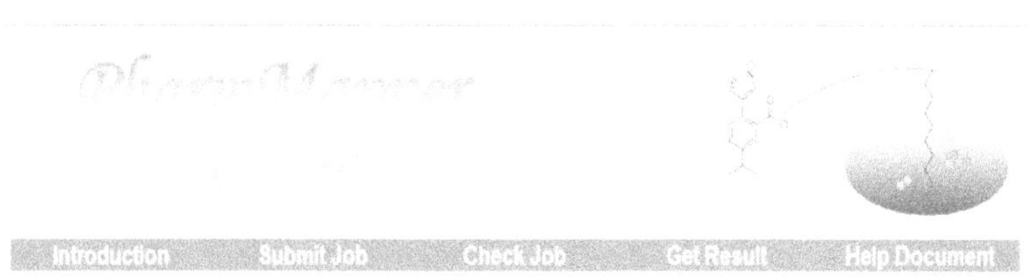

2. Click on 'Submit Job' option.
3. Submit query ligand in Tripos mol2 / MDL sdf file format

<table>
<tr><td colspan="2" align="center">**Step 1: Submit File**</td></tr>
<tr><td>Upload Query File</td><td>Browse...
Please submit Tripos mol2 or MDL sdf file!</td></tr>
<tr><td>Email Address (optional)</td><td></td></tr>
<tr><td>Job Description (optional)</td><td></td></tr>
</table>

Upload

4. Select the appropriate parameters (beginners can use default) and press submit button

<table>
<tr><td colspan="2" align="center">**Step 2: Submit Job**</td></tr>
<tr><td colspan="2" align="center">**Conformation Generation**</td></tr>
<tr><td>Generate Conformers</td><td>◉ Yes ○ No</td></tr>
<tr><td>Maximum Generated Conformations</td><td>300</td></tr>
<tr><td>Advanced Options</td><td>☐</td></tr>
<tr><td colspan="2" align="center">**Pharmacophore Mapping**</td></tr>
<tr><td>Select Targets Set</td><td>○ Human Protein Targets Only (2,241)
◉ All Targets (7,302)</td></tr>
<tr><td>Number of Reserved Matched Targets (Max 1,000)</td><td>300</td></tr>
<tr><td>Advanced Options</td><td>☐</td></tr>
</table>

Submit

5. In next step you will be directed to status page with Job ID

<table>
<tr><td>Introduction</td><td>Submit Job</td><td>Check Job</td><td>Get Result</td><td>Help Document</td></tr>
<tr><td colspan="5" align="center">**Submit Success**</td></tr>
</table>

Job ID   111213141419

111213141419

Check Status Now

6. Result page appears as follows

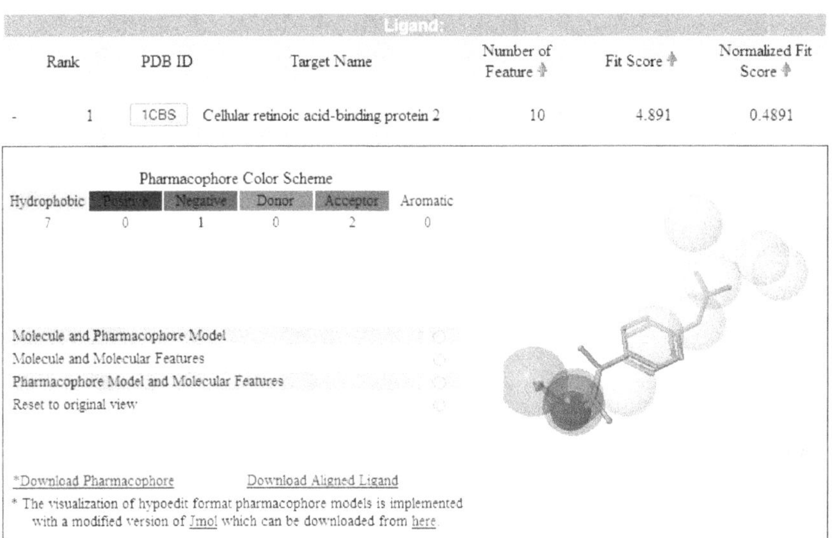

Result of 111213141419

Top 300 targets ranked by fit score in descending order

	Rank	PDB ID	Target Name	Number of Feature	Fit Score	Normalized Fit Score
+	1	1CBS	Cellular retinoic acid-binding protein 2	10	4.891	0.4891
+	2	1IHI	Aldo-keto reductase family 1 member C2	7	3.933	0.5618

7. By clicking on plus (+) symbol we can view pharmacophore model

Rank	PDB ID	Target Name	Number of Feature	Fit Score	Normalized Fit Score
1	1CBS	Cellular retinoic acid-binding protein 2	10	4.891	0.4891

Pharmacophore Color Scheme

Hydrophobic	Positive	Negative	Donor	Acceptor	Aromatic
7	0	1	0	2	0

Molecule and Pharmacophore Model
Molecule and Molecular Features
Pharmacophore Model and Molecular Features
Reset to original view

*Download Pharmacophore   Download Aligned Ligand
* The visualization of hypoedit format pharmacophore models is implemented
  with a modified version of Jmol which can be downloaded from here.

In PharmMapper server users are expected to upload the mol2 or Tris.mol format of the test molecule, customize the mapping parameters and submit a job. A job identity number, namely the JOB ID, is assigned to each job by the PharmMapper server. The user may use the JOB ID to check the status of the submitted job.

Input: PharmMapper interface is very simple. Its input form has only one mandatory field: A file with single drug-like molecule or natural product stored in Tris.mol format. The user must make sure the uploaded molecule has appropriate 3D structural information.

Output: A typical run of PharmMapper task takes 1–2 h, depending on the flexibility of the input molecule and filter parameters assigned. The output of a PharmMapper run is demonstrated in the form of a ranked list of hit target pharmacophore models that are sorted by fit score in descending order.

CHAPTER 12

MOLECULAR MODELING

The mission of medicinal chemist is to design and discover new chemical entities with drug-likeness. In molecular modeling, physical and computational creation of ligands, high affinity for the target and drug-likeness are considered. Molecular modeling helps understanding the types, nature and bonds involved in the atoms. Every molecule is characterized by a collection of atoms and collection of bonds. Distance between two atoms is known as bond length and angle between two atoms is known as bond angle. It plays important role in physical and chemical nature of drugs and physiological role. Key aspect of molecular modeling studies involves the calculation of the energy of conformations and its interactions.

Ball and stick models were used for long time to reveal the molecular nature of compounds. Computers became integral part in visualization and calculation of physicochemical properties of the molecules and are termed as 'molecular modeling'. This computational chemistry uses software (mathematical equation) for the design of molecules and is given the name computer aided drug design (CADD).

The major functions of molecular modeling process are listed below

1. Bio-physico chemical characterization
2. Generation of 3D structure of the molecule
3. Comparison between 3D structure of molecules (ligands and proteins)
4. Visualization of the molecule
5. Prediction of biological activity

Molecular modeling involves visualization of 3D structure of molecules, simulation, prediction and analysis of molecular properties.

12.1 Approaches in Molecular Modeling

Energy of the system is a function of thes type and number of atoms and their positions. In lead modification process, atoms / groups will be changed to increase the binding potential. The free energy change (ΔG) of a system is useful in assessing many aspects of the system. Decrease / increase in the target binding of ligand with respect to their structural modification can be analyzed knowing the free energy change of the complex.

$$\Delta G = \Delta H - T\Delta S$$

where ΔG = Change in free energy

ΔH = Change in enthalpy

ΔS = Change in entropy

T = Temperature

Molecular mechanics and quantum mechanics approaches are useful in calculating the free energy of the system.

Molecular mechanical method: Molecular mechanical methods use empirical force field calculations to estimate the free energy and are 10^4 fold faster than quantum mechanical methods. Molecular dynamics and monte carlo methods are useful in this connection.

Quantum mechanical method: Quantum mechanical methods are useful in lengthy calculations for small systems (10-100 atoms).

12.2 Molecular Mechanics

Molecular mechanics finds stable, low-energy conformations of molecules by changing their geometry at 0 °K. Hence this approach is called as energy minimization or geometry optimization. Molecular mechanics assist in drug receptor interaction analysis and 3D visualization (bioactive conformation) of molecules. The results obtained through molecular mechanics are more reliable and accurate. Molecular mechanics considers a molecule as a collection of atom held together by harmonic forces (bonds). These forces can be described by potential energy functions of bond length, bond angle, torsional angle and non-bonded interactions. These functions are collectively known as force field, and it estimates electronic effects of the molecule. The energy due to bonds, angles and torsional angle can be estimated using Hooke's law, van der Walls interactions are estimated using Lennard-Jones potential and coulombic forces assist in estimation of electrostatic interactions.

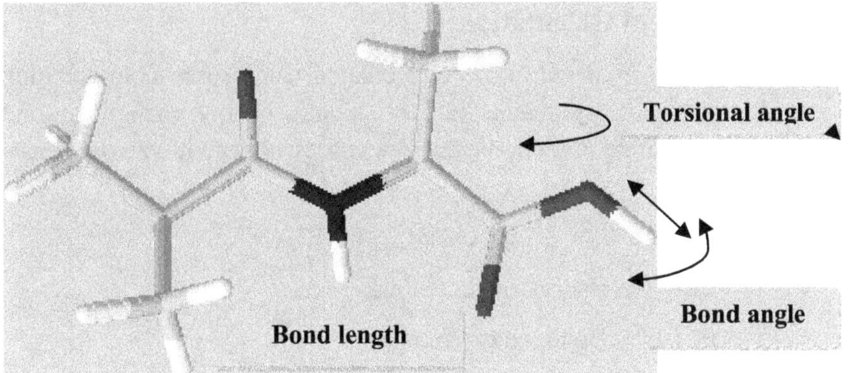

Molecular modeling usually carried out by molecular mechanics.

> Molecular mechanics calculates energy of the starting molecule.
> Molecular mechanics varies the bond length, bond angle and torsional angle to create new structure.
> Molecular mechanics finds energetically favourable conformation and then calculates the physical and chemical properties.

Molecular mechanics describes the energy of the whole system as the sum of inter and intra molecular interactions. A force field is an empirical fit to the potential energy of a molecular system. It uses molecular co-ordinates such as bond lengths, bond angle and torsional angle energies.

12.2.1 Energy Minimization

The goal of the energy minimization is to reduce the energy of high energy coordinates by optimizing the geometry. Energy minimization should be carried out once the structure is built. Because model construction process may result unfavourable bond length, bong angle and torsional angles. Unfavourable non-bonded interaction may also be present. The values of the relevant parameters together with the initial atomic coordinates are used to calculate total energy [E_{total}] of the molecule by the force field equation. The initial energy of the molecule is minimized by changing the values of the atomic coordinates until the minimum energy is obtained. Once the stable conformation is found, it is easy to calculate the physical and chemical properties. Molecular mechanics finds low energy conformations of a molecule by varying the geometry. The number of possible conformations increases with exponentially with the size of molecule, so it is not possible to locate the global minima.

12.3 Force Field Calculations

Total energy of a molecule can be calculated using force field equation by studying the energy change in bond length, energy change in bond angle, energy change in torsional energy, energy change in van der Waals interactions.

$$E_{total} = \epsilon\, E_{str} + \epsilon\, E_{bend} + \epsilon\, E_{torsion} + \epsilon\, E_{vdW}\; \epsilon E_{cou}$$

where E_{str} =   Energy of stretching

  E_{bend} =   Bond length change

  $E_{torsion}$ =   Change in the conformation

  ϵE_{cou} =   Electrostatic attraction

  E_{vdW} =   Van der waals force

Energy terms of molecular mechanics are explained by bonding interactions and non-bonding interactions.

12.3.1 Bonding Interactions

Bonding parameters can be classified into

Equilibrium type: It includes bond angle, bond length and are obtained from X-ray, neutron and electron diffraction studies.

Force constant: It can be obtained by microwave and IR spectral studies.

Energy of stretching: It describes the energy change as a bond stretches and contracts from its ideal unstrained length. Bond length should be near to the equilibrium bond length.

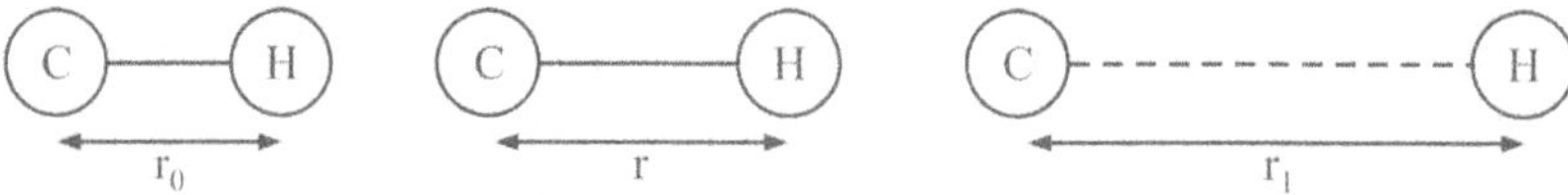

Bond stretching

The equation used to calculate bond energy change in case of bond between two atoms is given below.

$$E_{str} = 1/2K\left(r - r_0\right)^2$$

The equation used to calculate bond energy change in case of bond between three atoms is given below.

$$E_{str} = 1/2K_{(a-b)}\left(r_{a-b} - r_{0(a-b)}\right)^2 + 1/2K_{(b-c)}\left(r_{b-c} - r_{0(b-c)}\right)^2$$

where   K = Bond stretching force constant,

r_0 = contracted bond length,

r = actual bond length,

r_1 = unstrained bond length.

Bond Bending: It describes the energy change with respect to bending of bond angle from its ideal bond angle. Bond angle should be near to the equilibrium bond angle.

$$E_{ben} = 1/2\ K_\theta(\theta - \theta_o)^2$$

where K_θ = Angle bending force constant,

θ = actual bond length,

θ_o = unstrained bond angle.

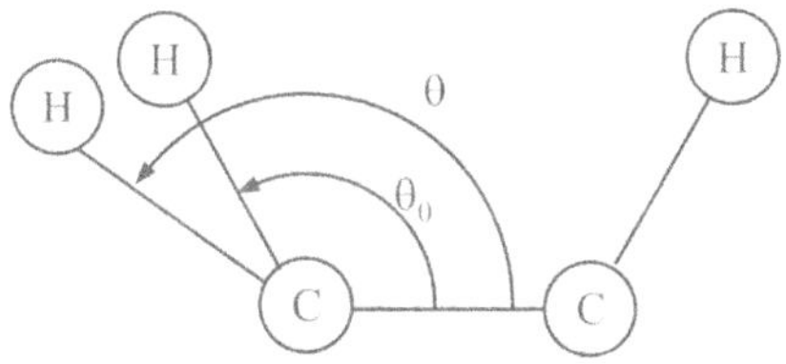

Bond angle

Torsion energy: It describes the energy change with respect to torsional angle change from its ideal torsional angle.

$$E_{tor} = 1/2\ K_\phi(1 + \cos\ (m(\phi - \phi_{offset})^2))$$

where K_ϕ = Torsional barrier constant,

ϕ = actual torsional angle,

ϕ_{offset} = unstrained bond angle.

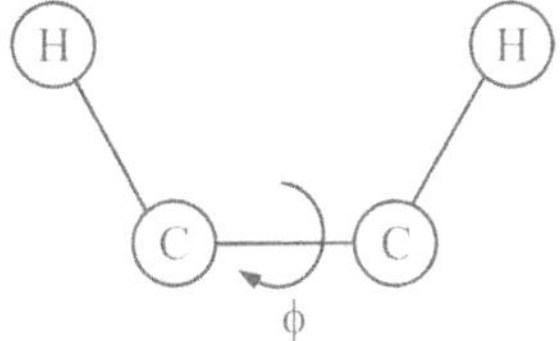

Torsional angle

12.3.2 Non-Bonded Interactions

They are usually smaller in magnitude, but have dominant effect because of their large number of atom pair. It explains the interactions between non-bonded atoms by considering electrostatic and van der waals interactions.

Electrostatic Interactions: Interactions between atoms present in the same or neighbouring molecules can be calculated using Coulombs law. The magnitude of the interaction is proportional to the atoms charges (q_i and q_j), inversely proportional to their separation (r_{ij}) and their dielectric constant (k).

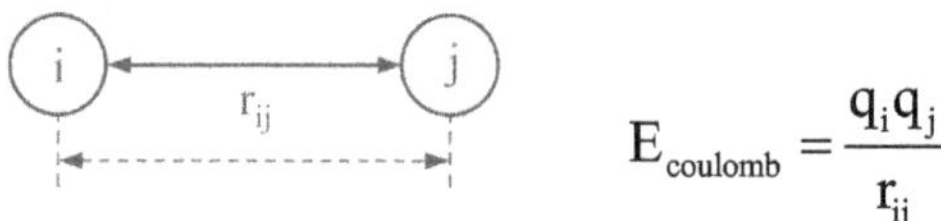

$$E_{coulomb} = \frac{q_i q_j}{r_{ij}}$$

Vander walls energy: Atoms are attracted by weak forces (Dispersive / London forces) and are repelled by (pauli exclusion principle) each other. The balance between attraction and repulsive forces generates van der walls interaction. The van der waals interactions are expressed by Lennard-Jones 6-12 potential. The vander waals interaction between two atoms [i and j] arises from a balance between repulsive and attractive forces. Atoms are attracted to each other by weak dispersion forces (London forces) and are repelled by each other because of the difference in quantum numbers. The attractive interactions are usually longer than the repulsion. But repulsive interaction becomes dominant when distance becomes short. Positioning of the atoms at the optimal distances stabilizes the system. In a long distance, attractive forces exists between all atoms and the forces become stronger linearly as $[1/r]^6$. In a close range repulsive forces predominates between atoms linearly as 1/r to the 12th power increases $[1/r]^{12}$.

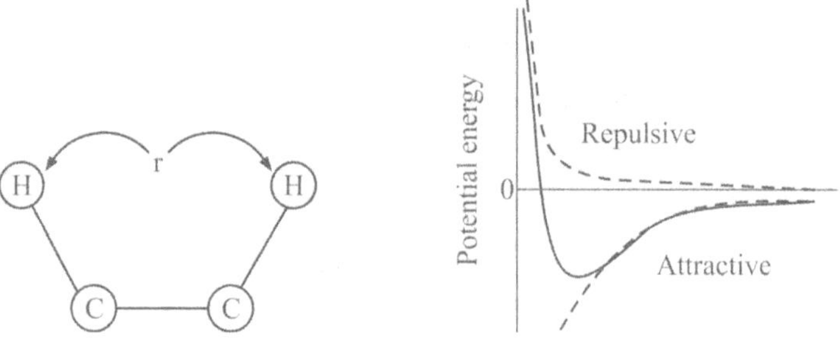

Van der waals effect

$$E_{vdw} = \varepsilon \left[\frac{\left(r_{min}\right)^{12}}{r} - \frac{2\left(r_{min}\right)^{6}}{r} \right]$$

The attraction forces between two atoms bring them together, and it reaches equilibrium distance. If the distance is further decreased between two atoms then they may overlap and this produces repulsion.

12.4 Energy Minimization Methods

1. Zero order / derivative technique - Simplex method
2. First order / derivative technique –
   (a) Steepest descent method (SD)
   (b) Conjucate gradient method (CG)/ powell method
3. Second order / derivative technique [Newton-Raphson method]

Zero order- simplex method: Identifies the regions of the lowest energy and useful mainly for the high energy molecules.

Steepest descent method (SD): This algorithm generates conformations with decreased energy. The path leading to minima is determined by using the previous value (in which the energy is decreased). In case the energy of the new conformation is decreasing, the process path will be continued until reaching the minima.

Conjucate gradient method (CG)/ powell: This algorithm accounts current gradient and previous in the conformational change. Hence it requires fewer calculations and is the method of choice for large systems

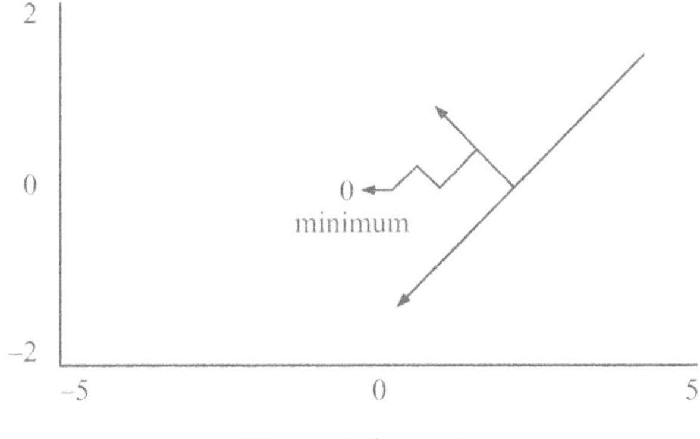

Steepest descent

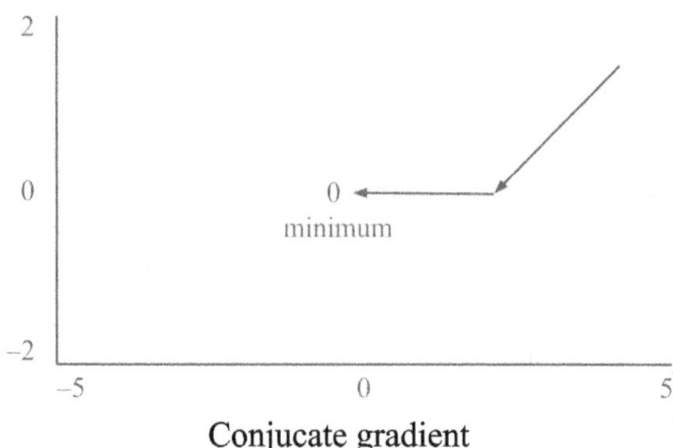

Conjucate gradient

12.5 Molecular Dynamics

Energy minimization in molecular mechanics is not a sophisticated one, because it stops as soon as it reaches first stable conformation it finds (it stops when a force field reaches nearest lowest energy [local minima]). Molecular dynamics is the computer simulation of molecular motions (folding process) helps in overcoming this limitation. Multiple energy minima can be bypassed by folding of a real molecule to global minimum.

The new generation simulation techniques (molecular dynamics) along with advanced computer hardware offer molecular modeling. Molecular modeling simulate, predict and analyse the bio-physicochemical properties of the molecules. These techniques considers the free energy of the system ($\Delta G = \Delta H - T\Delta S$) to explore the target binding potentials of the ligands. Decrease in the free energy of the molecule infers stronger target binding , whereas increase in the free energy refers to weaker binding. The enthalpy of the molecule decides its steric arrangement. The algorithm of the molecular dynamic tools estimates the free energy of the system. The physicochemical properties of the molecules can be calculated from this energy level.

12.6 Molecular Dynamic Simulations (MDS)

Molecular mechanics finds particular geometries and their associated properties by ignoring the time evolution of the system. Molecular mechanics (force field calculations) focuses on finding particular geometries and predicts properties based on stationary model. Atoms within molecule will vibrate differently at different temperatures. Molecular dynamics simulates molecular motion at high temperature, which help overcoming the energy barriers. MD simulations introduce heat into system and adjust velocities to maintain the temperature.

Time averaged structural and energetic properties, structural fluctuations and conformational transitions are accounted in molecular dynamics simulations. The temperature is expressed in terms of velocities. The velocities and forces acting on the each atom will be quantified by applying Newton's Law. MD simulations use classical physics and FF methods to study the atomic and molecular motions. The simulation of molecular motion at high temperature increases the probability of overcoming energy barriers. The possibility of sampling all possible minimum conformations without being trapped in local energy minimum increases. MD simulations by adding thermal energy overcomes the conformational barriers.

12.7 Quantum Mechanics

Drugs and their interaction with biological activity is responsible for the biological effect. Molecular orbital methods help understanding electron distribution. Quantum chemistry helps in this task and calculates the properties of the drug molecule. Quantum mechanics involves in the calculation of molecular orbital energies and calculates molecular geometry, energy, vibrational spectra, and electronegativity. The shapes and symmetries of Highest Occupied Molecular Orbital (HOMO) and Lowest Unoccupied Molecular Orbital (LUMO) help predicting the properties. Quantum mechanical calculations uses Schrödinger equation, which includes motion of the nucleus and electrons.

$$\hat{H}\Psi = E\Psi = (U+K)\Psi$$

where $\hat{H}$ = Hamiltonian (helps in the determination of energy)

Ψ (sigh) = Wave function

E = Total energy

U = Potential energy

K = Kinetic energy

The wave function (Ψ) describes the distribution of electrons in various orbitals (s, p, d, f and g). This equation explains the motion of the nucleus and electrons [distributions of electrons around molecules].

12.8 Quantum Mechanical Methods

1. Ab initio method

2. Density Functional Theory

3. Semi empirical molecular orbital methods

  (a) Complete neglect of differential overlap (CNDO)

  (b) Modified neglect of differential overlap (MNDO)

  (c) Perturbation configuration integration using localized orbital (PCILO)

Ab initio methods: It searches low energy (global) conformations of the molecules in 3(N-1) dimension [N= number of atoms in the molecule]. Then calculates the dipole moment, magnetic susceptibility, chemical shielding and electron affinities. The bio-physicochemical properties of the molecules can be predicted from the data generated.

Density Functional theory: In this method the energy of the molecules can be calculated based on their electron density. This approach is widely used in the energy calculations of proteins.

Semi empirical method: It involves in the conformational calculations through Complete Neglect of Differential Overlap (CNDO), Modified Neglect of Differential Overlap (MNDO) and Perturbation Configuration Integration using Localised Orbital (PCILO). The MOPAC program through Austin Model 1(AM1), Parameterised Model 3(PM3) and Modified Neglect of Differential Overlap (MNDO) calculates electronic configuration and predicts its properties.

12.9 Applications of Quantum Mechanics

Quantum mechanics can be used in the following operations.

1. Molecular orbital energy calculations
2. Geometry optimization
3. Dipole movement calculation
4. Transition state geometries and energies
5. Heat of formation (of specific conformation) calculation
6. Magnetic susceptibility prediction
7. Chemical shielding and chemical reactivity
8. Electron affinity calculation
9. Ionization potential prediction

12.10 Conformational Analysis

The computational process of identifying local minima, global minima and its bioactive conformation is known as conformational analysis. This plays important role in molecular modeling process. Molecules containing freely rotatable bonds can adopt many different conformations. Energy minimization generates chemically favourable conformations of the molecule. The conformation in which drug exhibits therapeutic potential is known as bioactive conformation. It may be a global minimum, local minimum or a transition state.

Conformation: Refers to both minima and maxima

Conformer: Refers to conformation of the molecule with minimum energy

12.10.1 Conformational Analysis Methods

- **Manual Method**

   Chemical intuition of the medicinal chemist plays a major role in this approach. It involves careful selection of possible conformation and estimation of its free energy after energy minimization. This method may ignore some of the molecular conformations, hence automated methods are developed.

- **Automated methods**

   Systematic method: It finds all minima within the defined search parameters. Success is a function of the number of increments used to explore each rotatable bonds. The method is applicable to molecules with less than 10 dihedral angles. Grid searching, torsion driving and constrained searching are some of the most commonly employed methods.

   Non-systematic method: This method is suitable for large molecules. Dynamics, stochasitic and distance geometry are the methods used for the computaion.

DOCKING

Drug activity is obtained through the molecular binding of the ligand to the binding sites of the receptor. Receptors do not recognize their ligands in terms of molecular frame works. The free energy difference between unassociated and associated states of the ligand with receptor decides the molecular recognition.

Molecular recognition plays a key role in promoting enzyme-substrate, drug-protein and drug-nucleic acid interactions. Hydrogen bonding, electrostatic, van der Waals and hydrophobic, interactions play key role in stabilizing associated structure. Detailed understanding of the nature of these interactions between the ligands and targets (protein/ nucleic acid) may provide potential drug leads. Docking includes searching, scoring and comparison of poses (conformations). Molecular docking is desired for predicting putative binding modes and affinities and are used in designing therapeutics.

Geometric and chemical complementarities of both ligand and receptor are essential for the biological effect. Prediction of intermolecular interaction is of vital importance for the development of new therapeutics. Computational methods are utilized to study the formation of intermolecular complexes. The computational process of searching ligand that is able to fit both geometrically and energetically to the binding sites of the target is known as docking.

Docking, a molecular modeling technique describes 'best-fit' orientation of a ligand and receptor protein (hand-in-glove). Docking is the process of fitting molecule into a model receptor binding site to predict possible ligand receptor interaction. It is a knowledge driven approach helps in predicting the binding pattern compounds to the target using computer programs. It enables medicinal chemist in predicting their biological activity potential and plays a major role in rational drug design.

13.1 Requirements

- 3D structure of ligand molecule in preferred format (sdf, MOL2, Tripos Mol2, etc.,)
- 3D structure of receptor protein in PDB format
- Softwares
  - Search algorithms- scoring function
  - Visualization tools
  - Analysers

13.2 Docking Types

13.2.1 Rigid Body Docking: The receptor and ligands are treated as rigid. Bond angles, bond lengths and torsion angles of the components are not modified at any stage of complex generation. Rigid body docking is inadequate, when substantial conformational change occurs within the components during complex formation.

13.2.2 Flexible-Ligand Docking: Receptor is kept rigid, whereas ligand is treated as flexible.

13.2.3 Flexible Docking: Docking procedures, which permit substantial conformational change on both receptor and ligand.

13.3 Molecular Docking Approaches

- **Geometry matching / shape complementary method:**

  Describes protein and ligand features, such as molecular surface
  1. Receptors molecular surface area is described in terms of its solvent accessible surface area
  2. Ligand molecular surface area is described in terms of its matching surface description

  Complenmentarity between two surfaces helps finding the complementary pose of the ligand and target

- **Simulation process:**
  1. Protein and ligand are separated by some physical distance
  2. Ligand finds its position into the protein active site after certain number of move in its conformation
  3. Conformational space consists of all possible orientaion and conformation of the protein pairs with ligand

4. Each snapshot of pair is referred as 'pose'

5. Moves incorporates rigid body transformations and torsional rotations

6. Each conformation contributes to energy

13.4 Protein-Ligand Docking

General steps

1. Preparation of the ligand

   - Geometry optimization
   - Energy minimization
   - Charge calculation

2. Preparation of protein

3. Docking calculation

4. Protein-ligand complex representation

13.5 Essential Components

Protein-Ligand consists of two essential components

- Sampling
- Scoring

Sampling: Generates putative ligand binding conformations of a protein. Two aspects of sampling are

1. Ligand sampling: The sampling algorithms generate putative ligand orientations around the binding site of the protein. There are three types of ligand sampling algorithms

   - Shape matching: The conformation of the ligand is normally fixed during shape matching process.

   - Systematic search: They are used for flexible-ligand docking, which generates all possible ligand binding conformations by exploring all degree of freedom of the ligand. Three types of systemic search methods are known and are

     (a) Exhaustive search

     (b) Fragmentation

     (c) Conformational ensemble

- Stochastic algorithm: Ligand binding orientations and conformations are sampled by making random changes to the ligand at each step in both the conformational space and the translational / rotational space of the ligand.

2. Protein flexibility: Ligand binding commonly introduces conformational rearrangements of the side chains of target. This can be grouped in to

- Soft docking: The simplest docking method provides computational efficiency and easiness. But applicable only for small conformational changes. It allows flexibility of the receptor and ligand structures through molecular relaxation.

- Side chain flexibility: In which back bones are fixed and side chains conformations are sampled.

- Molecular relaxation: It involves rigid body docking to place the ligand into the binding site and then relaxing the protein backbone and side chain atoms.

- Protein ensemble docking: Protein flexibility can be incorporated by utilizing ensemble of protein structures to represent different possible conformational changes.

13.6 Search Algorithms-Scoring Function

The evaluation and ranking of predicted ligand conformations is a crucial aspect of docking. Scoring functions considers the possible rotational and translational orientations of the ligand relative to the protein. Estimates the strength of the association between the 2 partners in the complex and helps in finding the binding mode and active conformation. The conformation with lowest energy is considered as the binding mode.

Pose generation: Number of poses (conformations) will be generated and evaluated in computational docking. The pose with lowest energy score will be considered as best fit and will be accepted for the activity prediction.

The scoring function is the key element in the protein-ligand docking and are grouped into three general classes

- Force-field based scoring function: They are based on decomposition of the ligand energy into individual terms such as van der waals, electrostatic, bond stretching, bond bending, bond torsional energies of inter-and intra molecular interactions.

$$E_{total} = \epsilon\, E_{str} + \epsilon\, E_{bend} + \epsilon\, E_{torsion} + \epsilon\, E_{vdW}\, \epsilon E_{cou}$$

where E_{str} = Energy of stretching;

   E_{bend} = Bond length change;

   $E_{torsion}$ = Change in the conformation;

   ϵE_{cou} = Electrostatic attraction;

   E_{vdW} = Vander waals force   [refer 12.3]

- Empirical based scoring function: The binding energy score will be calculated by summing up enthalpic and entropic interactions. It includes electrostatic, hydrophobic-hydrophilic and hydrophobic-hydrophobic interactions.

$$\Delta G_{bind} = \Delta G_{H\text{-}bonding} + \Delta G_{metal} + \Delta G_{Lipo} + \Delta G_{rot}H_{rot} + \Delta G_o$$

   ΔG_{bind} = Estimated free energy of binding;

   $\Delta G_{H\text{-}bonding}$ = Contribution of H-bonding to ΔG_{bind};

   ΔG_{metal} = Contribution of metal interaction to ΔG_{bind};

   $\Delta G_{rot}H_{rot}$ = Contribution of frozen-rotatable ligand bonding to ΔG_{bind};

   $\Delta G_{rot}H_{rot}$ = Contribution of non-specific interaction to ΔG_{bind}

- Knowledge based scoring function: It works based on the information derived from database protein-ligand complexes. They rely on pairwise atom potentials calculated from statistical analysis of bonds between ligand and protein atoms. It correlates statistical information about the ligand-protein binding and free energy of binding.

- Consensus docking: This technique improves the probability of finding a correct solution by combining multiple scoring functions.

13.7 Receptor Structure

The quality of the receptor (target) structure plays a central role in the success of docking calculations. The higher resolution of the crystal structure of protein produces better docking results. Resolution is a reciprocal term, where high resolution is expressed as small number and large number denotes lower resolution. Generally resolution of 2-3 Å is achieved in biomolecule.

13.8 Solvent Effect

Water influences biochemical reactions and ligand-receptor binding. Solvent energy plays pivotal role in the qualitative understanding of the drug-receptor interaction. Improvements in the ranking of ligands can be achieved by using ligand solvation energy. Solvent energy is the energy released due to attractive dispersion and electrostatic forces and entropy of water.

In particular solvent energy plays major role in case of docking small molecules to nucleic acids. Numerous models such as continuum model, discrete model and hybrid model were developed to study the solvent effect. Implicit solvent models are routinely used in this connection.

13.9 Molecular Docking Applications

Docking helps in the generation of lead compounds for the design of therapeutics

1. Lead identification: Screening libraries of database molecules *in silico* to identify lead molecules for further development into potential drug candidates
2. Lead optimization: Structural optimization of lead molecule to enhance their potency

13.10 Major Problems Associated With Docking

1. Receptor structures are complicated; they frequently change shape and solvent structure upon binding to a ligand.
2. The number of possible conformations rises exponentially with the number of rotatable bonds.
3. Calculating the differential affinity between two related ligands using thermodynamic methods is time consuming.

13.11 Docking Server

Docking server is a web based molecular docking program useful in the high throughput screening. It allows efficient and robust docking calculations by integrating several softwares.

Features

- High throughput screening
- Docking for known binding sites

- Calculation of inhibition constant, binding geometry and secondary interactions
- Determination binding sites

Steps

1. Preparation of the ligand
   - Geometry optimization
   - Energy minimization
   - Charge calculation
2. Preparation of protein
3. Docking calculation
4. Protein-ligand complex representation

Preparation of ligands

Ligands can be drawn using Java applet or uploaded in appropriate file format (MDLmol, Sybyl mol2, PDB, Hyperchem Hin, Smiles format, SDF format)

Parameters Selection:

1. Desired pH
2. Molecular mechanics / semiempirical quantum chemical calculation parameters
3. Rotatable bonds and atom types

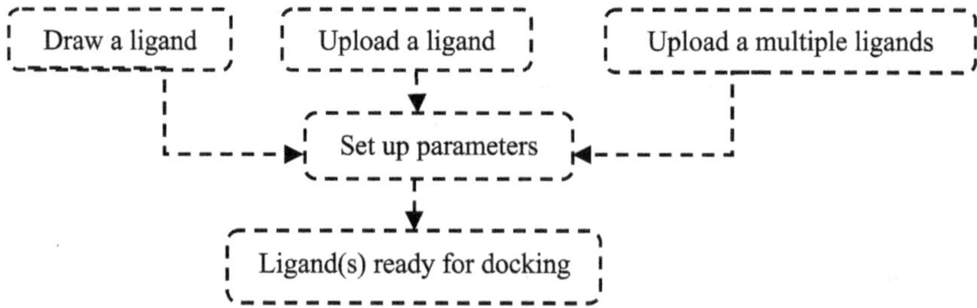

Preparation of Proteins

3D protein structures can be uploaded or directly downloaded to docking server from Protein Data bank (PDB) by providing PDB ID.

Parameters Selection

1. Protein chain, hetero atoms, ligands and water selection

2. Simulation box setup

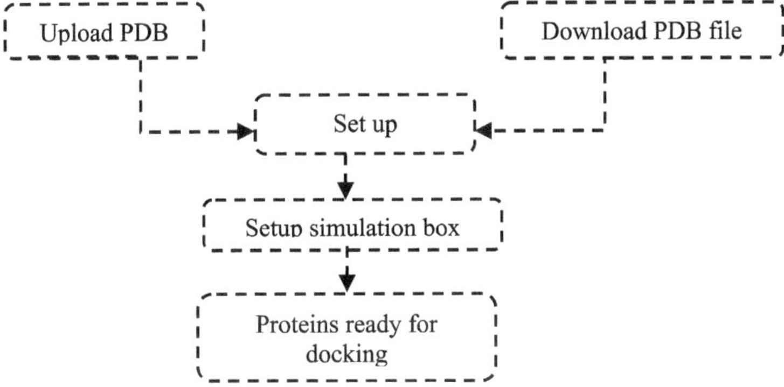

Ligand-Protein Docking Calculation

Protein, ligand and required parameters should be selected.

Parameters Selection:

- Protein, ligand, simulation type, number of runs and number of evaluations selection.

Results evaluation

Secondary ligand-protein interaction can be analysed to know how good the dock.

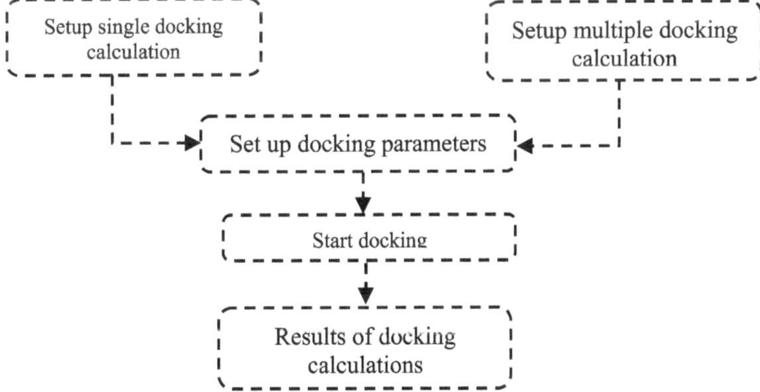

http://www.dockingserver.com/web/docking/

Step-1: Click DOCKING link in main page

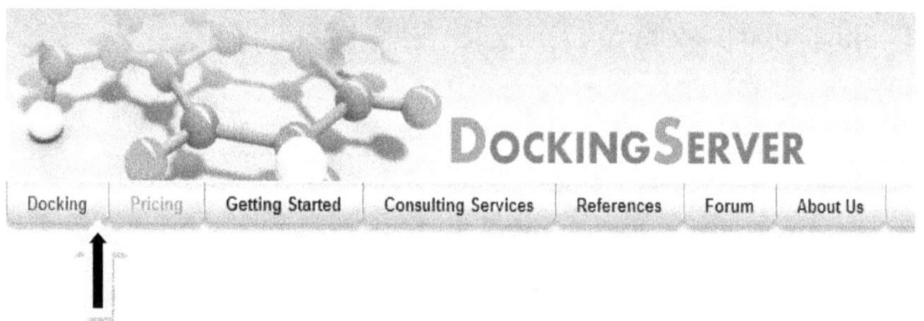

Step-2: Click MY PROTEINS link and use upload or download option to load protein

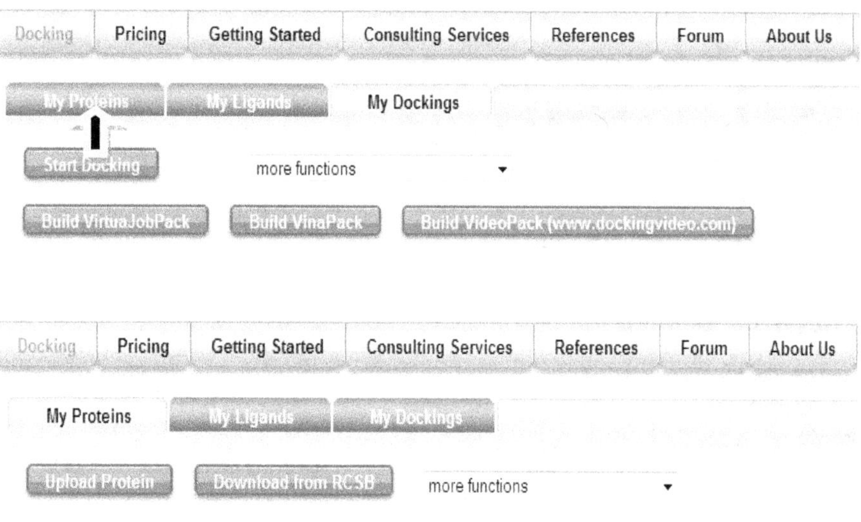

Step-3: Enter PDB ID or protein name to download protein from PDB

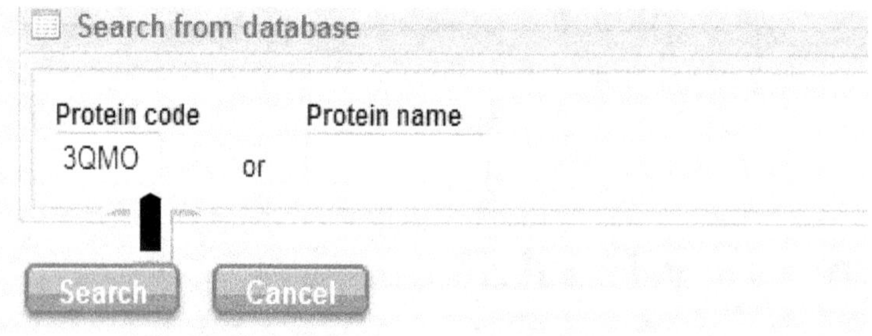

Step-4: Select and download the protein from list

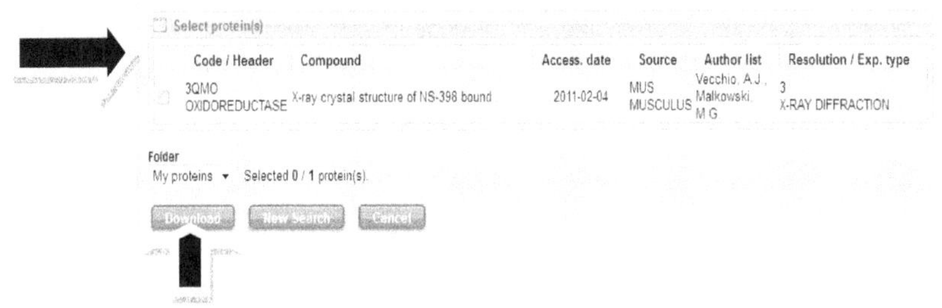

Step-5: Process the protein preparation step

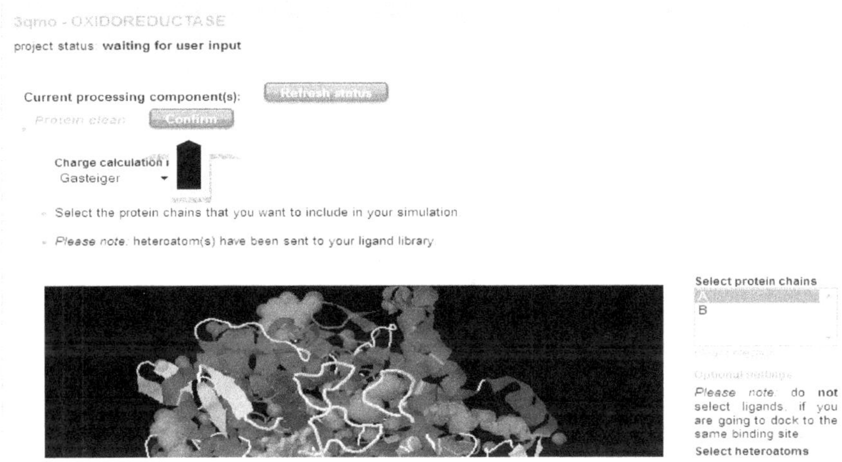

3qmo - OXIDOREDUCTASE

project status: **waiting for user input**

Current processing component(s):   Refresh status

Protein clean   Confirm

Charge calculation:
Gasteiger   ▾

- Select the protein chains that you want to include in your simulation

- *Please note:* heteroatom(s) have been sent to your ligand library

Select protein chains

A
B

Optional settings

Please note: do **not** select ligands, if you are going to dock to the same binding site

Select heteroatoms

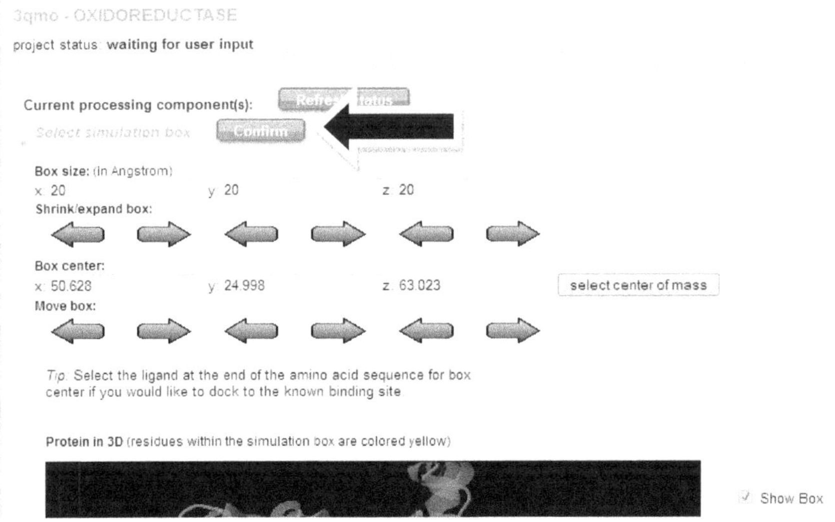

3qmo - OXIDOREDUCTASE

project status: **waiting for user input**

Current processing component(s):   Refresh status

Select simulation box   Confirm

Box size: (in Angstrom)
x: 20   y: 20   z: 20
Shrink/expand box:

Box center:
x: 50.628   y: 24.998   z: 63.023   select center of mass
Move box:

Tip. Select the ligand at the end of the amino acid sequence for box center if you would like to dock to the known binding site

Protein in 3D (residues within the simulation box are colored yellow)

✓ Show Box

Step-6: Use My Ligands link to save ligand molecule

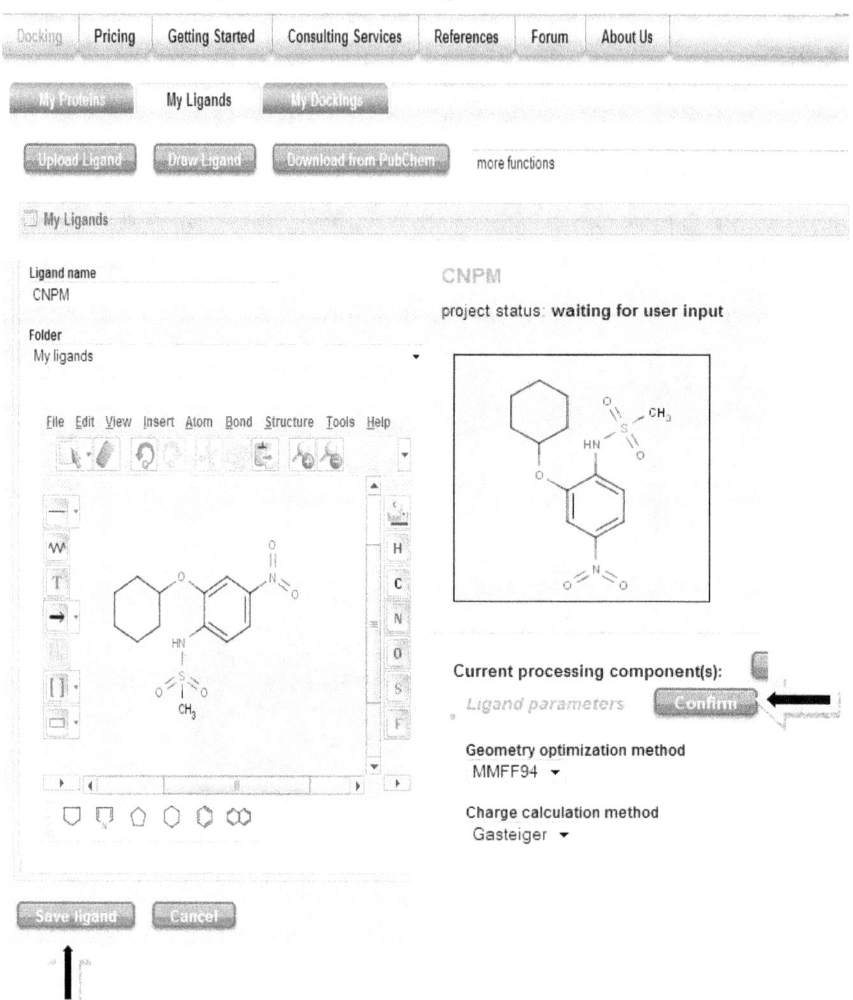

Step-6: Select ligand from MY LIGANDS

Step-7: Click STRAT DOCKING LINK to proceed with docking

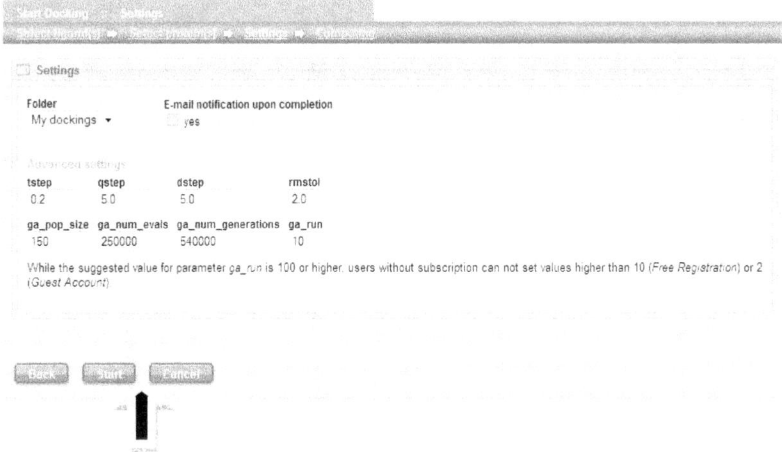

Step-8: Result page of docking procedure appears

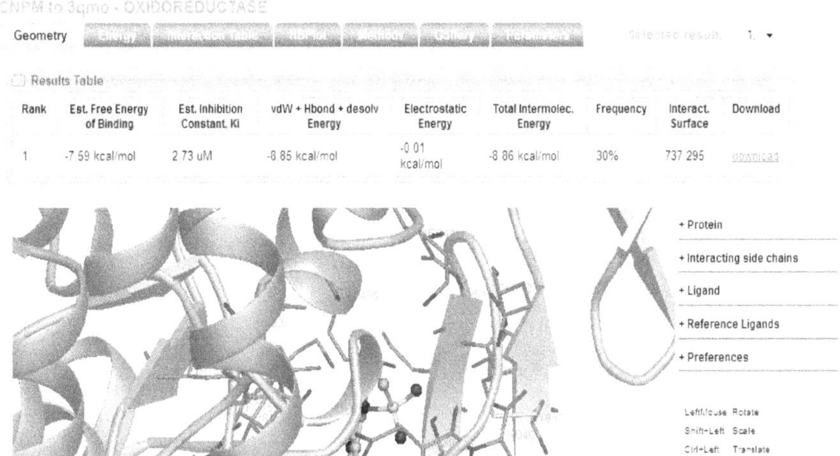

Rank	Est. Free Energy of Binding	Est. Inhibition Constant. Ki	vdW + Hbond + desolv Energy	Electrostatic Energy	Total Intermolec. Energy	Frequency	Interact. Surface	Download
1	-7.59 kcal/mol	2.73 uM	-8.85 kcal/mol	-0.01 kcal/mol	-8.86 kcal/mol	30%	737.295	DOWNLOAD

13.12   Swiss Dock

Swiss Dock, a web based molecular modeling tool developed by molecular modeling group of Swiss Institute of bioinformatics. Modeling is based on the software EADock DSS, which generates many binding modes for the ligand and target. The binding modes with most favorable energies can be visualized.

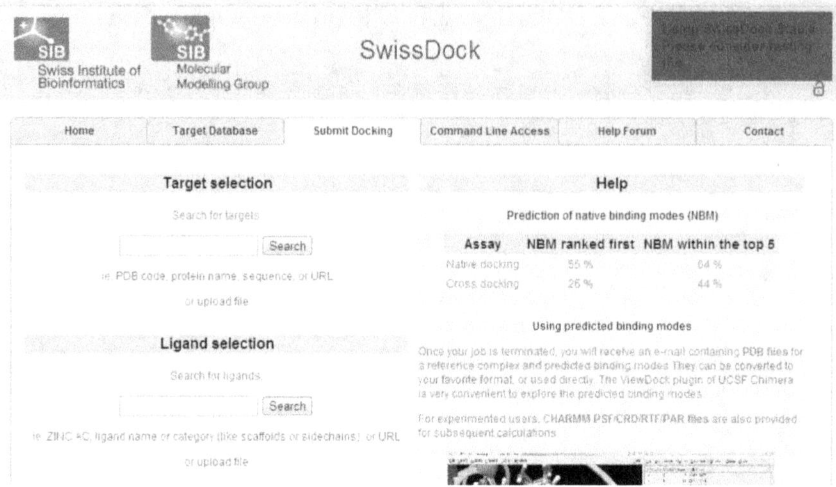

13.13 Autodock

Autodock is an computational tool aid in bioactive agents development, by predicting the interaction of small molecules on macromolecules. it is developed by Molecular Graphic laboratory, Scripps research Institute, La Jolla, USA. It uses Monte Carlo annealing technique (Metropolis method) for configuration exploration. It calculates the energy of the molecular complex by using grid based molecular affinity potentials. Autodock consists of two main components: autogrid: describes the grid of protein (binding site), autodock: performs the docking of ligands on pre-calculated grids of protein.

13.14 ArgusLab

ArgusLab is a free molecular modeling, graphics and drug design software tool. It is developed by Mark A Thompson, Planaria Software LLC, Seattle, WA. An efficient shape based algorithm is used and flexible ligand docking is possible, where the ligand is described as a torsion tree and grids are constructed that overlay the binding site.

<h1>CHAPTER 14</h1>

ARGUSLAB

The theoretical prediction of molecular properties are valuable tool in drug design program. ArgusLab is free software package useful in this regard (molecular modelling studies), which provides molecular sketching with template library. It has the provision to handle entire periodic table through Universal Force Field (UFF). Molecular mechanics based geometry cleaning is an another important feature of this software. Semiempirical methods such as Extended Huckel Theory (EHT), Austin Model 1(AM1), Parametric Model 3 (PM3) and Modified Neglect of Di-atomic Overlap (MNDO) along with Hartree-Fock model performs geometry optimization of the sketched molecules and calculates quantum chemical descriptors. These methods enable visualization of molecular orbitals and electron density surface, and calculation of electrostatic potentials.

EHT is an extension of the Huckel π electron approximation and treats all valance electrons present in a molecule. The MNDO and AM1 methods requires relatively shorter computational times. AM1 method provides good descriptions even for anions and hydrogen bonded systems. Hartree-Fock is wave function based method, which calculates the molecular electronic structure. Quantum chemical descriptors calculation helps in the prediction of molecular bonding interaction (binding energy) and toxicity level in biophase.

Working with ArgusLab

ArgusLab interface consists molecular display (black window), a progress report section (lower) and molecular tree view (left). Molecular tree view can switched to builder tool kit.

14.1 Binding Energy Calculations

The knowledge of the shape and electron density of the molecule assess the binding nature of the ligand to the target. All chemical interactions are either electrostatic or covalent and orbitals are involved in covalent interactions. According to the frontier molecular orbital theory (FMO), interaction between two orbitals depends on their energies associated with the Highest Occupied molecular orbital (E_{HOMO}) and Lowest Unoccupied Molecular orbital (E_{LUMO}). E_{HOMO} explains the basicity of hydrogen bond acceptor and E_{LUMO} explains the covalent acidity of the proton of a hydrogen bond donor.

E_{HOMO} is related to ionization potential of the molecule and measures the molecules tendency to be attacked by the electrophiles. E_{LUMO} is related to electron affinity of the molecule and measures the molecules tendency to be attacked by the nucleophiles. HOMO-LUMO gap models the stability of the molecule in chemical interactions. All these will help in the prediction of molecule biological interactions and thus its activity.

Ligand preparation: Pencil dot option in the tool bar can be used for constructing the molecule (by default it codes carbon). Fragment library also can be used for constructing the molecule. Atoms can be joined by using bond option in the tool bar. Right mouse button is for atom mode by default, using this atom type can be viewed and atom hybridisation (Sp3 and Sp2) and aromaticity can be changed. Through right click or hybridization option of edit link can be used to convert the non-aromatic molecule into aromatic.

To the constructed molecule hydrogen has to be added followed by geometry cleaning, this saves the molecule in specified location (agl, pdb, cml format). Alternatively molecules sketched using other tools in suitable formats can be imported in to display window.

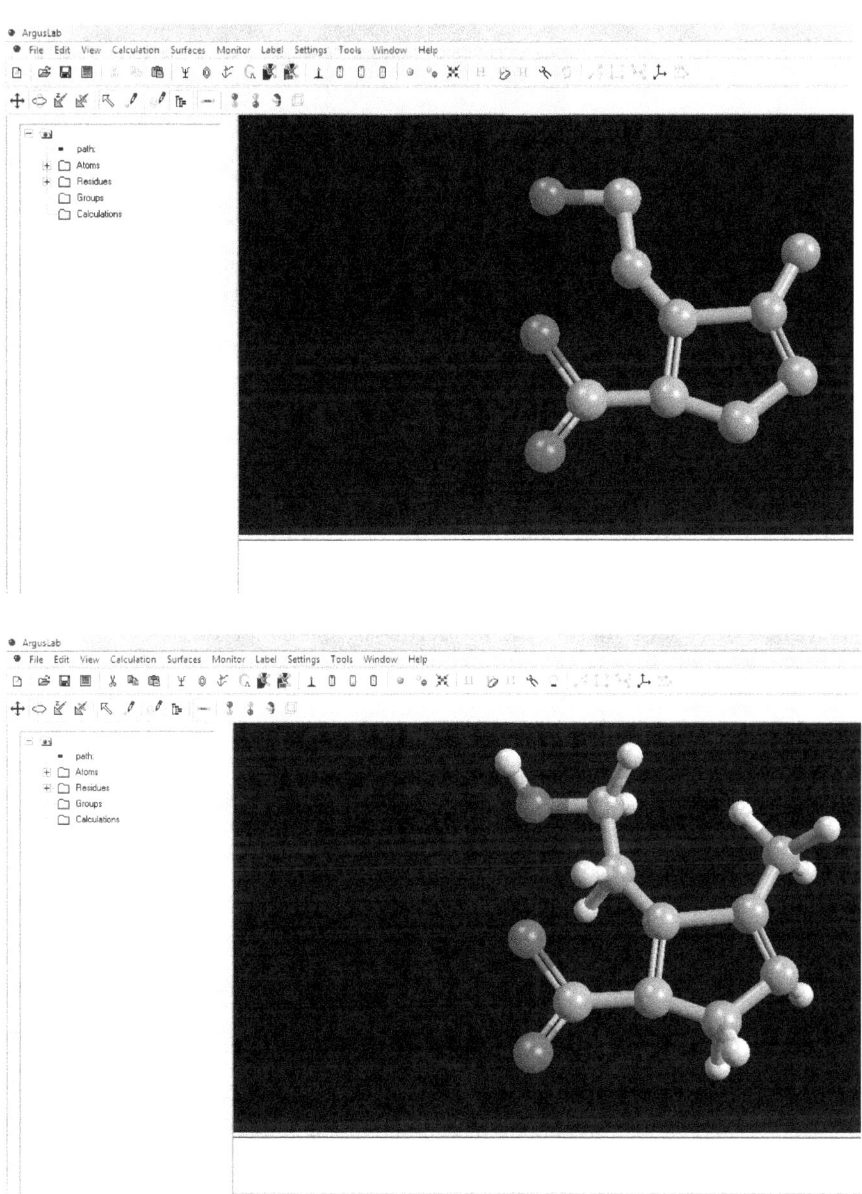

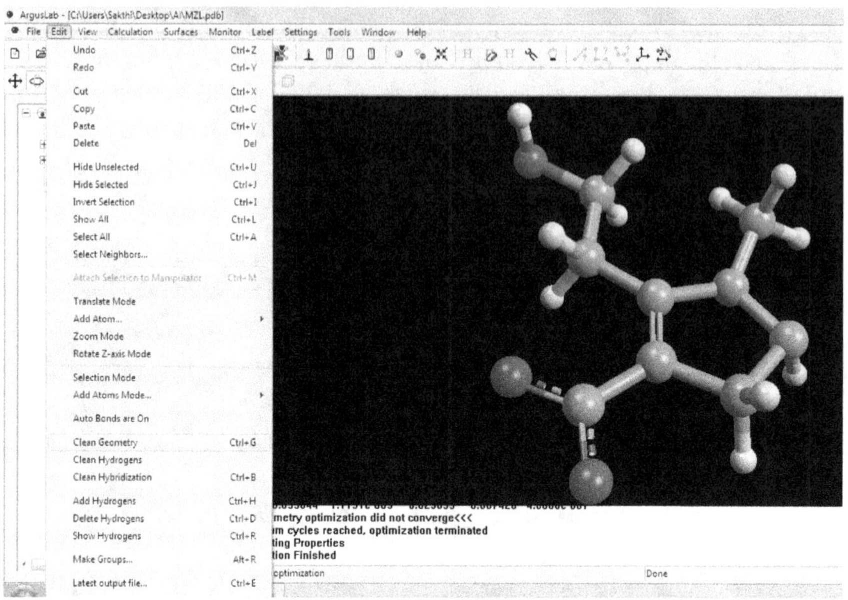

Molecular Property calculations: Energy option of calculation tool can be used calculate the dipole moments, mulliken charges, ADO charges, Wiberg Bond order, HOMO, LUMO and electron density. Selecting suitable parameters of QM-Hamiltonian and MM-Hamiltonian along with Hartree-Fock model derive the properties of the molecules.

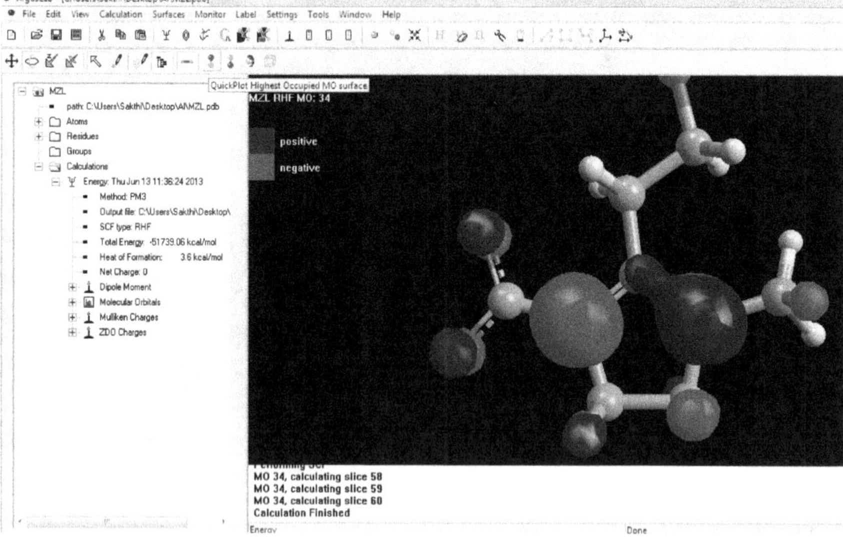

14.2 Docking Simulations

ArgusLab works through two docking engines such as ArgusDock and GADock. Shape Dock approximates exhaustive search and requires <30 seconds for 10-15 torsions in a laptop computer. GA dock works through Lamarckian genetic algorithm. As Score is the score measures the energy of the interaction and is based on terms taken from HPScore of Xscore.

Ligand preparation: Ligands can be sketched using draw mode / using templates, alternatively it can be imported in suitable format.

Geometry optimization: Hamiltonian QM (EHT, AM1, PM3), Hamiltonian MM (UFF, AMBER), Hartree-Fock SCF (with Max iterations-200, convergenge 10^{-10} kcal/mol, RHF [closed cell] / UHF [open cell]). Geometry search (Steepest descent / BFGS). Bunsen burner option can be used instead.

Target preparation: Import the protein databank file in .pdb format through OPEN option of tool bar. Switch to molecular tree view option and expand the tree PDB $\rightarrow$Residues $\rightarrow$ Misc. Right click Ligand and select 'Make a Ligand Group from this Residue' option (ArgusLab will generates a new group with new name). Expand Groups and right click on New Ligand and 'Make BindingSite Group for this Group'. Binding site box can be set according to the knowledge derived from literature (Grid generation).

Docking: Open 'Calculation option' from tool bar and expand 'Dock a ligand' option. Select 'ligand', 'binding site' and other parameters such as Docking Engine. Press 'Start' button to initiate the docking simulation. At the end of the operation results will appear in 'Progress report section' and docking pose will appear in 'molecular display window'.

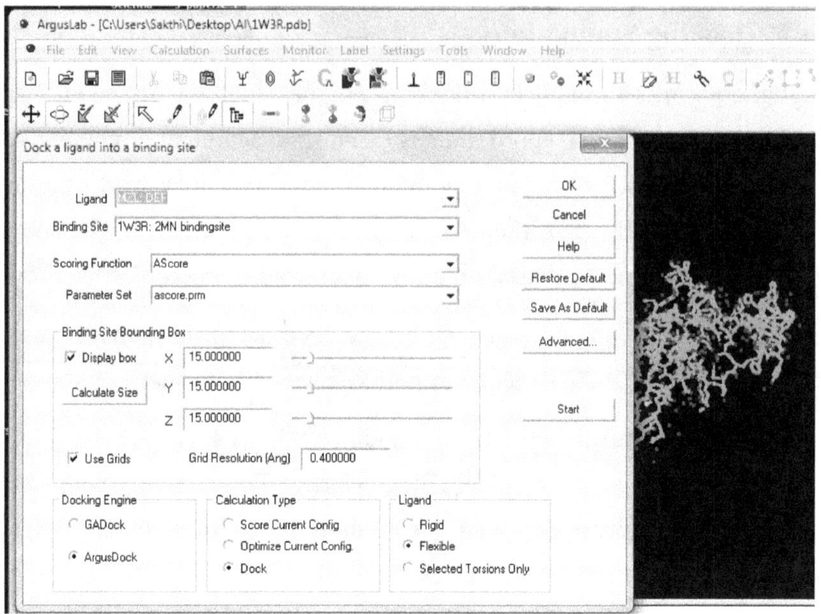

Viewing the results: After docking in molecular tree under Groups new ligand option (3 2MN) will appear. Right click on 3 2MN and view 'Hydrogen bonds'. Molecules can be placed in centre of the window by using the option centre. RMSD difference between X-ray and docked ligand can be calculated using 'Calculate RMSD position between two similar groups' option of Groups link of Tree view.

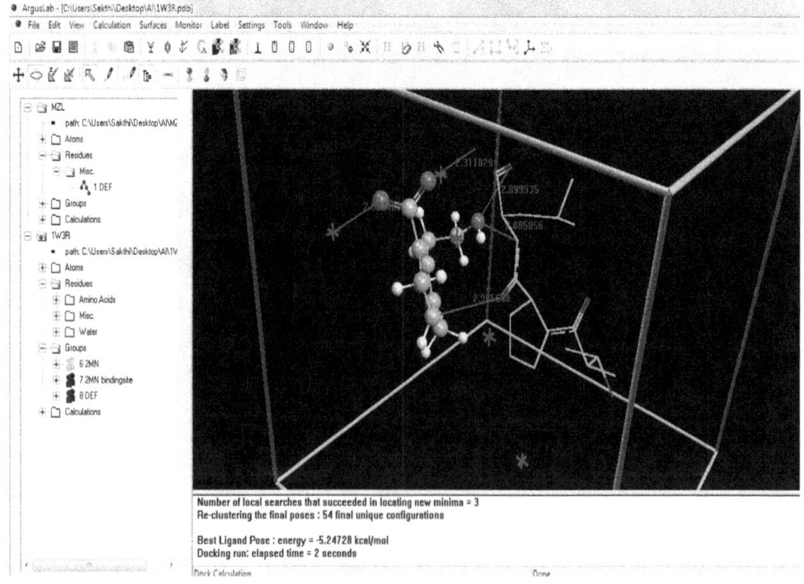

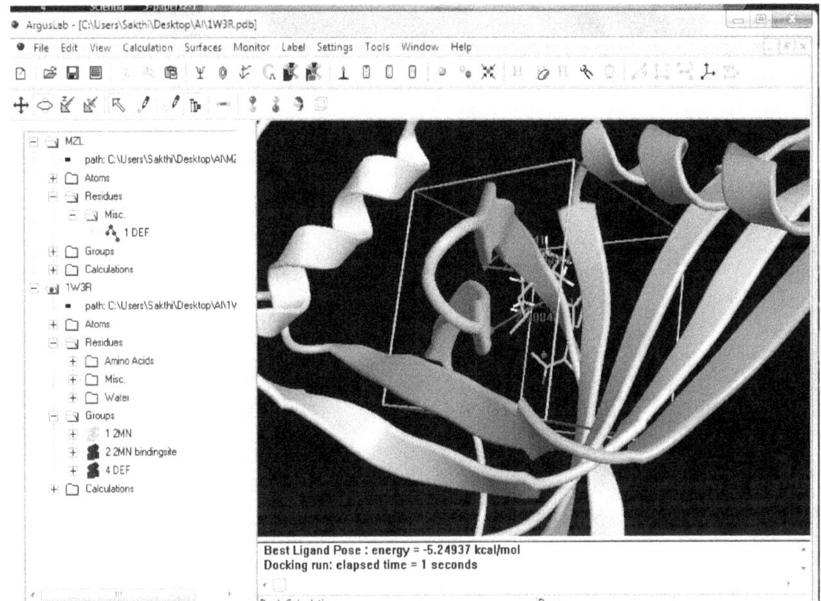

Saving the results: The obtained results can be saved in suitable format (*.agl, *.pdb) for the further analysis.

Capturing the image: Export option of file tool can be used to save the result views in either *.bmp / *.jpg / *.tiff format.

BIOINFORMATICS

Field of science in which biology, computer science and information technology merge into a single discipline.

- Interface between biological science and computational science
- Deals with organization, storing, retrieving, querying and interpretation of set of biological data
- Plays major role in target identity with the help of molecular biology and biophysical techniques

Bioinformatics includes 3 major sub-disciplines

1. Development of algorithms and statistics
2. Analysis and interpretation of data
3. Development and implementation of tools

Bioinformatics is a management information system, searches biological databases, compares sequences and predicts structure of the protein and its functional role and termed as homololgy modeling.

CHAPTER 15

BIOLOGICAL DATABASES

Biological database (heart of bioinformatics) is a large, organized body of persistent data, usually associated with computerized software designed to update, query and retrieve components of the data. These databases include both "public" repositories of gene data like GenBank or the Proteins Data bank (PDB) and private databases. Biological databases are grouped into:

1. Sequence databases
2. Structure databases

15.1 Sequence Databases

Most biological databases consists nucleotide and amino acid sequence information, taxonomic information such as the structural and biochemical characteristics of organisms. Each sequence of nucleotides and amino acids represents a particular gene or protein respectively. The fields of biology and chemistry have facilitated an increase in the speed of sequencing genes and proteins.

The requirements of researchers to benefit from all these informations are:

1. Ready access to the collected pool of sequence information.
2. A way to extract sequences of interest to a given researcher.

   Nucleotide sequence databases

GenBank	http://www.ncbi.nlm.nih.gov/Genbank/
EMBL	http://www.ebi.ac.uk/embl
DDBJ	http://www.ddbj.nig.ac.jp
Ensembl	http://www.ensembl.org
UniGene	http://www.ncbi.nlm.nih.gov/UniGene/

Protein sequence databases

SwissProt	http://www.expasy.ch/sprot/
PIR	http://pir.georgetown.edu
PFAM	http://www.sanger.ac.uk/Software/Pfam
	http://www.cgr.ki.se/Pfam
Interpro	http:// http://www.ebi.ac.uk/interpro/
Prosite	http://expasy.ch/prosite/

Genomics databases

Human	http://www.ncbi.nlm.nih.gov/genome/guide/
Nucleic acid search	http://www.oup.co.uk/har/database/c/
Mol Biol Net	http://www.molbiol.net/

15.1.1 Sequence Formats

Most sequence analysis programs require DNA / Protein sequences file in a particular format (eg: FASTA format). The nomenclature committee of the International Union of Biochemistry (IUB) has established a standard single-letter code to represent bases in nucleic acids. The Joint International Committee has established single-letter amino acid codes. For computer analysis of sequences it is more convenient to use these single-letter codes, especially in case of amino acids where three letter codes (codons) are used normally. Different sequence analysis software uses different sequence formats in ASCII file format.

GenBank sequence format

- The GenBank format is a standardised informational format developed by NCBI.

- It is human readable and convey both bibliographic and feature information about a sequence.

- GenBank records are delimited by a pair of forward slashes // on a single line.

EMBL Sequence format

- The EMBL format was developed by European Bioinformatics Institute (EBI) and is used by several major databases including EMBL and SwissProt.

- It is a human readable format and not geared towards parsing. EMBL is line based and consists of a two letter code followed by three spaces.

- Each line in the record must have two letter identifier including blank lines with the exception of the sequence section.

- The sequence section begins with the sequence header, denoted by a line containing the two letter code SQ.

- The sequence header is followed by a set of sequence lines and the record ends with two letter code //.

SwisProt Sequence format

It is very similar to the EMBL format and provides more information about the physical and biochemical properties of the protein.

FASTA sequence format

FASTA format is a text-based format for representing protein and nucleotide sequences using standard IUB / IUPAC single- letter codes. A sequence in FASTA format begins with > symbol followed by single line description. In case of single-letter code lower-case letters are accepted and are mapped into upper-case. A single hyphen or dash represents a gap in the sequence.

CODATA sequence format

- It is also known as Protein information Resource (PIR) format, has been used by the National Biomedical Research Foundation (NBRF) / Protein information Resource (PIR) and other programs.

- It resembles FASTA format by the presence of > symbol at initial, but it differs from FASTA by the presence of character P for complete sequences or F for fragments and 1 for linear or 2 circular sequences.

- A semicolon and four to six character unique name for the entry follows this.

- There is also an essential second line with the full name of the sequence, a hyphen and species of origin.

Abstract Syntax Notation (ASN.1) sequence format

- ASN.1 is a formal data description language that has been developed by the computer industry.

- It has been adopted by NCBI to encode data such as sequences, maps, taxonomic information, molecular structure and bibliographic information.

- It includes information regarding literature references, function of the sequences, locations of mRNAs, coding region and important mutations.

AceDB sequence format

- It is an genome information system which stores and displays multiple types of genomic data

- Data is stored in a set of structured binary files and the data model specifies a tree for each object class based upon tag-value pairs

- Data is imported and exported through text files called ace files i.e with the extension.ace

Genetics Computer Group (GCG) sequence format

- Information about the sequence in the GenBank entry is included first.

- A line of information about the sequence, data and a check sum value follows this.

- Lines of information are terminated by two period, which mark the end of information and start of the sequence on the next line.

Plain / ASCII staden sequence format: It includes only the sequence with no other accessory informations

General feature format: Used by EMBOSS suite of sequence analysis program

XML sequence format: It is widely used for sharing genome data between computer locations

Sequence Format Convertor

READSEQ: It is an extremely useful sequence formatting program, recognizes a DNA / protein sequence files in any of the format and write a new file with an alternative format. Data files that have multiple sequences also can be converted.

SEQIQ: Sequence conversion program for nix machine.

GCG suite

- 'From' programs convert sequence files from GCG format into the named format FROMEMBL, FROMFASTA, FROMGENBANK, FROMIG, FROMPIR, FROMSTADEN.

- 'To' programs convert the alternative format in to 'GCG' format are TOFASTA, TOIG, TOPIR, TOSTADEN.

- GETSEQ: Converts a simple ASCII file (received from remote PC) to GCG format.

- REFORMAT: Formats GCG file.

- SPEW: Sends GCG file as an ASCII to a remote PC.

  There are no programs to convert to GenBank and EMBL format.

15.2 Structure Databases

Proteins are essential constituents of bioloical function and are composed of L-α-amino acids by peptide bonds. Peptides with less than 50 amino acids are known as polypeptides and more than 50 amino acid residues are known as proteins. The proteins often exist with non-polypeptide cofactors. The proteins fold into one or more specific spatial conformations attributed by covalent (disulphide) and non-covalent (ionic, hydrogen and hydrophobic bonds) interactions. The biomolecular structure of protein is responsible for its function and is referred as bioactive conformation. Protein structure determination requires techniques like sequencing, gel electrophoresis, X-ray crystallography, dual polarization interferometery, nuclear magnetic resonance (NMR) spectroscopy and electron microscopy.

Primary structure

The linear sequence of amino acids joined together by peptide bonds are termed as primary structure of protein. Peptide bond is covalent in nature and has partial double bond character. it is produced by the link between carboxyl group of one amino acid and amino group of another. The two ends of the polypeptide chain are C-terminus (carboxyl terminus) and N-terminus (amino terminus). The significant number of primary sequence change (mutation) affects the protein function. Substitution of chemically similar amino acids (valine with isoleucine – both are hydrophobic) is conservative. Amino acids residues, which are significantly less stringent are known as variable. The important protein sequence databases include National Institute of biotechnology Information (NCBI), European Bilogy Laboratory Data Library (EMBL), Protein Information Resource (PIR) and UniprotKB of swissprot.

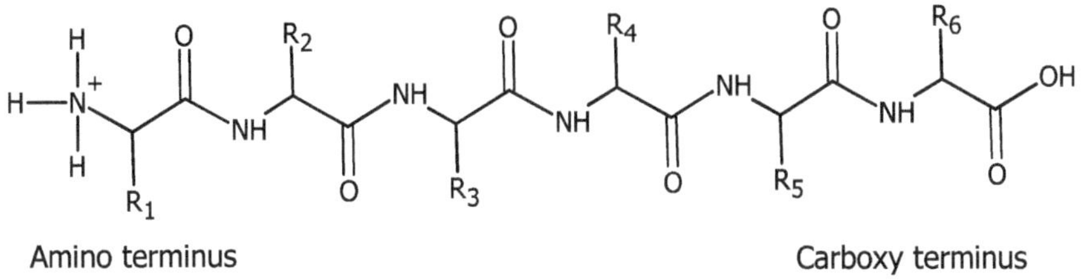

Fig. 15.1 Primary structure of protein.

Secondary Structure

It refers to highly regular folding of regions of polypeptide chains and consists of α-helix and β-pleated sheet. These patterns are due to the rotation angle about Cα-C [ϕ (phi)] and angle Cα-N [ψ (psi)].

1. α-helix (spiral): It is a cylindrical, rigid, rod-like helical arrangement of the amino acids in the polypeptide. It is produced by the hydrogen bonds between -NH group of amino acid and -C=O group of amino acid four residues away. In a α- helix there are 3.6 amino acids per turn of the helix (0.54 nm, 5.4 Å). The distance of one amino acid residue is 0.15 nm (1.5 Å).

2. β-pleated sheet (folds): It is the fully extended conformation and hydrogen bonds between adjacent polypeptides (between -NH group and -C=O group adjacent amino acid) stabilises this structure. If the adjacent polypeptide runs in same direction then it is called as parallel β-pleated sheet and opposite are known as anti-parallel β-pleated sheet. Super secondary structures (motifs) are produced by packing side chains from adjacent secondary elements close to each other. All β-sheet strands are twisted in right handed sense and contain 2-15 strands.

   α-helix and β-pleated sheet form recognizable super secondary motifs (β-α-β, two strands of β- sheet connected by α-helix)

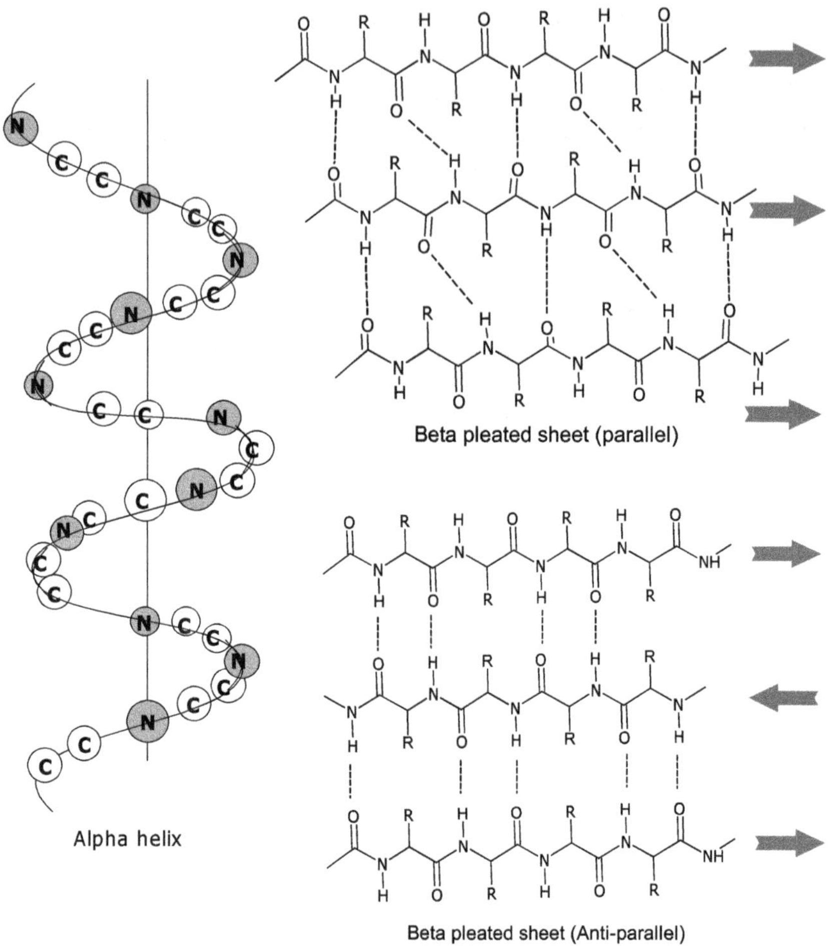

Fig. 15.2 Secondary structure of protein.

Tertiary Structure

It refers to the spatial arrangement of the amino acids present in the polypeptide. The covalent (disulphide) and non-covalent (ionic, hydrogen and hydrophobic bonds) interactions stabilises the structure. These interactions also play major role in the generation of bioactive conformations. This functional and three dimensional (3D) structural unit is called as polypeptide.

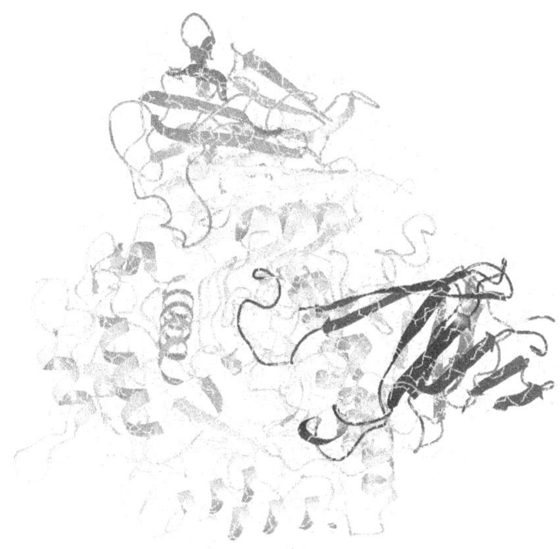

Fig. 15.3 Tertiary structure of protein.

Quaternary Structure

The 3D structure of proteins having more than one polypeptide chains are known as quaternary structure. These polypeptides are held together by covalent and non-covalent interactions. Each chain of polypeptide is known as oligomers / subunits /monomers.

Structure database keeps 3D structures of biomolecules obtained from X-ray crystallography and NMR spectroscopy. The image of protein and nucleic acid structures has become a common feature of biochemistry text books and research articles. The data stored in the structure database records represents a practical summary of the experimental data. Each biomolecular structure provides potentially critical information regarding the function of any given protein sequence.

15.2.1 3D Molecular Structure Data

2D structures of the molecules are not sufficient enough to explain the properties of a molecule 3D structure are important. For the proper understanding of the structure and its property 3D structure can be obtained databases. Protein structure databases useful in bioinformatics are

PDB	http://www.rcsb.org/pdb
CATH	http://www.biochem.ucl.ac.uk/bsm/cath

SCOP	http://scop.mrc.imb.cam.ac.uk/scop
DALI	ekhidna.biocenter.helsinki.fi/dali/start
MMDB	http://www.ncbi.nlm.nih.gov/Structure/ MMDB/mmdb.shtml

15.3 Protein Data Bank (PDB)

PDB is developed by Brookhaven National Laboratories and is managed by the Research Collaboratory for Structural Bioinformatics (RCSB). It contains information regarding all 3D structures of proteins, nucleic acids, carbohydrates and a variety of other complexes experimentally determined by X-ray crystallography and NMR spectroscopy. RCSB-PDB includes sequence details, atomic coordinates, crystallization conditions, 3D structure neighbors, compute methods, geometric data, structural factor, 3D images, etc. A unique 4 character alphanumeric code is given to proteins called as PDB-ID or PDB code. (eg:1PRG for PPAR gamma)

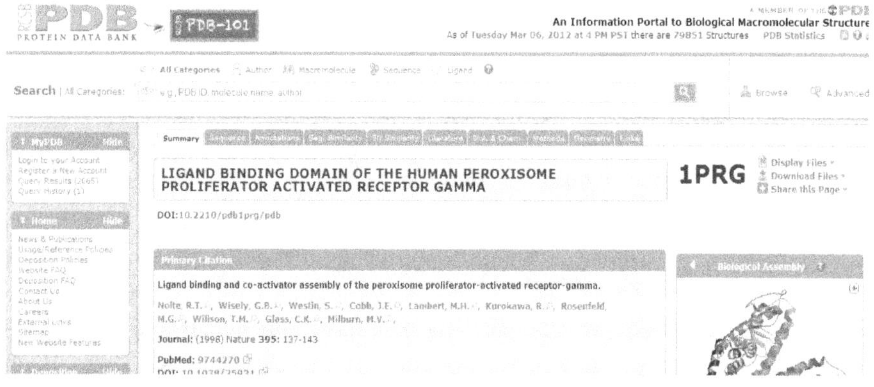

15.3.1 Search Methods

1. By providing PDB ID
2. By searching the text found in PDB files
3. By searching against specific fields of information – Search against deposition data or author etc.

15.3.2 PDB Sequence Format

- PDB record consists of 12 sections that range from descriptive titles and remarks to structure descriptions including atomic coordinates.

- Positions 1 through 6 of each line contains a line identifier, position 9 and 10 is the continuation marker and position 11 through 70 contains the actual data.

15.3.3 PDB Informations on Protein

- **Summary:** It contains a complete description of the protein includes the authors who worked on it, journal in which it is published, PubMed ID, abstract of the research details. It also provides molecular descriptions like classification, structure weight, number and type of chains, fragments associated to it, organism from which it is isolated, UniprotKB details.

- **Sequence:** It gives FASTA format of the protein sequence and annotations (in SCOP, CATH, PFAM, Interpro, SAP).

- **Annotations:** It contains a detailed profile about the protein includes domaininfo, class (alpha and beta proteins, peptides), fold, super family, family, domain and species.

- **Sequence alignment:** PDB also provides tool for sequence alignment of protein sequences.

- **3D similarity:** Similar 3D structures for the entry PDB-ID can be identified for the homology analysis.

- **Literature:** It provides details about the research team, journal in which it is published, MeSH details and related articles from PubMed central.

- **Biology and chemical report:** It provides complete details regarding the biology and chemical nature of the molecule.

- **Methods:** Includes the methods applied in 3D structure prediction.

- **Geometry:** It provides details about bond length, bond angle and dihedral angle of protein along with its graphical representations such as Ramachandran plot.

15.4 CATH

CATH is a hierarchical classification of protein domain structures, which clusters proteins at four major levels:

Class: Similar secondary structure content (all α, all β, α / β etc)

Architecture: Major structural secondary elements in similar arrangement

Topology: Probable common ancestor

Homologous super family: Indicative of demonstrable evolutionary relationship

The boundaries and assignments for each protein domain are determined using a combination of automated and manual procedures which include computational techniques, empirical and statistical evidence, literature review and expert analysis.

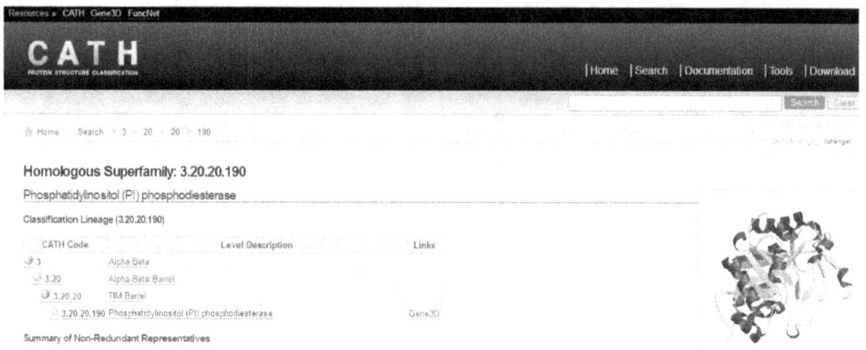

15.5 Structural Classification of Proteins (SCOP)

The SCOP database is a largely manual classification of protein structural domains based on similarities of their amino acid sequences and three-dimensional structures. SCOP utilizes four levels of hierarchic structural classification.

1. **Class** - general "structural architecture" of the domain

    –   **Class α:** Comprises a bundle of α-helices connected by loops on the surface of the protein.

    –   **Class β:** Comprises anti parraller β sheets (eg: enzymes, antibodies)

    –   **Class α / β:** Comprises mainly paraller β sheets with intervening helices

    –   **Class α + β:** Comprises mainly segregated α-helices and anti-parallel β sheet

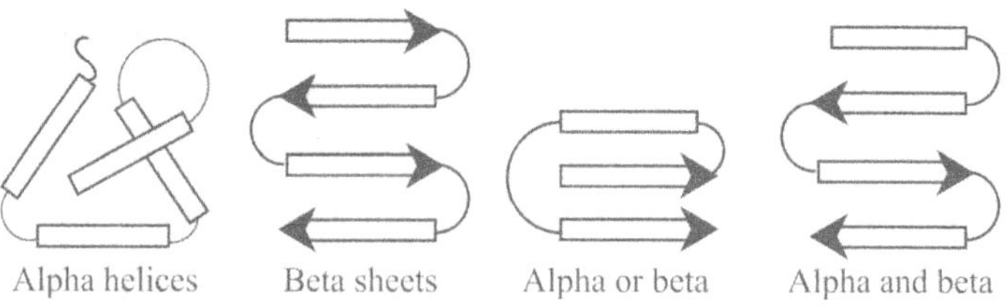

   – **Multi domain (α and β):** Compare domains of more than one
     of the above 4 classes

2. **Fold** - similar arrangement of regular secondary structures but
   without evidence of evolutionary relatedness

3. **Superfamily** - sufficient structural and functional similarity to infer
   a divergent evolutionary relationship but not necessarily detectable
   sequence homology

4. **Family** - sequence similarity can be detected.

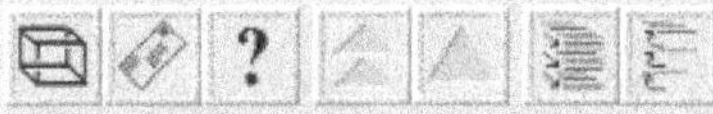

Structural Classification of Proteins

Superfamily: PLC-like phosphodiesterases

Superfamily

Lineage:

1. Root: scop
2. Class: Alpha and beta proteins (a/b) [51349]
   Mainly parallel beta sheets (beta-alpha-beta units)
3. Fold: TIM beta/alpha-barrel [51350]
   contains parallel beta-sheet barrel, closed; n=8, S=8; strand order 12345678
   the first seven superfamilies have similar phosphate-binding sites
4. Superfamily: PLC-like phosphodiesterases [51695]
   Superfamily

Families:

1. Mammalian PLC [51696] (2)
2. Bacterial PLC [51699] (2)
3. Glycerophosphoryl diester phosphodiesterase [89508] (4)
   Pfam 03009

15.6 DALI / FSSP

Proteins are classified based on the structural alignment of all pair wise
combinations of the proteins in the PDB by DALI.

15.7 Molecular Modeling Database (MMDB)

It is an integral part of NCBI Entrez information retrieval system.
MMDB records are in ASN.1 and PDB format files also are obtained

from MMDB. MMDB records have value-added information compared with the original PDB entries. Search filed includes PDB and MBD ID codes, free text from the original PDB remark records, author name and other bibliographic fields. Proteins of known structures in the PDB have been categorized into structurally related groups in MMDB.

15.8 Spatial Arrangement of Backbone Fragments (SABF)

SABF provides a protein database categorized on the basis of structural similarity.

15.9 DNA Databank

A DNA databank is essentially a storage facility that maintains DNA extracted from a variety of sources including blood, saliva, hair, skin, muscle and liver, etc. DNA databanks can serve a variety of purposes that include screening for disease gene- genetic diseases, paternity testing, identity matching for criminal investigations, genetic fingerprinting for criminology and research-related studies.

DNA databases available in the worlds are

1. Combined DNA Index System (CODIS)
2. GenBank - NCBI
3. United Kingdom National DNA Database
4. Californian DNA database (included in CODIS).
5. National Criminal Investigation DNA Database (NCIDD)

Combined DNA Index System (CODIS): The Combined DNA Index System (CODIS) is a DNA database funded by the United States Federal Bureau of Investigation (FBI).

GenBank: GenBank is a National Institutes of Health (NIH) genetic sequence database and is a comprehensive public database of nucleotide and protein sequences with supporting bibliographic and biological annotation. GenBank is the fastest growing repositories of known genetic sequences. It has a flat structure that is an ASCII text file, readable by both humans and computers. In addition to sequence data, GenBank files contain information like accession numbers and gene names, phylogenetic classification and references to published literature. GenBank contains 22.6 billion nucleotide bases from 18.2 million different sequences and a new release is made every two months. It is a part of International Nucleotide Sequence Database Collaboration, which comprises the DNA DataBank of Japan (DDBJ), European Molecular Biology Laboratory (EMBL) and GenBank at NCBI.

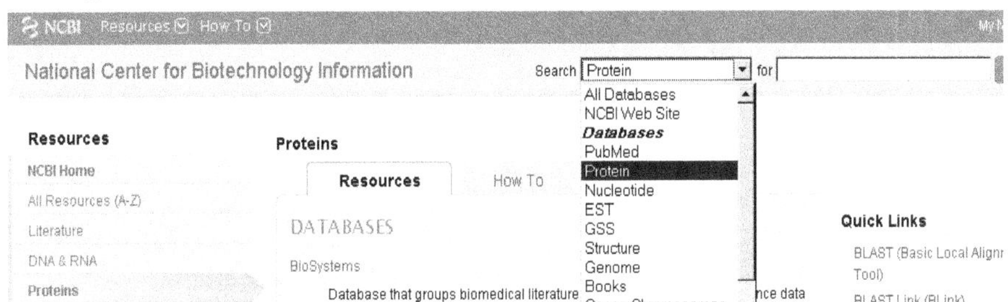

European Molecular Biology Laboratory (EMBL): The EMBL Nucleotide Sequence Database is a comprehensive database of DNA and RNA sequences collected from the scientific literature and patent applications and directly submitted from researchers and sequencing groups. Data collection is done in collaboration with GenBank and DNA Database of Japan (DDBJ).

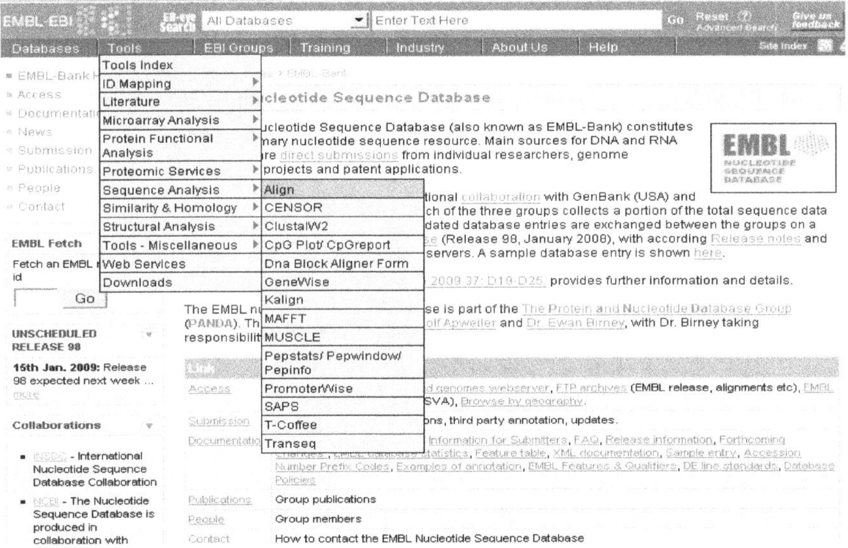

DNA Database of Japan (DDBJ): DDBJ is sole DNA data bank in Japan and it is established by National Institute of Genetics, Japan. It is functioning as the one of the international DNA database. It includes the functions of EMBL and NCBI through the collaboration (international databank collaboration). Public gene expression database CIBEX is available through DDBJ.

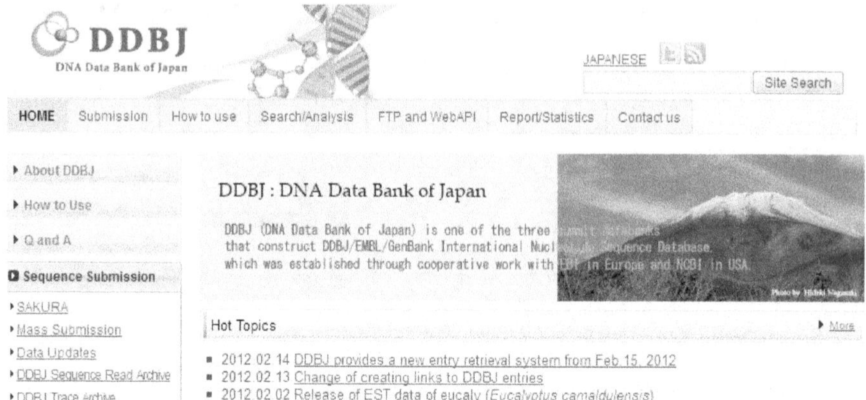

SwissProt: SwissProt is the curated protein sequence database established by department of Medical Biochemistry of the University of Geneva [Swiss Institute of bioinformatics (SIB)] and the EMBL data entry library. SwissProt provides a high level of annotations such as functions, domain structure, post transitional modifications (PTMs), variants of the proteins. SwissProt entries are produced from translocations of sequences in EMBL extracted from the literature or submitted directly by researchers. SwissProt entries are copyrighted but available freely to academia. SwissProt has distinct criteria and they are as follows

1. Annotation: It contains two classes of data

   - Core data: Consists of sequence data, citation information and taxonomic data

   - Annotation: Consists of functions, domain, PTMs, secondary and quarternary structure of proteins. Similarities to other proteins and disease associated with deficiencies of the proteins also can be viewed.

2. Minimum redundancy: Protein sequence data from different literature reports are merged to reduce the redundancy.

3. Integration: It offers high levels of integration with other databases and also has a very low level of redundancy (less identical sequences). It is cross referenced with 30 different databases.

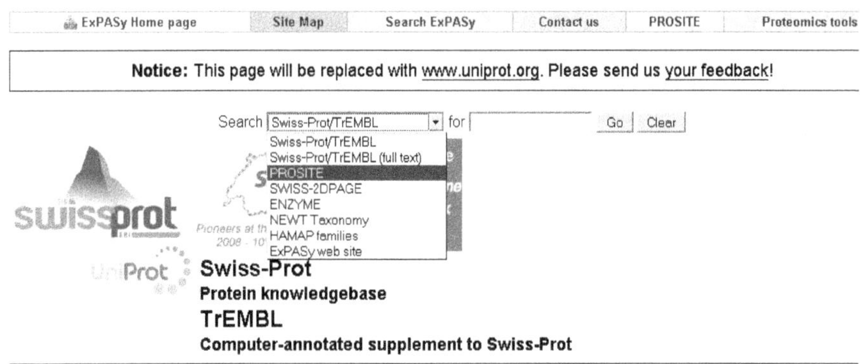

The UniProt Knowledgebase consists of:

- **UniProtKB/Swiss-Prot**; a curated protein sequence database which strives to provide a high level of annotation (such as the description of the function of a protein, its domains structure, post-translational modifications, variants, etc.), a minimal level of redundancy and high level of integration with other databases [More details / References / Linking to Swiss-Prot / User manual / Re changes / Disclaimer].
- **UniProtKB/TrEMBL**; a computer-annotated supplement of Swiss-Prot that contains all the translations of EMBL nucleotide seque entries not yet integrated in Swiss-Prot.

TrEMBL: TrEMBL is a computer annoted supplement of SwissProt developed jointly by SIB and EBI. It contains all the translations of EMBL nucleotide sequence in SwissProt format excluding coding sequences which are included in SwissProt. Entries in TrEMBL are progressively merged with SwissProt entries.

Protein Information Resource (PIR): PIR is established by National Biochemical Research Foundation (NBRF) and provides protein database and analysis tools on molecular evolution, functional genomics and computational biology. PIR in collaboration with Munich Information Center for Protein Sequences (MIPS) and Japan Information Database developed PIR International Protein Sequence Database (PIR-PSD). PIR-PSD is a comprehensive, non-redundant, expertly annotated and fully classified sequence database. The primary data sources for PSD are GeneBank / EMBL / DDBJ translations, published reports and direct submissions to PIR.

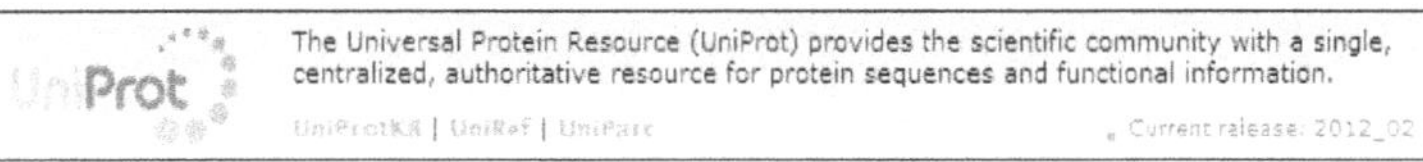

PIR has four distinct sections

PIR-1	It contains fully classified and annotated entries
PIR-2	It includes preliminary entries
PIR-3	It includes unverified entries which have not been reviewed
PIR-4	Conceptual translations of artifactual sequences Conceptual translations of sequences that are not transcribed or translated Protein sequences or conceptual translations that are extensively genetically engineered Sequences that are not genetically encoded and not produced on ribosome

PFAM: PFAM is a database of multiple alignments of protein domains / conserved protein regions and profiles Hidden Markov Model (HMM). Profile HMM is useful in determination of the protein family and deals sensibly with multi domain protein. PFAM is composed of two parts

PFAM A: Contains curated families with associated profile HMMs and it is useful in alignment and database search.

PFAM B: Sequence segments that are not included in PFAM A are clustered automatically

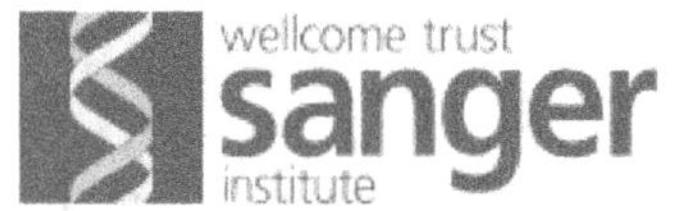
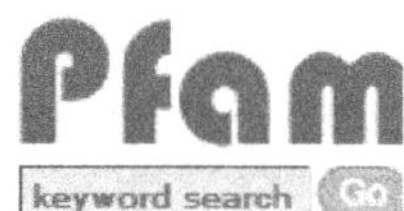

HOME | SEARCH | BROWSE | FTP | HELP | ABOUT

Pfam 26.0 (November 2011, 13672 families)

The Pfam database is a large collection of protein families, each represented by **multiple sequence alignments** and **hidden Markov models (HMMs)**. More...

QUICK LINKS	YOU CAN FIND DATA IN PFAM IN VARIOUS WAYS...
SEQUENCE SEARCH	Analyze your protein sequence for Pfam matches
VIEW A PFAM FAMILY	View Pfam family annotation and alignments
VIEW A CLAN	See groups of related families
VIEW A SEQUENCE	Look at the domain organisation of a protein sequence
VIEW A STRUCTURE	Find the domains on a PDB structure
KEYWORD SEARCH	Query Pfam by keywords
JUMP TO	enter any accession or ID Go Example

Enter any type of accession or ID to jump to the page for a Pfam family or clan, UniProt sequence, PDB structure, etc.

Or view the help pages for more information

INTERPRO

It is the most efficient and reliable database provides internal consistency and checks and deeper coverage. It is found useful in genome analysis.

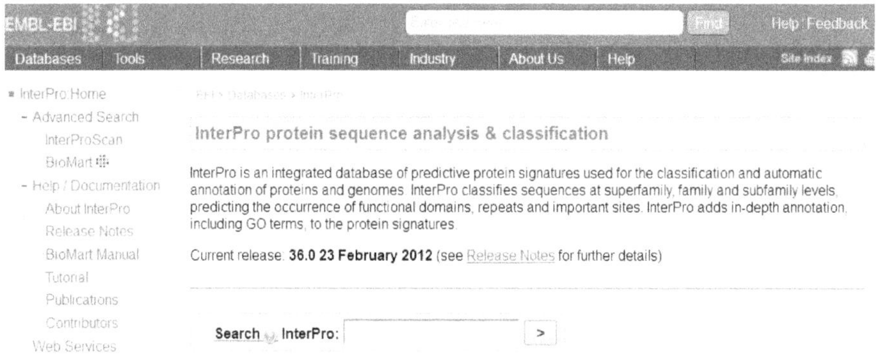

PROSITE: Prosite is the database of biologically significant sites and patterns. It determines the function of proteins transcribed from genomic or cDNA sequence. It contains as many biologically meaningful patterns and profiles as possible and are highly specific. It includes concise description of the protein family / domain along with summary of the development of pattern or profile.

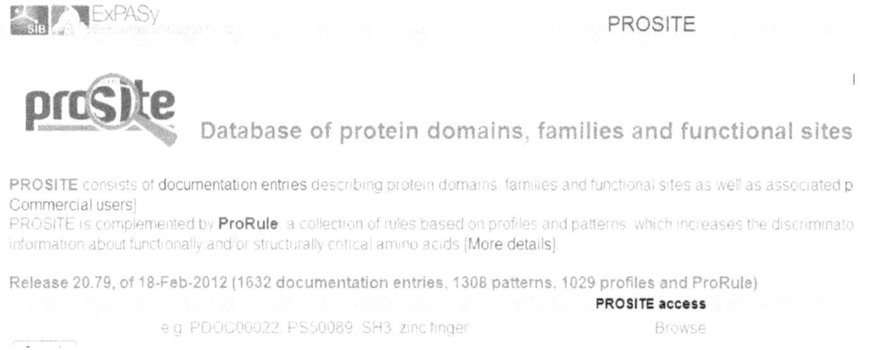

## CHAPTER 16

BIOPHYSICAL TECHNIQUES

The most commonly used method in the investigation of molecular structure are X-ray crystallography, nuclear magnetic resonance spectroscopy and electron microscopy.

16.1 X-ray Crystallography

Accurate knowledge of molecular structure is a pre requisite for rational drug design. X-ray crystallography studies provide unambiguous, accurate and reliable 3D structure with absolute configuration of a molecule. This method revealed the structures of vitamin, DNA, protein and drugs. Size and shape of the receptor (receptor mapping) and conformational analysis of the drug molecule can be done through this method.

Most of the protein structures (>80 %) available today are determined through X-ray crystallography technique. The crystal structure of the protein scatters the X-rays onto electronic detector. After each blast of X-rays (few seconds to several hours) crystals will be rotated to get desired orientations. This enables the capturing of crystal scattering in three dimensions. Distance between atoms will be measured in angstroms. X-ray crystallographers have solved structures of proteins up to 2,500 kilodaltons.

16.2 NMR Spectroscopy

Protein NMR spectroscopy is the important technique in structural biology and serves in drug design. NMR spectroscopy characterizes the structure and molecular dynamics of the target and ligand molecules. It provides insight into the ligand-target complex and found useful in rational drug development process. NMR spectroscopy is well suited when crystals of molecules are not available (X-ray crystallography requires crystals). NMR structures show significant pH variation and the protein backbone may display considerable motion and unfolding at different pH.

NMR spectroscopy lags behind X-ray crystallography in the size of the structure it can handle. The largest structures NMR spectroscopist has determined are 30 to 40 kilodaltons (270 to 360 amio acids). NMR reveals how the macromolecules interact with ligands. Multi-dimentional NMR combines several sets of experiments, which spreads out the data into discrete spots. The location of each spot indicates unique properties of one atom in the sample.

16.3 Electron Microscopy

Protein structures are usually determined from either 2D crystals and polyhedrons. Electrons can be used in these situations, because these electrons interact more strongly with than X-rays. X-ray will travel through 2D crystals without diffracting and cannot be used to form image of the crystal, where as electrons form image. The strong interactions between electrons and protein forms thick crystals (>1 μm). A common problem to X-ray crystallography and electron crystallography is they damage organic and protein molecules.

<h1>CHAPTER 17</h1>

MOLECULAR BIOLOGY

Molecular biology knowledge is required for the better understanding of bioinformatics and homology modelling. The central dogma of molecular biology includes DNA replication, transcription and translation. Two major divisions of molecular biology are

- Genomics
- Proteomics

17.1 Genome Analysis

Totality of genetic information in an organism is known as 'genome' and the study of genome is known as 'genomics'. Genomics deals with the systematic use of genome information to provide answers in biology and medicine. Genomic information is generally coded in double stranded DNA, but in viruses coded in single stranded DNA / RNA. Genomics has the potential of offering new therapeutic methods for the treatment of some diseases, as well as new diagnostic methods.

17.2 Structural Genomics

This genome-based approach involves the analysis of macromolecular structure (particularly proteins) using computational tools and theoretical frameworks. The goal of structural genomics is to obtain accurate three-dimensional structural models for all known protein families, protein domains or protein folds. This high-throughput method combines experimental and modeling approaches. Structural alignment is a tool of structural genomics, and attempts to determine the structure of every protein encoded by the genome. The availability of large number of sequenced genomes and previously-solved protein structures allows scientists to model protein structure on the structures of previously solved homolog's. In addition to elucidating protein functions, structural genomics can be used to identify novel protein folds and potential targets for drug discovery.

17.3   Functional Genomics

Functional genomics aid in understanding the function of genes and other parts of the genome. It utilizes vast wealth of data produced by genome sequencing projects to describe genome function. It uses high-throughput techniques (DNA microarrays, proteomics, metabolomics and mutation analysis) to describe the function and interactions of genes. Functional genomics focuses on the dynamic aspects such as DNA replication, gene transcription, translation, and protein-protein interactions. It gives insights in to the function of DNA at the levels of genes, RNA transcripts, and protein products. Functional genomics involves studies of natural variation in genes, RNA, and proteins.

17.4   DNA Replication

DNA replication occurs during S phase of the cell cycle, during this phase the enzymes (DNA polymerase) responsible for DNA synthesis are adequate in quantities. It involves several enzymatic reactions and proof reading procedures in order to ensure genetic stability (fidelity) and is co-ordinated with cell growth and division. A newly synthesized DNA molecule contains one newly synthesized material and one old strand (template). DNA replication begins at fixed points on the chromosome and involves DNA strand unwinding, incorporation of nucleotide precursors and renaturation of replicated molecules. All the 3 process occur at the environment known as origin of replication (replication fork).

Components of DNA Replication

1. DNA helicase: It catalyses the ATP dependent unwinding of double strand DNA.

2. RNA primer: 10-200 residues length oligonucelotides.

3. Primase: It helps in the initiation of DNA synthesis.

4. DNA polymerase: It catalyses the DNA synthesis, generates phospho diester bond between deoxy ribonuceotide. 3^1 exonucleases (DNA polymerase I) serves as a "proofreading" function and 5^1 exonucleases (DNA polymerase I) involve in DNA repiar. DNA polymerase III plays major role in nucleotide incorporation during replication.

5. Single strand binding proteins (SSBPs): SSBPs are known as T4 protein, helix destabilizing protein.

6. Topoisomerase: It provides a swivel mechanism for relieving the stress.

7. DNA ligase: It co-valently closes nicks in double strand DNA, activated by lysine residue adenylation.

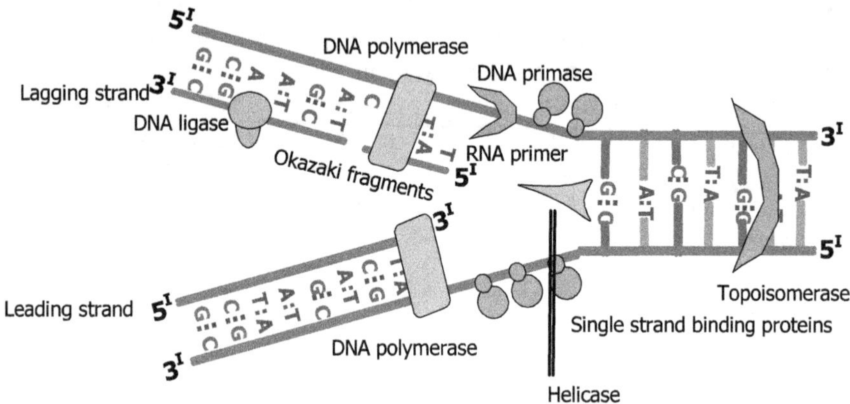

Fig. 17.1 DNA replication process.

DNA replication is more accurate than any other enzyme catalyzed reaction and requires activated deoxy ribonucleoside-5-triphosphate as substrate.

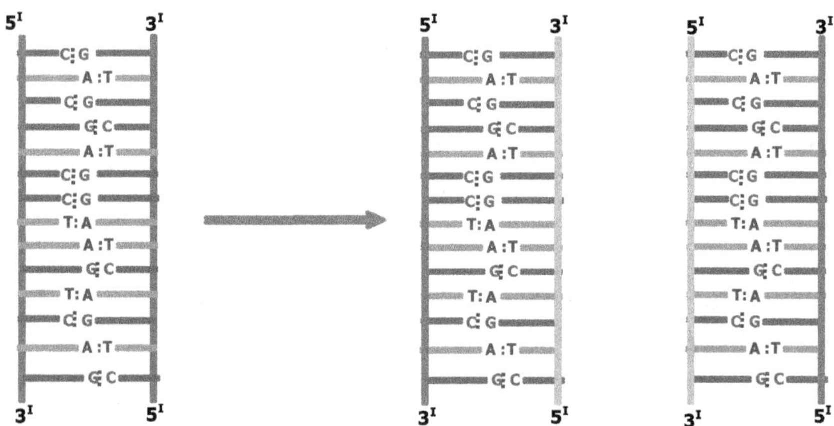

Fig. 17.2 Replicated DNAs.

DNA replication is discontinuous; one strand grows in the direction of fork movement and the other strand in opposite direction.

Process of Replication

Chain initiation: The AT base pair rich region is preferable for DNA replication, because of lesser hydrogen bonding than CG base pairs and which facilitates the unwinding (dsDNA cleavage) process. Unwinding process produces replication bubbles, which occurs at every 10 nucleotide residue.

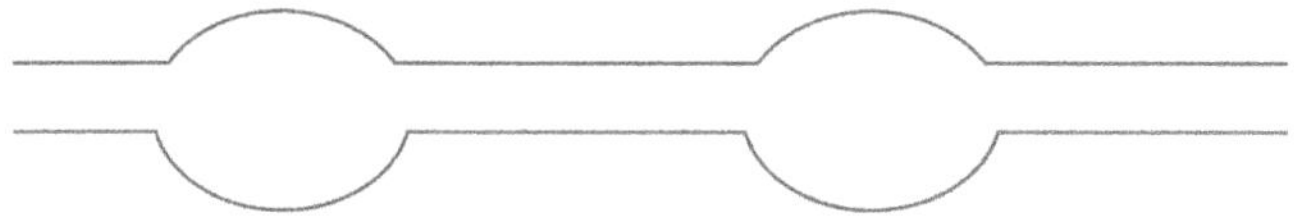

Fig. 17.3 Replication bubbles.

Chain elongation: DNA polymerase involve in the insertion of complementary nucleoside to the template strand. This chain elongation process occurs in two directions. One chain elongates in the direction of replication fork and is called as leading strand (5^1-3^1). The other chain elongates in the opposite direction and is called as lagging strand (3^1-5^1). The 3^1 hydroxyl group of the deoxy ribonucelotide phosphate (RNA primer) will be attacked by 3^1 phosphate of dNTP. It liberates the pyrophosphate and forms phosphodiester bond between two nucleosides. Then the attached nucleoside will pair with complementary base in the template through hydrogen bonds (A and T through two H-bonds and C and G through three H-bonds).

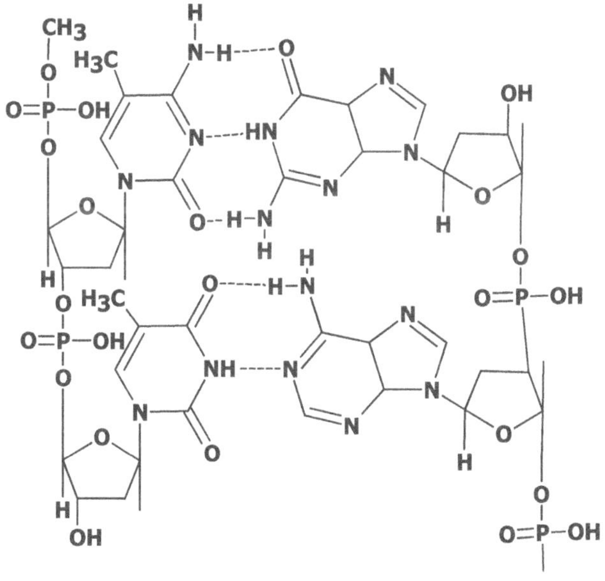

Fig. 17.4 Base pairing of AT and CG through H-bonding.

17.5 Transcription

Transcription is the process by which a molecule of DNA is copied into a complementary strand of RNA, messenger RNA (mRNA). The strand code for RNA molecule is called as template and other one is called as coding strand. The template for one gene may behave as coding strand for other gene and vice versa. mRNA acts as a messenger between DNA and the ribosomes, in which protein synthesis effects. RNA polymerase binds to promoter region, which upstream from coding region. RNA polymerase attaches to DNA at a special sequence that serves as a "start signal". Promoter region contains TATA box (Pribnow Box / Hogness box) and TGTTGACA region (CATT box). The TATA box contains AT rich bases (TATAAT), which is 10 bases upstream and CATT box is 35 bases upstream from transcription start site.

RNA polymerases unwind about 17 base pairs and cleave dsDNA in to ssDNA, one strand serves as a template and other as coding strand. The RNA bases attach to the complementary DNA template, thus synthesize mRNA. The protein ρ (rho) is responsible for the termination of chain elongation. Then RNA polymerase detaches from the DNA and attaches to new molecule.

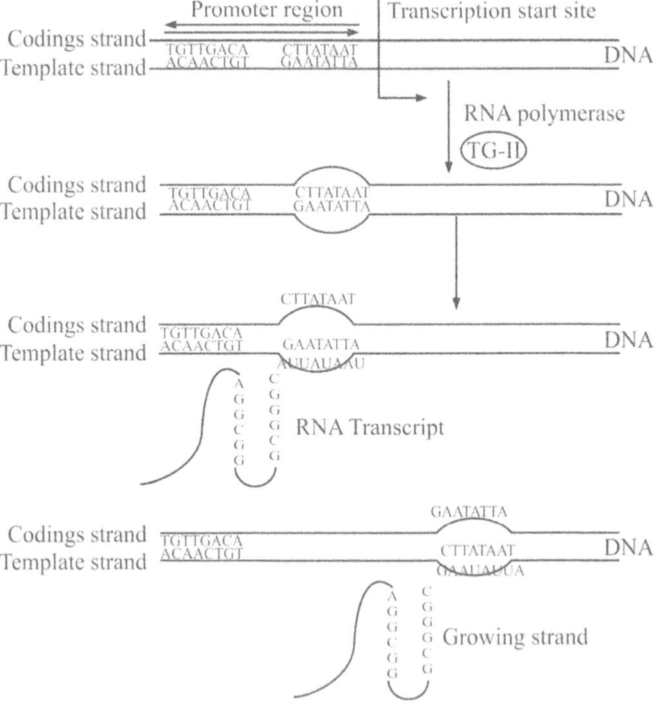

Fig. 17.5 DNA transcription process.

All eukaryotic RNA (mRNA, 5S RNA tRNA) will undergo extensive processing such as capping, nucleolytic and ligation reactions, terminal additions and nucleotide modification in nucleus. Capping ensures RNA stability, includes the removal one of the terminal phosphate group by RNA phosphatase. Guanylyl transferase adds GTP to the remaining phosphate groups and generates 5^I-5^I triphosphate linkage. Methyl transferase further methylates nitrogen of guanine. The cap structure binds to cap binding protein (CBP 20 and CBP 80) and forms complex, which influences the process of splicing.

The mRNA formed contains both amino acid coding portion (exons) and intervening sequences (introns). Splicing is molecular process involves the joining of these exons catalysed by spliceosome. Small nuclear ribonucleoproteins (SnRNPs) and the spliceosome bind to exon-intron borders. It is a transestrification process whereby two exons are joined to give complete coding base containing strand.

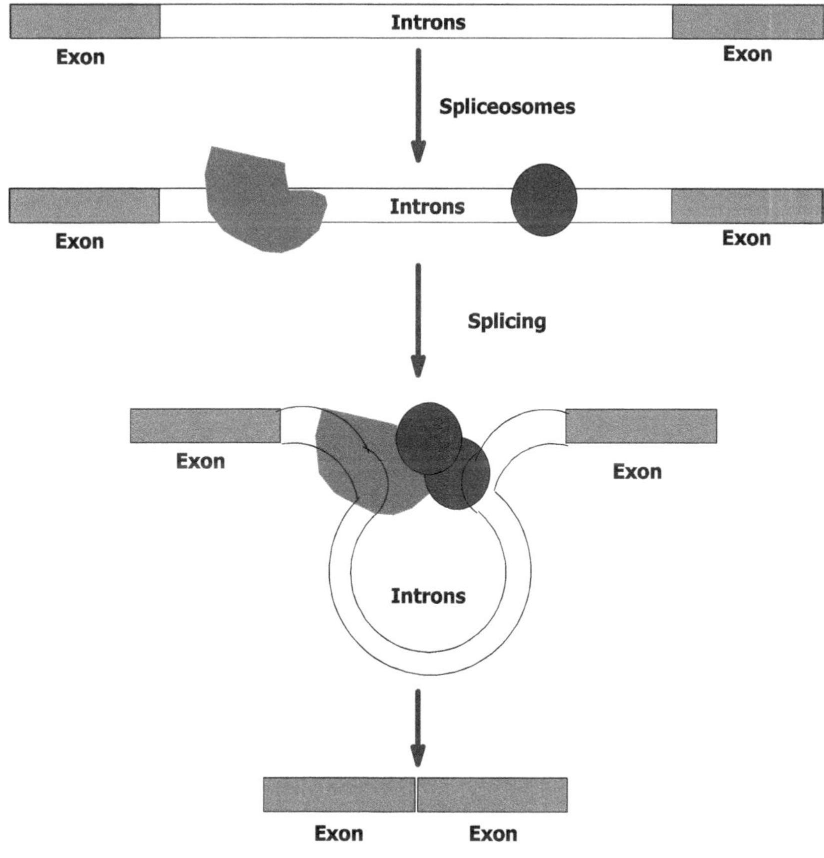

Fig. 17.6 Process of splicing.

17.6 Translation

Translation is the process of decoding mRNA molecule into a polypeptide chain or protein. Each combination of 3 nucleotides on mRNA is called a codon (three-letter code). Each codon specifies a particular amino acid that is to be placed in the polypeptide chain (protein). Four bases in different combination produces 64 codons (4^3, $4 \times 4 \times 4$). Out of which 61 codons specify particular amino acids, there are many codons they specify same amino acids. The codon AUG specifies for amino acid methionine is known as initiator codon, which initiates the protein synthesis mechanism. Three codons UAA, UAG and UGA are called as terminator codons.

The translation mRNA into amino acids require adapter molecule, and tRNA serves for this purpose. Specific tRNA synthetase through ATP dependent mechanism transfers specific amino acid tRNA molecule. The 40S ribosome attaches to mRNA attaches to the mRNA with the aid of 7-methyl guanosine triphosphate (7-CH$_3$ GTP) and initiation factor-I (IF-I). IFs release favors the attachment of 60S ribosome and generates 80S ribosome (complete ribosome). The 80S ribosome contains peptidyl site (site P) and amino acyl site (site A). Anticodon of tRNA (peptidyl tRNA) attaches to the first codon (AUG) in site P and amino acyl tRNA interacts with GTP and Elongation factor-I (EF-I) present in site A. The α-amino group of peptidyl tRNA forms peptide bond with aminoacyl tRNA present in A site. The newly formed tRNA then displaces the existing tRNA from site P and another amino acyl tRNA enters into site A and the chain elongation process continues until it encounters the terminator codons.

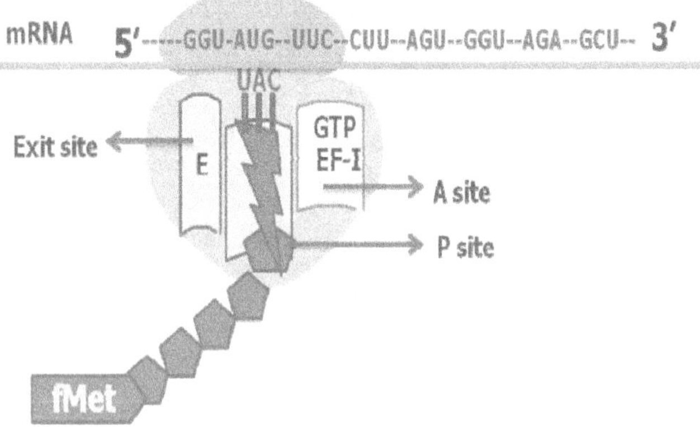

Fig. 17.7 Protein synthesis initiation.

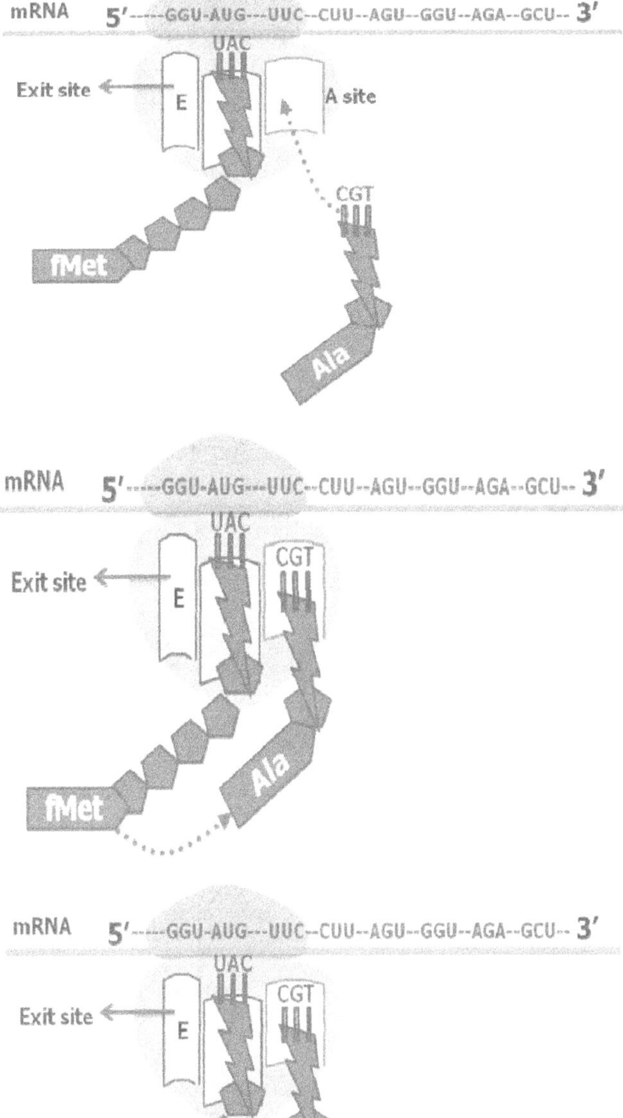

Fig. 17.8 Protein synthesis elongation.

17.7 Recombinant DNA (rDNA) Technology

To understand a complex biological process, a biochemist isolates and studies the individual components *in vitro*. rDNA involves isolation and manipulation of DNA to make chimeric molecules and making identical copies (cloning).

Steps involved in DNA cloning

1. Isolation of chromosomal DNA
2. Cutting DNA at precise locations
3. Selecting small molecule of DNA capable of self replicating – cloning vectors
4. Joining two DNA fragments covalently
5. Moving recombinant from test tube to host cell
6. Selecting / identifying host cell containing recombinant DNA

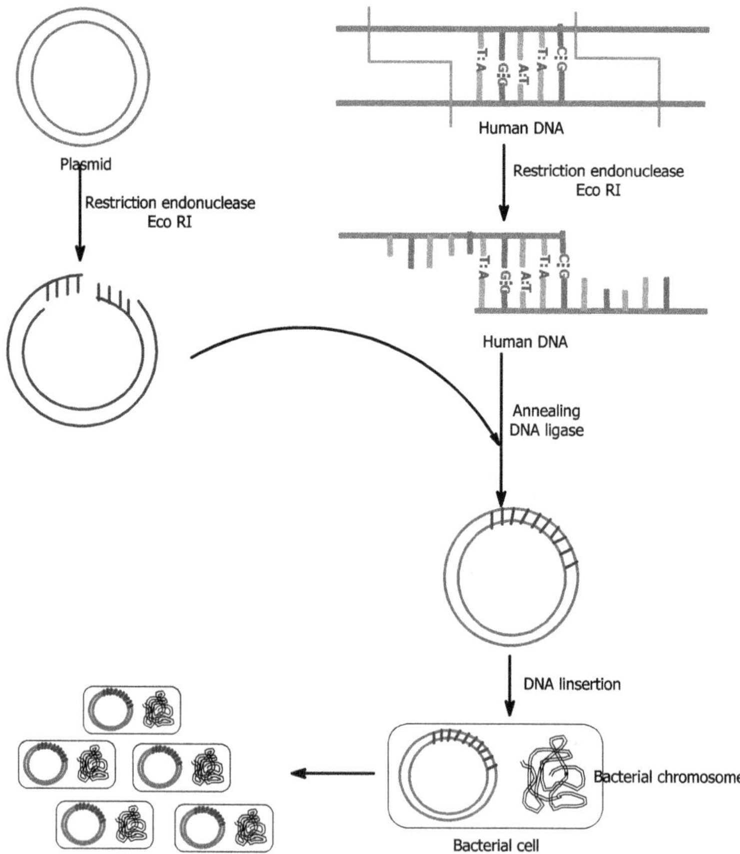

Fig. 17.9 Pathway of DNA cloning.

Components of Cloning

- Restriction endonuclease: It cuts DNA into short pieces in a sequence specific manner, generates a set of smaller fragments and protects host bacterial DNA from foreign organisms.

- Cloning vectors: Cleaved and enriched DNA fragments (by gel electrophoresis) are then joined to cloning vectors, which is digested by the same restriction endonuclease. They allow amplification of inserted DNA segments. The commonly used cloning vectors are

  - Plasmids: Plasmids are small circular DNA (cDNA) molecules that replicate independently of chromosomal DNA.

  - Bacteriophages: It contains linear DNA molecules into which foreign DNA can be inserted and replicated. This permits cloning of DNA fragments up to 23, 000 bp for *in vitro* packaging.

  - Cosmids: Cosmids are extracted from bacteria and mixed with restriction endonucleases. Fragments from 30-46 kb can be accommodated and it combines essential elements of a plasmid and Lambda systems.

  - Bacterial Artificial Chromosomes (BACs): Plasmids designed for cloning very long DNA segments (1,00, 000 – 3,00,000 bp)

  - Yeast Artificial Chromosomes (YACs): YACs are constructed by recombinant DNA (rDNA) techniques from a yeast centromere.

- DNA ligase: DNA ligases joins DNA segments into cloning vectors by catalysing the formation of phosphodiester bonds. Both sticky and blunt ends can be ligated by covalent bonding and this hybrid combination of two molecules is called as recombinant.

- Host cell: Moving recombinant from test tube to host cell for the replication.

- Selecting / identifying host cell containing recombinant DNA.

Chapter 18

HOMOLOGY MODELING

Homology modeling (HM) or comparative modeling attempts to predict protein structures on the strength of a protein sequence similarity to another protein of known structure. Threading and *ab initio* methods also useful in protein structure prediction, but homology modeling is widely accepted. The structure of protein is essential for substrate specificity, stability and interaction with other protein and determines its function. The most accurate structure prediction method is homology modeling; it uses the information from homologous structures to predict the tertiary structure.

HM predicts three-dimensional (3D) structure of the target protein based on sequence alignment. It qualitatively describes the nature of the relationship between two or more proteins (description about common evolutionary origin) and also known as knowledge based modeling. HM is based on the fact that structural conformation of a protein is more highly conserved and small changes in sequence results in variation in the 3D structure. Many proteins (whose 3D structures are not resolved) shares significant sequence similarity to a protein of known 3D structure. If one protein sequence shows significant homology (i.e identical residues or significant similarity) to another protein of known 3D structure, then a fairly accurate model of that protein 3D structure can be obtained via homology modeling.

A set of proteins that are hypothesized to be homologous, then their 3D structure are conserved to greater extent. Identical protein sequences results in identical 3D structures, but the reverse is not true. There is no two sequences have clear sequence similarity and dissimilar 3D structure. Thus it is generally assumed that a common ancestor always implies a common structure. Experimental structures are available for small number of sequenced proteins. 3D structure prediction greatly helps unravelling its function, binding mechanism and aids in virtual screening.

206

Basis of homology modeling is

1. Similar sequences adopt identical structures

2. The 3D structure of protein is depends upon its amino acid sequence

3. Knowledge of protein sequence helps predicting the construction of the protein

As structural genomics continue to deposit representative 3D structures of proteins, homology modeling will play an increasing role in structure based drug design (SBDD).

18.1 Steps Involved in Homology Modeling

1. Identification of known 3D structures of a related protein (template)

    The first step in building model involves identification of one or more proteins of known 3D structures that are similar to the query sequence. Usually in comparative modeling the template is chosen by virtue of having the highest level of sequence similarity with the target protein. Identification of known 3D structures of a related protein can serve as a template.

2. Sequence alignment of target and template proteins

    - It involves the generation of an accurate sequence alignment of the query protein to the template protein.

    - BLAST or FASTA programs help determining the identity between two sequences.

    - Homologous proteins will be used when there is difficulty in aligning two sequences.

    - Multiple sequence alignment program (CLUSTALW) helps in finding conserved regions (homologous sequences). This approach is suited for proteins with low (< 40 %) identities.

3. Model building for the target, based on the 3D structure of the template and the alignment

    - Models build with 50 % sequence identity are accurate enough for drug discovery applications.

    - Pairwise alignment tool implement dynamic programming methods to search for optimum alignment (local / global) between pair of sequences. This approach is useful to search database for homologous sequences.

4. Refinement, validation and evaluation of models

Percentage identity between template and target protein contributes to the errors in the model

- If percentage identity is > 90 %, it gives more accurate model.

- Percentage identity in the range of 50-90 % produces minimum errors.

- Less than 25 % percentage identity leads to significant errors in the model.

Hence verification of the model is an essential step in the homology modeling. The quality of the model is dependent upon the number of residue identies in common between the two proteins, expressed as root mean square deviation (RMSD). It can be done through general check for the normality of bond length, bond and torsion angles of experimentally determined structures. Force field methods are useful in this process. The most important factor in the assessment of constructed models is scoring function. The Ramachandran plot is most powerful determinant of the quality of the model.

Sequence alignment plays an important role in developing homology model. These steps are repeated until satisfactory results are obtained. Multiple sequence alignment align several sequences to identify conserved regions. It predicts functional sites, protein function as well as aid in phylogenetic analysis.

18.2 Software Tools for Homology Modeling

MODELLER and SwissModel are the two important modeling tools available for the prediction of the 3D structure of proteins.

18.3 Applications of Homology Modeling

Homology modeling is widely used in structure based drug design process and it includes the following.

- HM helps in understanding the effects of mutation.
- HM identifies active and binding sites on protein.
- HM helps identifying ligands for a given binding site (data mining).
- HM models substrates specificity and predicts antigenic epitopes.
- Explains the protein-protein docking simulations.

<h1>CHAPTER 19</h1>

SEQUENCE SIMILARITY

Biological sequences that are similar (not identical), provides useful information to help discover functional, structural and evolutionary relationship. A character or string in one sequence is said to be identity, when it is shared between sequences of two species. The degree to which two sequences (species) share identities is indicated by similarity. In general sequence determines shape and shape determines function. Sequence similarity discovers and validates similarity in shape and function of different sequences.

Sequence of the gene of interest is compared to every sequence in a sequence database

- Alignment with best matching sequences are scored and shown
- If more than 50 % of the query sequence is identical with the database proteins, then the prediction is very strong

Some of the related terms used in sequence similarity process are

Homologous: Genes from different organisms having similar sequences because of the common ancestor gene.

Orthologous: Similar sequences in different organisms, which have arisen due to speciation event and it retains their functionality throughout evolution.

Paralogous: Similar sequences in same organism, due to gene duplication with divergent function.

Xenologous: Similar sequences due to horizontal transfer of genetic material through symbioses and virus-induced transduction between unrelated organisms (don't share evolutionary origin).

Analogous: Similar sequences in same organism derived from convergent evolution.

Resemblance of two sequences from different organisms is based on the hypothesis, that all genetic material had one ancestor.

19.1 Sequence Alignment

Searching for a series of individual CHARACTERS or PATTERNS that are present in the same order in the set of sequences is referred to as sequence alignment. An arrangement of two sequences of DNA / RNA / protein helps in to identifying the region of similarity. The degree of similarity determines their functional, structure or evolutionary relationship. Gaps are inserted considering the possibility of mutational change (insertion / deletion in either of two sequences) to maximise the similarity. One which exhibit the most significant similarities and least differences are called as optimal alignment. It allows us to extrapolate quantitative expressions of inter-relatedness and to infer possible structural, functional or evolutionary relationships. An alignment of two residues might be viewed as reflecting a common evolutionary origin.

19.2 Why ALIGN Sequences?

19.2.1 Significance of Alignment

- Common ancestral sequence may have similar secondary and 3D structure, gene regulation and biochemical function.

- Best possible / optimal alignment derives functional information, structural information and evolutionary information

19.2.2 Important Terms in Alignment

- **Identity:** Two proteins that have a certain number of amino-acids in common at aligned positions considered as match.

- **Similarity:** Residues will be replaced by other residues of similar physico-chemical properties, due to mutations (conservative) also considered as match.

- **Homology:** Proteins are evolutionarily related and from a common ancestor.

  Similarity and homology are two complementary terms and must not be confused.

19.3 Methods of Sequence Alignments

There are four methods

1. Brute force: Trivial method

2. Dot Matrix: Useful for simple alignment and does not produce optimal alignment

3. Dynamic programming: Produces optimal alignment and provides global / local alignment

4. Heuristic method: Fast computational method includes BLAST, FASTA

CHAPTER 20

DOT MATRIX

Dot matrix is the most important technique for sequence alignment. Similarity between two sequences can be detected as a diagonal on an identity matrix. Graphic similarity comparisons use the power of the human researchers to discern patterns in the data. Dot plot analysis is a method tries to locate possible alignment of characters between the two sequences after comparing two sequences. Dot plots of sequence similarity are created using a matrix where the rows in the matrix corresponding to the characters in the 1st sequence and the columns in the matrix correspond to the characters in the 2nd sequence. Whenever a match is found a dot is placed on the corresponding position in the matrix.

Dot matrix is used for comparing two sequences of very much alike and to check their possible alignment.

20.1 Procedure

One sequence (sequence A) is listed across the top of the matrix and the other (sequence B) is listed down the left side. Starting from the first character in sequence B, the comparison moves across the page and places a dot / mark in a column, where the character in A and B are same. The second character in sequence B is compared in a similar manner and the process is continued until all the characters are done. Number of identities or similarities based on scoring matrix is useful in calculating score. Region of similar sequence is revealed by a diagonal row of dots / marks. Isolated dots are known as 'random matches' and are not significant. Detection of matching regions may be improved by filtering out random matches in a dot matrix.

Sequence 1 = G A A T T C C G
Sequence 2 = G A A T C G A

(A)

(B)

	G	A	A	T	T	C	C	G
G	X							X
A		X						X
A		X	X					
T				X	X			
C						X	X	
G	X							X
A		X	X					

20.2 Applications

- Dot matrix analysis reveals the presence of insertions / deletions and repeats.
- Useful in finding direct / inverted repeats in protein and DNA sequences.
- Reveals the presence of repeats of the same sequence character many times.
- Helps in predicting region in self complementary RNA.

20.3 Dot Matrix Programs

- DOTTER - for UNIX-X and Windows
- COMPARE and DOT PLOT
- EMBOSS
    - DOTMATCHER - aligns sequences using scoring
    - DOTUP - finds common words in the sequences
    - DOT PLOT - finds common pattern in the sequences
- Though PALIGN is not a Dot Matrix program it can be used

20.4 Experimental Procedure for Dot Matrix Analysis

1. Open the URL page http://myhits.isb-sib.ch/cgi-bin/dotlet for dot matrix program.

2. Take your sequences or download FASTA format of a protein/ nucleotide sequences.

3. Enter the 1st sequence and 2nd sequence by using browser.

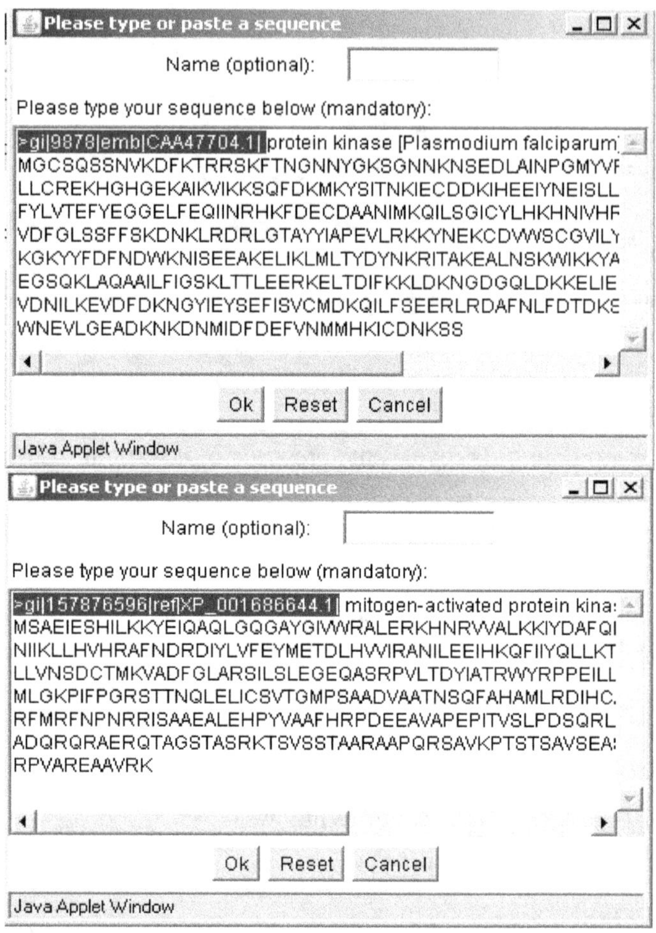

4. Select the parameters.

5. Finally click "compute"

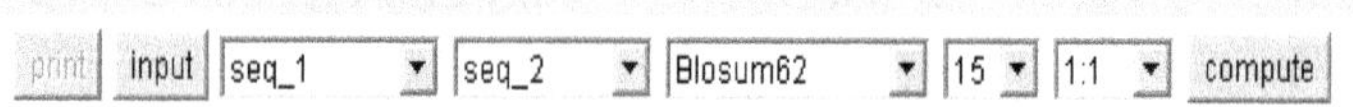

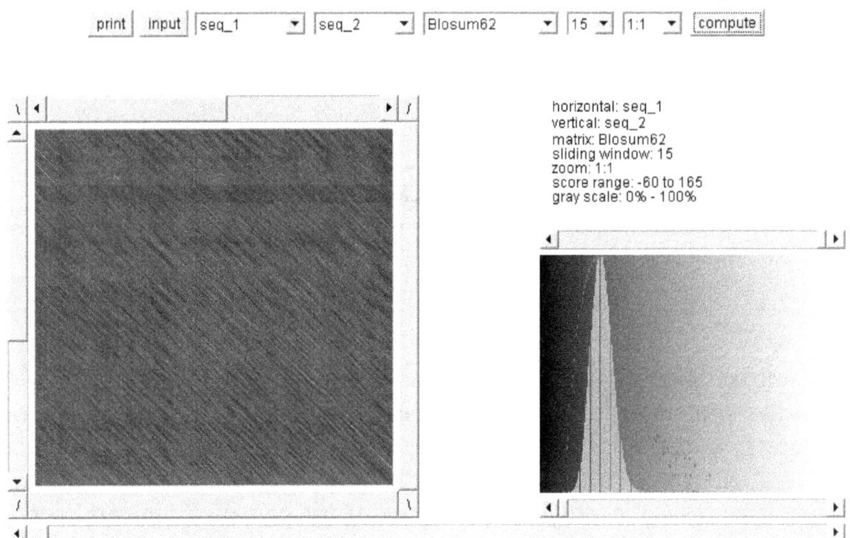

seq_1 8
GIEMBCAAPROTEINKINASEPLASMODITMFALCIPARTMMGCSQSSNVKDF
GIREFXPMITOGENACTIVATEDPROTEINKINASEPROTEINKINASELEIS
seq_2 8

## CHAPTER 21

DYNAMIC PROGRAMMING

Dynamic programming (DP) is a computational method which is used to align two protein or nucleic acid sequences by comparing every piece of characters in the 2 sequences. DP aligns two sequences by beginning at the ends of the two sequences and attempt to align all possible pairs of characters. Dynamic program compares every pair of characters in the two sequences and generates best or optimal alignment. It is highly computational demanding method. The latest algorithmic improvements and ever increasing computer capacity make possible to align a query sequence against a large DB in a few minutes.

The sequences to be aligned are arranged across a row and column of rectangular matrix. The score is calculated for each position of the matrix according to possible events

1. Replacement / conservation of the residue
2. Insertion in sequence A / sequence B

The alignment procedure depends upon scoring system, which can be based on probability that

1. A particular DNA /amino acid pair is found in alignments of related proteins
2. The same DNA / amino acid pair is aligned by chance
3. Introduction of a gap would be a better choice as it increases the score.
4. The ratio of the first two probabilities is usually provided in an amino acid substitution matrix.
5. There are many such matrices, two of them PAM and BLOSUM are considered later.

Uses scoring schemes for matches, mismatches and gaps. The score for the gap introduction and its extension is also calculated from the matrices and represent a prior knowledge and some assumptions.

21.1 Types of Dynamic Programming

- Global alignment program which works on Needleman-Wunsch algorithm
- Local alignment which works on Smith-Waterman algorithm

  Both algorithms are derived from the basic dynamic programming algorithm.

21.2 Steps in Dynamic Programming

- Initialization
- Scoring – Matrix fill
- Trace back – optimal alignment

21.3 Dynamic Programming for Global Alignment

21.3.1 Initialization Step

Let us consider the following two sequences for the alignment

Sequence 1 = G A A T T C C G T T A

Sequence 2 = G G A T C G A

1. Create a matrix with X +1 Rows and Y +1 Columns
2. Arrange one of the sequence (Seq 1) across the column and second one (Seq 2) across the rows
3. The 1st row and the 1st column of the score matrix are filled as multiple of gap penalty

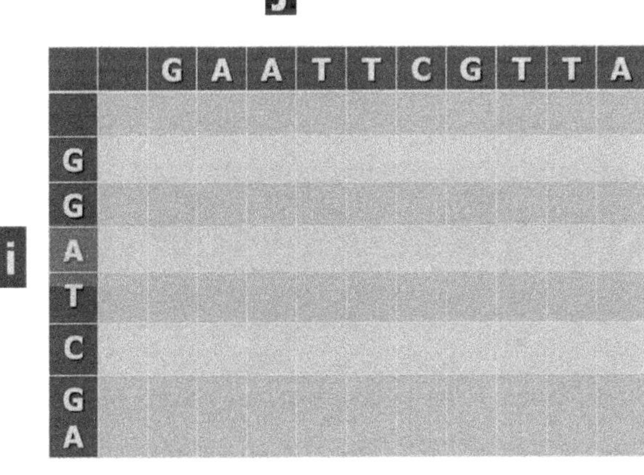

j

		G	A	A	T	T	C	G	T	T	A
	0	-4	-8	-12	-16	-20	-24	-28	-32	-36	-40
G	-4										
G	-8										
A	-12										
T	-16										
C	-20										
G	-24										
A	-28										

(The left-margin label **i** runs down the row labels.)

21.3.2 Scoring -Matrix Fill Step

The formula given below is used in the calculation of scores for each matrix depending upon the nature whether it is a match, mismatch or gap.

$$S_{i,j} = \text{Max } \{\text{Score diagonal, Score left, Score up}\}$$

$$= \text{Max } \{S_{i-1,j-1} + S(a_i,b_j),\ S_{i,j-1} + W,\ S_{i-1,j} + W\}$$

$S_{i,j}$ = Similarity score achieved at (i, j);

$S(a_i,b_j)$ = Match / mismatch

$S_{i,j-1}$ = Go left; $S_{i-1,j}$ = Go above;   W = gap

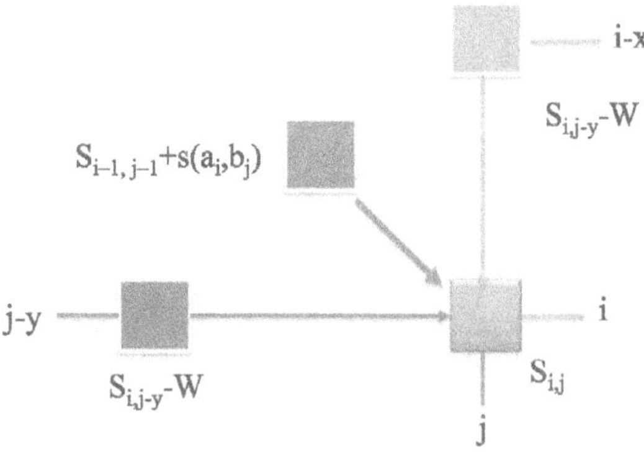

Fig. 21.1 Formal description of dynamic programming algorithm.

The score values for each category is assigned as follows

Match   =   5;   Mismatch = - 3;   Gap = - 4

Score diagonal (SD) $=$ $S_{i-1,\,j-1} + s(a_i, b_j)$,

Score left (SL) $=$ $S_{i,\,j-1}$ $+ W$

Score up (SU) $=$ $S_{i-1,\,j}$ $+ W$

   $S_{i,\,j}$ = **Max {Score diagonal, Score left, Score up}**

For matrix $S_{1,1}$

Score diagonal (SD)	Score left (SL)	Score up (SU)
$= S_{i-1,\,j-1} + s(a_i, b_j)$,	$= S_{i,\,j-1} + W$	$= S_{i-1,\,j} + W$
$= S_{1-1,\,1-1} + 5$	$= S_{1,\,1-1} + (-4)$	$= S_{1-1,\,1} + (-4)$
$= S_{0,0} + 5$	$= S_{1,0} + (-4)$	$= (-4) + (-4) =$ **-8**
$= 0 + 5 =$ **5**	$= (-4) + (-4) =$ **- 8**	$= (-4) + (-4) =$ **- 8**

   $S_{i,j} = S_{1,1}=$ Max { Score diagonal, Score left, Score up} $=$ **5**

For matrix $S_{1,2}$

Score diagonal (SD)	Score left (SL)	Score up (SU)
$= S_{i-1,\,j-1} + s(a_i, b_j)$,	$= S_{i,\,j-1} + W$	$= S_{i-1,\,j} + W$
$= S_{1-1,\,2-1} + (-3)$	$= S_{1,\,2-1} + (-4)$	$= S_{1-1,\,2} + (-4)$
$= S_{0,1} + (-3)$	$= S_{1,1} + (-4)$	$= (-8) + (-4) =$ **-12**
$= 0 + (-4) =$ **5**	$= 5 + (-4) =$ **1**	$= (-4) + (-4) =$ **- 8**

   $S_{i,j} = S_{1,1}=$ Max {Score diagonal, Score left, Score up} $=$ **1**

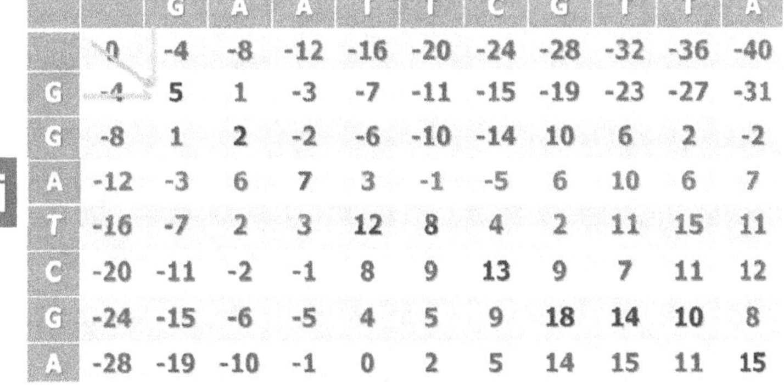

		G	**A**	**A**	**T**	**T**	**C**	**G**	**T**	**T**	**A**
		0	-4	-8	-12	-16	-20	-24	-28	-32	-36	-40
G		-4	5	1	-3	-7	-11	-15	-19	-23	-27	-31
G		-8	1	2	-2	-6	-10	-14	10	6	2	-2
A		-12	-3	6	7	3	-1	-5	6	10	6	7
T		-16	-7	2	3	12	8	4	2	11	15	11
C		-20	-11	-2	-1	8	9	13	9	7	11	12
G		-24	-15	-6	-5	4	5	9	18	14	10	8
A		-28	-19	-10	-1	0	2	5	14	15	11	15

(row index i; column index j)

21.3.3 Trace Back Step

- There are likely to be multiple maximal alignments. The trace back step determines the actual alignment(s) that result in the maximum score. Trace back starts from the last cell, i.e. position X, Y in the matrix, gives alignment in reverse order.

- There are three possible moves: diagonally (toward the top-left corner of the matrix), up, or left.

- Trace back takes the current cell and looks to the neighbor cells that could be direct predecessors.

- The algorithm for trace back chooses as the next cell in the sequence one of the possible predecessors.

		G	A	A	T	T	C	G	T	T	A
		0	-4	-8	-12	-16	-20	-24	-28	-32	-36	-40
G	-4	5	1	-3	-7	-11	-15	-19	-23	-27	-31
G	-8	1	2	-2	-6	-10	-14	10	6	2	-2
A	-12	-3	6	7	3	-1	-5	6	10	6	7
T	-16	-7	2	3	12	8	4	2	11	15	11
C	-20	-11	-2	-1	8	9	13	9	7	11	12
G	-24	-15	-6	-5	4	5	9	18	14	10	8
A	-28	-19	-10	-1	0	2	5	14	15	11	15

21.4 Dynamic Programming for Local Alignment

- Smith-Waterman algorithm performs a   local alignment on two sequences

    - Useful for dissimilar sequences that are suspected to contain regions of similarity or

      Similar sequence motifs within their larger sequence context

- The best alignment over the conserved domain of two sequences

21.5 Comparison with DOT MATRIX

Alignment generated by dynamic program can be compared to the dot matrix alignment

- To know whether the longest regions are being matched or not

- It reveals that whether insertion and deletion are located in the reasonable places or not.

## CHAPTER 22

HEURISTIC METHOD

Heuristic method is also known as "tried and true method". The name 'word' or 'k-tuple' method is given because it searches for identical short stretches of sequences (word / 'k-tuple). Identified k-tuples will be joined into alignment by using dynamic program. Heuristic methods are faster (~50 times) than dynamic programming and finds related sequences from database. It includes

BLAST   -   Basic Local Alignment and Search Tool

FASTA   -   FAST Approximation

SSEARCH -   Sequence SEARCH

BLAST is popular among all due to their availability through www.

22.1 Steps

1. Finds list of words / k-tuples

   (short string of (row) of sequence letters, usually 3 for proteins and 5-15 for nucleic acid)

2. Compares 'k-tuples' (word list) to the database sequences

3. Finds list of high scoring segment pairs (HSP)

   (HSP is a high scoring word that is found in a query and in a database sequence)

4. Chooses maximal segment pair (MSP)

5. Joins these words / k-tuples into an alignment by the DP method (Align 2 sequences)

ANPCCSNPCQNRGECMSTGFDQYKCDCTRTGFYGENCTTPEFLTRIKLLKPTPNTVHYILTHF

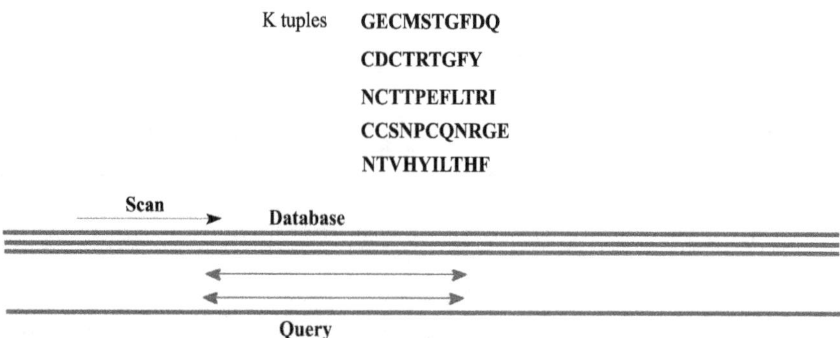

22.2 Basic Local Alignment and Search Tool (BLAST)

Basic Local Alignment and Search Tool (BLAST) is used for alignment of protein/nucleotide sequences and helps

1. To detect related proteins

2. To study the relationship between the sequences

22.2.1 Varients of BLAST

BLASTP: Compares query protein sequence against a database protein sequences

BLASTN: Compares query nucleotide sequence against a database nucleotide sequences

BLASTX: Compares a nucleotide query sequence translated in all reading frames against a protein sequence database.

TBLASTN: Compares a protein query sequence against a nucleotide sequence database dynamically translated in all reading frames

TBLASTX: Compares translated nucleotide query sequence against the translated nucleotide sequence database. The tblastx program cannot be used with the nr database on the BLAST Web page because it is computationally intensive

Megablast

- Megablast is useful for nucleotide only and it is optimized to align very similar sequences.

- Used to compare 2 large sets of sequences, 10 times faster than other variants.

- Mega BLAST uses linear gap penalty.

Contiguous megablast: It is suitable for nearly identical sequences.

Discontiguous megablast: Cross-species comparison can be effected by using discontinuous megabalst.

PSI-BLAST (Position Specific Iterated BLAST)

- Instead of using single amino acid at a given position in the query sequence it is better to use a combination of amino acids known to be present at the same position in that protein and related ones

- The search of sequence database will be there by expanded to include additional related sequences that might otherwise missed

Method for finding related sequences in a database

- Distant homology detection
- Domain identification
- Evolutionary analysis
- Sequence clustering
- Target selection

PHI-BLAST --Pattern Hit Initiated BLAST

- Combining matching of regular expression pattern with a position specific protein search

- PHI locates other protein sequences containing the regular expression pattern and homologous to query protein sequences

22.3 Experimental Procedure for BLAST Runs

Basic Local Alignment and Search Tool (BLAST) is used for sequence similarity searching of both proteins and nucleotides. Alignment of protein / nucleotide sequences helps

1. To detect related proteins
2. To study the relationship between the sequences

22.3.1 Selecting the BLAST Program

The BLAST search page allows us to select BLAST program (from several different programs).

1. Open the Basic BLAST search database page from National Centre for Biotechnolgy Information (NCBI).

2. From the "Program" Pull down menu select the appropriate program.

nucleotide blast	Search a **nucleotide** database using a **nucleotide** query *Algorithms:* blastn, megablast, discontiguous megablast
protein blast	Search **protein** database using a **protein** query *Algorithms:* blastp, psi-blast, phi-blast
blastx	Search **protein** database using a **translated nucleotide** query
tblastn	Search **translated nucleotide** database using a **protein** query
tblastx	Search **translated nucleotide** database using a **translated nucleotide** query

22.3.2 Entering Sequence

The BLAST accepts input sequences in three formats;

- FASTA sequence format
- NCBI accession number
- Gene identity number (GI)

FASTA format: Fasta format is a standard input format for the sequence alignment. It contains one-line header followed by line of sequence data. Nucleotide / protein sequences in FASTA formatted files are processed by a line starting with a symbol " > ". First word on this line is the name of the sequence, rest of the line is a description of the sequence and remaining lines contains the sequence itself.

Accession or GI number: Accession number or the Gene idendity number of a sequence in GenBank, can be used instead of using FASTA format. It is a unique identity for particular sequence that is string of letters. The accession number consists of two letters followed by the six digits.

Eg:NP_628159   GI:21222380 phosphodiesterase [Streptomyces coeli-color A3(2)]

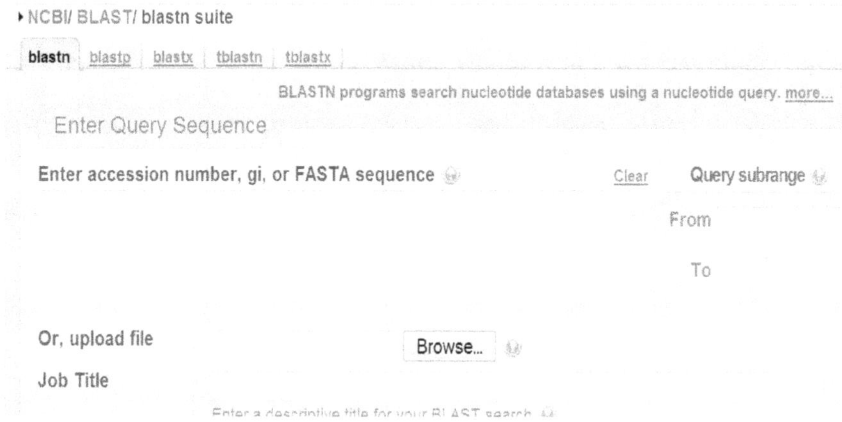

22.3.3   Selecting the BLAST Database

Database	Description
nr	Non-redundant GenBank CDS translations+PDB+SwissProt+PIR+PRF
swissprot	Last major release of the SWISS-PROT protein sequence database (no updates).
patents	Protein sequences derived from the Patent division of GenBank.
pdb	Sequences derived from the 3-D structure Brookhaven Protein Data Bank.
alu	Translations of select Alu repeats from REPBASE, suitable for masking Alu repeats.

Several NCBI databases are available to compare query sequences. Some databases are specific to proteins or nucleotides and cannot be used in combination with certain BLAST programs. (for example a blastn search against Human genome plus transcript (G+T), NCBI genomes and PDB etc., BLAST P search against PDB [Protein data bank], Swissprot protein databases.)

Proteins databases

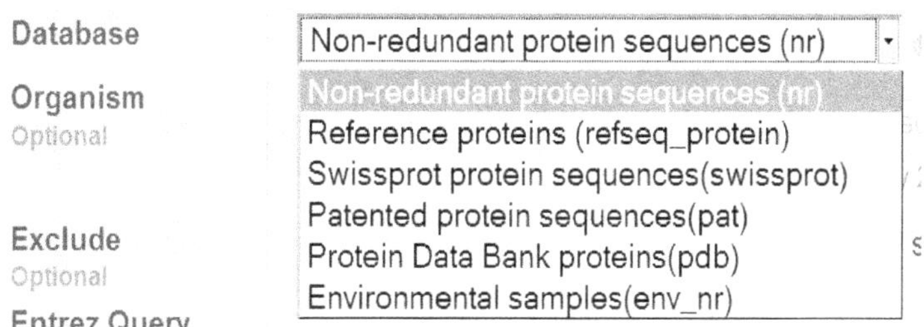

Nucleotide databases

Database	Description
nr	All non-redundant GenBank+EMBL+DDBJ+PDB sequences. (but no EST, STS, GSS, or HTGS sequences)
dbst	Non-redundant database of GenBank+EMBL+DDBJ EST Divisions.
dbsts	Non-redundant database of GenBank+EMBL+DDBJ STS Divisions.
est_others	The non-redundant database of GenBank+EMBL+DDBJ EST Divisions all organisms except mouse and human.
pdb	Sequences derived from the 3-dimensional structure of proteins.
htgs	High Throughput Genomic Sequences.

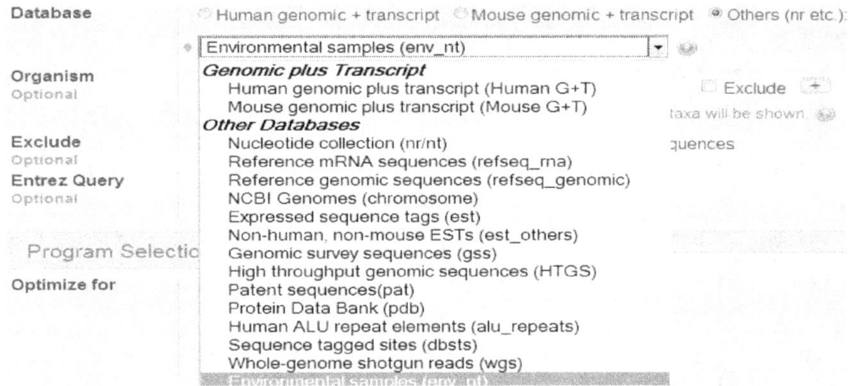

Organism: The organism of our interest can be specified in a given coloumn.

Entrz query: BLAST results can be limited to the results of query against the database. Eg: Glucokinase NOT HSP-1. This will limit a BLAST search to all glucokinase except in HSP-1

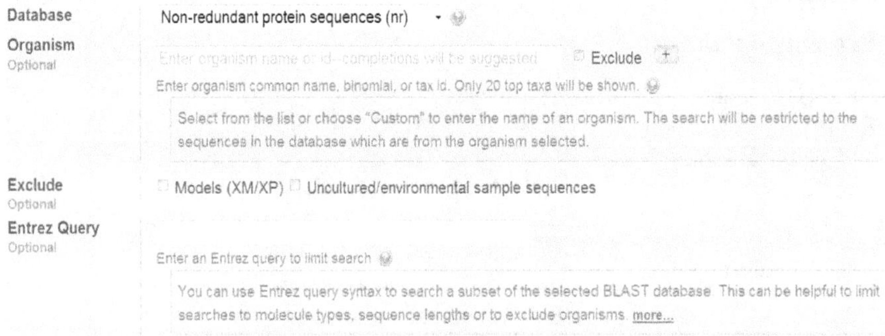

22.3.4 Algorithm Selection

There are different types of algorithms available for different types of BLAST program

Algorithm for proteins

- Blastp (protein-protein BLAST)
- PSI-BLAST (Position-Specific Iterated BLAST)
- PHI-BLAST (Pattern Hit Initiated BLAST)

Algorithm for nucleotides

- Highly similar sequences (megablast)
- More dissimilar sequences (discontinuous megablast)
- Somewhat similar sequences (blastn)

22.3.5 Algorithm Parameters Selection

General parameters (for both proteins and nucleotides):

- Max target sequences: Select the minimum number of aligned sequences to display
- Short queries
- Expect threshold
- Word size

Scoring parameters for proteins:

- Matrix
- Gapcosts
- Compositional adjustments

Scoring parameters for nucelotides:

- Match / mismatch scores
- Gapcosts

Filters and masking

- Filter : Low complexity regions
- Mask : Mask for lookup table only

Mask lower case letters

22.3.6 Run BLAST

- Click on BLAST option to run the search

22.4 Interpretation

Blast version number, sequence database and query sequence can be identified.

1. References for that particular sequence can be viewed in result page.

2. Below this graphical representation will be displayed

Color key for alignment scores

| <40 | 40-50 | 50-80 | 80-200 | >=200 |

Query

| | | | | | | |
0   20   40   60   80   100   120

- Query sequence on the top
- Each bar appears below that represents the portion of another sequence similar to query sequence

   Red bar – most similar sequence

   Pink bar – similarity is there

   Green bar – not impressive at all

   Black / blue bar – bad score.

3. The score of database sequences in bits score and expectation value (E value) of alignment can be viewed.

   Bits score: The value 'S' derived from the raw score in which the statistical properties of the scoring system used have been taken into account.

   Expectation value (E value): The number of different alignment with scores equivalent to or better than 'S' that are expected to occur in a database search by chance.

   Lower the E value, higher the significance in similarity.

   An assessment of their statistical significance, based upon the extreme value distribution, called E values. The E value is dependent on:
   - Length of the query sequence
   - Size of the database
   - Raw score

4. Gapped alignment between query and subject sequence are shown

5. **Bits = (λ × raw score – ln k) / Ln 2**

6. % identity, % positive and % alignment also seen.

7. As a general rule 25 % identity over a stretch of 100 residues can be considered to be good evidence of common ancestry for two sequences.

22.5 Fast Approximation (FASTA)

FASTA is a powerful tool for scanning databases to find sequences that are similar to a query sequence. FASTA is a useful program for rapid alignment of pairs of protein and DNA sequences. Generally best to make protein-protein comparisons but can also compare DNA sequence to DNA databanks. FASTA starts by making generalization from the idea of dot plots. FASTA algorithm divides the query sequence into overlapping words usually of length two for protein or six for nucleic acid. In a dotplot regions of similarity between 2 sequences show up as diagonals. FASTA essentially calculates sum of the dots along each diagonal, and FASTA uses a word based method. It looks for matching sequence pattern or words called "k-tuples". Based in these word matches it builds local alignment.

- Instead of comparing individual residues in the 2 sequences FASTA searches for matching sequence "patterns" and "words" called "k-tuples"

- For DNA search, FASTA is theoritically better able than BLAST to find matches

22.5.1 Steps

- Identifies regions shared by 2 sequences, that have the highest density of single residue identities (k-tup=1) or 2 consecutive identies (k-tup=2).

- Rescans the best regions identified by using PAM-250 matrix.

- Determines if gaps can be used to join the regions identified in step-2, and similarity score for the gapped alignment.

- Constructs an optimal alignment of the query sequence and the library sequence and FASTA uses hash coding method.

- A look up table shows the positions of each sequence word of length of k , constructed for each sequence.

- The relative position of each word in the two sequences is then calculated by subtracting the position in the first sequence from that in the second.

- The k-tuple length is defined and usually 1 or 2 for protein sequences and 5 to 20 for nucleotides.

Position	1 2 3 4 5 6 7 8 9 10 11
Protein 1	n c s p t a
Protein 2	

Amino acid	Position		Off set
	Protein 1	Protein 2	Pos A – Pos B
a	6	6	0
c	2	7	-5
k		11	
n	1		
p	4	9	-5
r		10	
s	3	8	-5
t	5		

22.5.2 FASTA Variants

FASTA	Compares protein sequence to another protein sequence / protein sequence library
TFASTA	Compares protein sequence to DNA sequence
LFASTA	Identifies one or more regions of similarity between 2 sequences
PLFASTA	Present dot matrix plot of regions of sequence similarity between 2 sequences
FASTX and FASTY	Translate a probe DNA sequence and compares to a protein sequence database
TFASTX and TFASTY	Compares a protein sequence to a DNA sequence database

FASTX and TFASTX allows only frame shift between codons

FASTY and TFASTY allows substitutions and frame shift within codon

FASTA 3: FASTA has gone through a series of updates and enhancement leading to version 3, denoted FASTA 3. FASTA 3 has improved methods of aligning sequences and of calculating the statistical significance of alignment and can detect distantly related sequences.

FASTX 3 and FASTY 3 compares DNA sequences to protein sequence database. FASTX 3 is simpler, faster and allows frame shift only between codons. FASTY 3 is slower, but produces better alignment with poor quality sequences because frame shifts are allowed within codons.

22.6 Experimental Procedure for FASTA Run

FASTA similarity search can be run using EBI supported FASTA / SSEARCH / GGSEARCH / GLSEARCH programs.

- FASTA: Provides heuristic search with protein query
- FASTX / FASTY: Translates DNA query and runs FASTA
- SSEARCH: Performs optimal alignment with local alignment program
- GGSEARCH: Performs optimal alignment with global alignment program
- GLSEARCH: Performs optimal alignment for global query with local alignment program

22.6.1 Steps Involved in Similarity Search using FASTA

1. Open www.ebi.ac.uk/Tools/sss/fasta

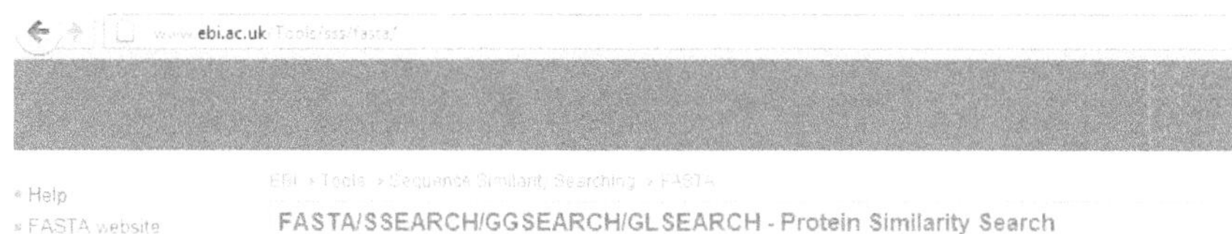

2. Select the appropriate protein database

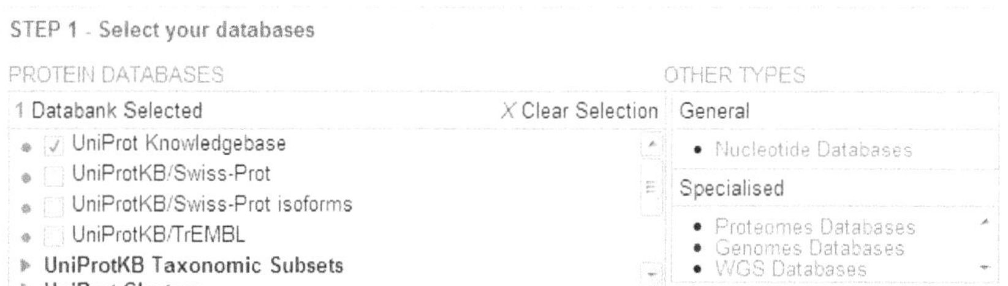

3. Select the type of sequence (protein / DNA / RNA) and enter sequence of suitable format in the clip board

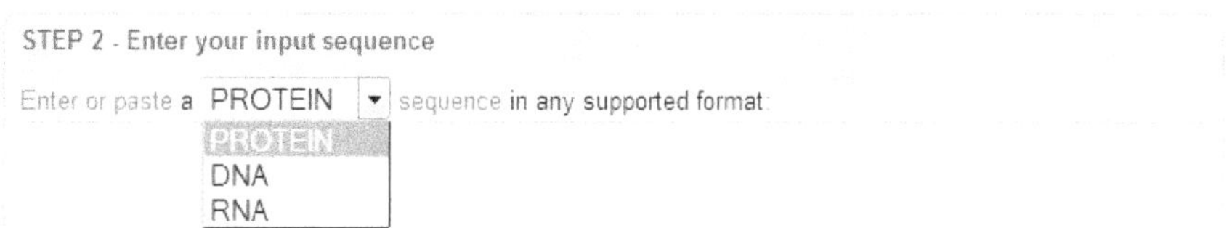

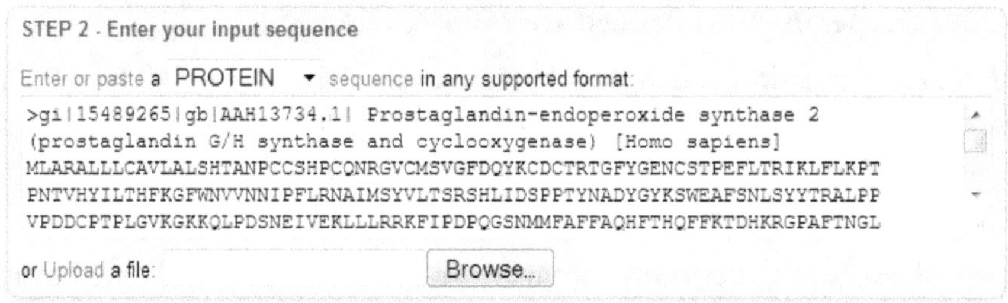

4. Set the parameters

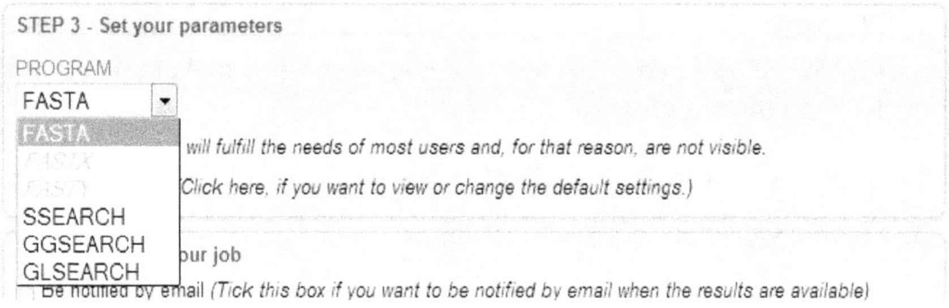

5. Press submit button to run FASTA

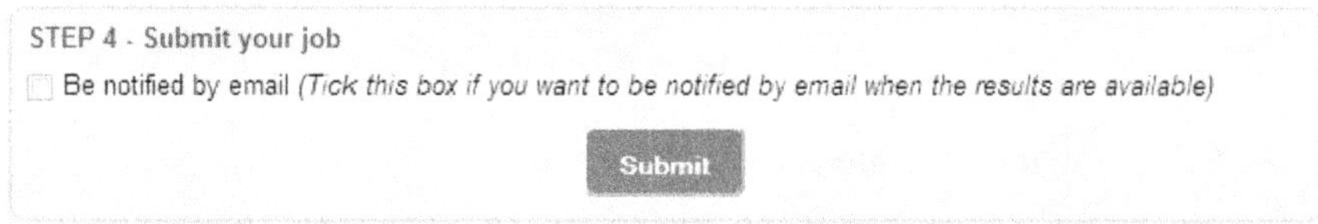

6. Analyse the results

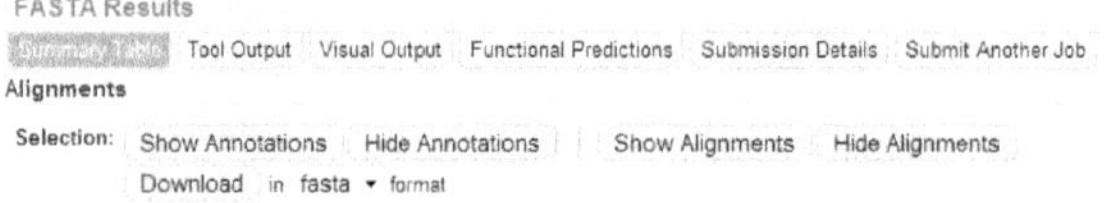

FASTA Results

Summary Table | Tool Output | Visual Output | Functional Predictions | Submission Details | Submit Another Job

Alignments

Selection: Show Annotations   Hide Annotations   Show Alignments   Hide Alignments
Download in fasta ▼ format

Clear Selection   Select All   Invert Selection

Algn	DBID	Source	Length	Score	Identities	Positives	E()
☑ 1	SP:PGH2_HUMAN	Prostaglandin G/H synthase 2 OS=Homo sapiens GN=PTGS2 PE=1 SV=2 *Cross-references and related information in:* ► Gene Expression ► Nucleotide Sequences ► Genomes ► Ontologies ► Enzymes ► Protein Families ► Literature ► Reactions, Pathways & Diseases ► Macromolecular Structures ► Protein Sequences	604	4137	100.0	100.0	0.0
☑ 2	TR:F7BVZ9_MACMU	Uncharacterized protein OS=Macaca mulatta GN=PTGS2 PE=4 SV=1 *Cross-references and related information in:* ► Genomes ► Protein Families ► Literature ► Ontologies	604	4068	98.2	98.7	0.0
☑ 3	TR:F7HZJ7_CALJA	Uncharacterized protein OS=Callithrix jacchus GN=PTGS2 PE=4 SV=1 *Cross-references and related information in:* ► Nucleotide Sequences ► Genomes ► Protein Families ► Ontologies	606	3981	95.7	98.8	0.0
☑ 4	SP:PGH2_RABIT	Prostaglandin G/H synthase 2 OS=Oryctolagus cuniculus GN=PTGS2 PE=2 SV=1 *Cross-references and related information in:* ► Nucleotide Sequences ► Genomes ► Ontologies ► Enzymes ► Protein Families ► Literature	604	3808	88.9	97.8	0.0
☑ 5	TR:Q8SPQ9_CANFA	Cyclooxygenase 2 OS=Canis familiaris GN=Cfa 3449 PE=2 SV=1 *Cross-references and related information in:* ► Nucleotide Sequences ► Genomes ► Ontologies ► Protein Families ► Literature	604	3798	90.1	97.7	0.0
☑ 6	TR:A8QIU4_FELCA	Cyclooxygenase 2 OS=Felis catus PE=2 SV=1 *Cross-references and related information in:* ► Nucleotide Sequences ► Ontologies ► Protein Families ► Literature	604	3793	90.1	97.4	0.0
☑ 7	TR:Q8SPR3_PIG	Prostaglandin G/H synthase-2 OS=Sus scrofa GN=PGHS-2 PE=2 SV=1	604	3786	89.5	97.4	0.0

FASTA Results

Summary Table   Tool Output   Visual Output   Functional Predictions   Submission Details   Submit Another Job

Alignments

Selection: Show Annotations   Hide Annotations   Show Alignments   Hide Alignments

Download   in fasta ▾ format

Clear Selection   Select All   Invert Selection

Align.	DB:ID		Source
☑ 1	SP:PGH2_HUMAN		Prostaglandin G/H synthase 2 OS=Homo sapiens GN=PTGS2 PE=1 SV=2

Cross-references and related information In:
▶ Gene Expression ▶ Nucleotide Sequences ▶ Genomes ▶ Ontologies ▶ Enzymes
▶ Protein Families ▶ Literature ▶ Reactions, Pathways & Diseases
▶ Macromolecular Structures ▶ Protein Sequences

```
>>SP:PGH2_HUMAN P35354 Prostaglandin G/H synthase 2 OS=Homo
sapiens GN=PTGS2 PE=1 SV=2 (604 aa)
 initn: 4137 init1: 4137 opt: 4137  Z-score: 4965.1  bits: 928.8 E(17449634):    0
Smith-Waterman score: 4137; 100.0% identity (100.0% similar) in 604 aa overlap (1-604:1-604

                10        20        30        40        50        60
gi|154  MLARALLLCAVLALSHTANPCCSHPCQNRGVCMSVGFDQYKCDCTRTGFYGENCSTPEFL
        ::::::::::::::::::::::::::::::::::::::::::::::::::::::::::::::
SP:PGH  MLARALLLCAVLALSHTANPCCSHPCQNRGVCMSVGFDQYKCDCTRTGFYGENCSTPEFL
                10        20        30        40        50        60

                70        80        90       100       110       120
gi|154  TRIKLFLKPTPNTVHYILTHFKGFWNVVNNIPFLRNAIMSYVLTSRSHLIDSPPTYNADY
        ::::::::::::::::::::::::::::::::::::::::::::::::::::::::::::::
SP:PGH  TRIKLFLKPTPNTVHYILTHFKGFWNVVNNIPFLRNAIMSYVLTSRSHLIDSPPTYNADY
                70        80        90       100       110       120

               130       140       150       160       170       180
gi|154  GYKSWEAFSNLSYYTRALPPVEDDCPTPLGVKGKKQLPDSNEIVEKLLLRRKFIPDPQGS
        ::::::::::::::::::::::::::::::::::::::::::::::::::::::::::::::
SP:PGH  GYKSWEAFSNLSYYTRALPPVEDDCPTPLGVKGKKQLPDSNEIVEKLLLRRKFIPDPQGS
         ...       ...       ...       ...       ...       ...
```

FASTA Results

Summary Table   Tool Output   Visual Output   Functional Predictions   Submission Details   Submit Another Job

Fast Family and Domain Prediction

Download in SVG format   Switch to Subject Sequence View

FASTA (version: 36.3.5a Jun, 2011(preload8))
Database: uniprotkb
Sequence: gi|15489265|gb|AAH17734.1| Prostaglandin-endoperoxide synthase 2 (prostaglandin G/H synthase and cyclooxygenase) [Hom
Length: 604

Launched Mon, Oct 17, 2011 at 11:24:11
Finished Mon, Oct 17, 2011 at 11:27:36

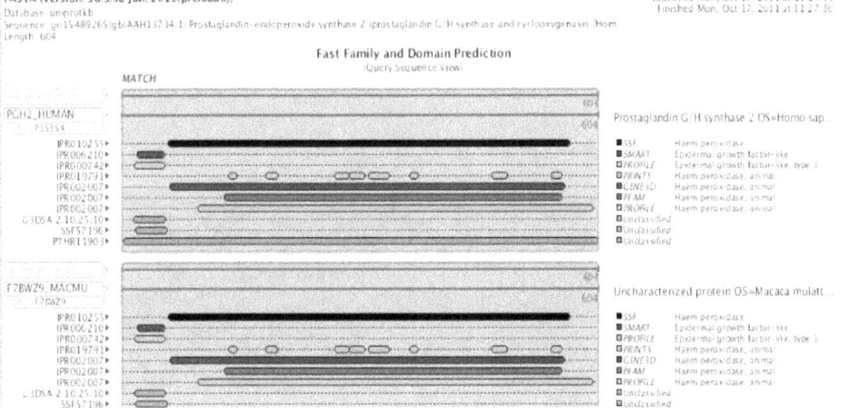

22.7 Differences between FASTA and BLAST

FASTA	BLAST
For DNA searches FASTA is theoretically better able than BLAST	BLAST is faster than FASTA
Searches for all matching words	Searches for most unusual or high scoring words
FASTA 3 calculates statistical parameters from unrelated sequences	Calculates the parameters for the scoring matrix and gap penalty combination
Low complexity region gives high scoring matches	Facility to remove low complexity regions

CHAPTER 23

SEQUENCE COMPARISON METHODS

Sequence comparison methods are of two broad categories

1. Pairwise method- two sequences are compared.
2. Multiple sequence alignment method- models or profiles are built and compared either with other sequences or profiles.

These can be classified further as

1. Global alignment
2. Local alignment

23.1 Global Alignment

- Global alignment method compares two sequences over their entire lengths.
- Global alignment method maximizes region of similarity and minimizes gaps.
- Global alignment method uses Needleman-wunsch dynamic program algorithm.

```
L G P S S K Q T G K G S - S R I S D N
|       |     | | |       |       |
L N - I T K S A G K G A I T R  L I D A
```

In the above example entire length of sequence is considered for sequence alignment.

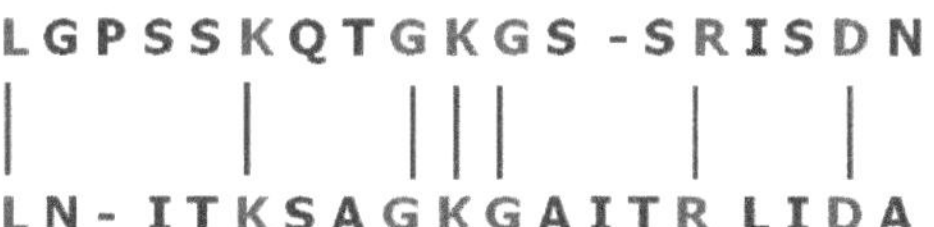

When there is no gap inserted, the amount of similarity is observed less. But when gap is introduced in the sequence A, sequence similarity is found to be maximum.

```
1  AGGATTGGAATGCT.CAGAAGCAGCTAAAGCGTGTATGCAGGAT?GGAATTAAAGAGGAGGTAGACCG      67
   |||||||||||||| |||||||||||||||||||||||||||||||:||| ||||||||||||||||:||
1  AGGATTGGAATGCTACAGAAGCAGCTAAAGCGTGTATGCAGGAT?GGAATTAAAGAGGAGGTAGACCG      68
```

Databases

http://www.igh.cnrs.fr/bin/align-guess.cgi

http://www.gcg.com

http://bioweb.pasteur.tr/docs/EMBOSS/needle/html

23.2 Local Alignment

- Local alignment compares two sequences over particular length.
- Local alignment uses Smith-waterman dynamic program algorithm.

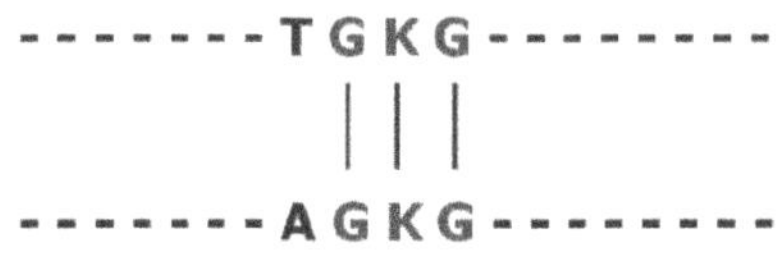


```
1  AGGATTGGAATGCTCAGAAGCAGCTAAAGCGTGTATGCAGGATTGGAATTAAAGAGGAGGTAGACCG...   67
   ||||||||||||||   |       |       |   |||  ||    |  |      |  ||
1  AGGATTGGAATGCTAGGCTTGATTGCCTACCTGTAGCCACATCAGAAGCACTAAAGCGTCAGCGAGACCG   70
```

Databases

http://www.ncbi.nlm.nih.gov

http://www.ncbi.nlm.nih.gov/IEB/Research/Aconibly

http://www.ebi.ac.uk/emboss/align

http://us.expasy.org/

http://genome.cs.mtu.edu/align/align.htm

23.3 Interpretation

- Mismatches can be interpreted as point mutations.
- Gaps are considered as indel (insertion / deletion of residue in either of two sequences) type of mutation.
- The presence or absence of conservative substitutions suggest that those characters has structural or functional importance.

23.4 Pairwise Alignment

Pairwise alignment is used to identify regions of similarity that may indicate functional, structural and evolutionary relationship between two biological sequences (protein/ DNA).

23.5 Experimental Procedure for Pairwise Alignment Program (NCBI Blast)

23.5.1 Aim

1. To become familiar with protein and nucleotide sequence alignment using NCBI BLAST.

2. To acquire knowledge of using various flavours of BLAST (PSI-BLAST, MegaBlast etc.,)

23.5.2 Steps

1. Open the URL page http://www.ncbi.nlm.nih.gov/blast/Blast.cgi for BLAST program.

2. Choose BLAST program from basic BLAST list.

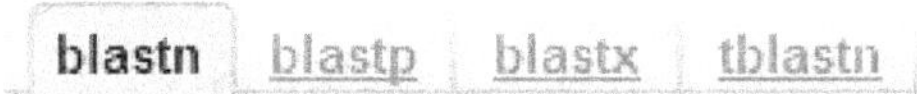

3. Retrieve FASTA format of protein / nucleotide sequence from http://www.ncbi.nlm.nih.gov/protein or http://www.ncbi.nlm.nih.gov/ nucleotide and place it in a box. (other protein/ nucleotide databases also can be used).

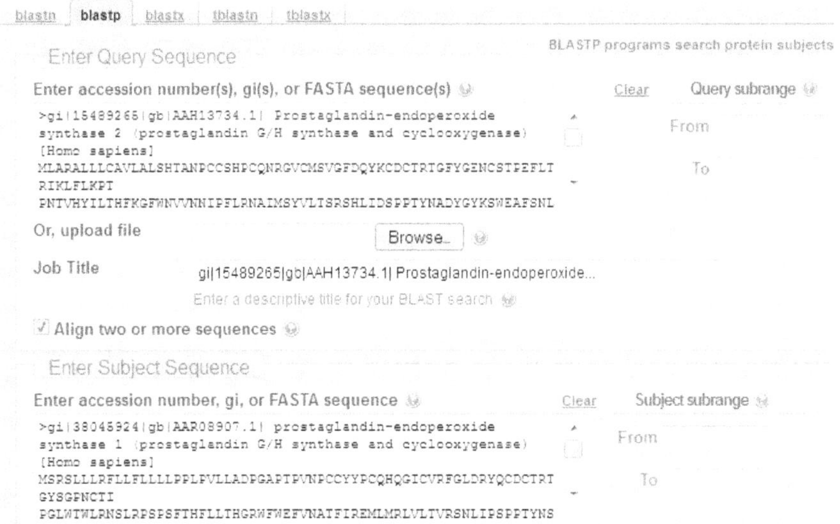

4. Accession number or GI number of particular sequence can also be placed in given box or we can enter the sequence manually.

5. Query subrange and subject subrange can be set for producing optimal alignment.

6. Choose search set parameters and refine the search.

For proteins

Database   Non-redundant protein sequences (nr)   ▾

Organism
Optional   Enter organism name or id--completions will be suggested   Exclude +

Enter organism common name, binomial, or tax id. Only 20 top taxa will be shown.

Select from the list or choose "Custom" to enter the name of an organism. The search will be restricted to the sequences in the database which are from the organism selected.

Exclude
Optional   Models (XM/XP)   Uncultured/environmental sample sequences

Entrez Query
Optional   Enter an Entrez query to limit search

For nucleotides

Choose Search Set

Database   ⦿ Human genomic + transcript   ○ Mouse genomic + transcript   ○ Others (nr etc.)

Human genomic plus transcript (Human G+T)   ▾

Exclude
Optional   Models (XM/XP)   Uncultured/environmental sample sequences

Entrez Query
Optional   Enter an Entrez query to limit search

7. Select the parameters

   Algorithm for proteins

   (i)   BlastP

   (ii) PSI blast

   (iii) PHI blast

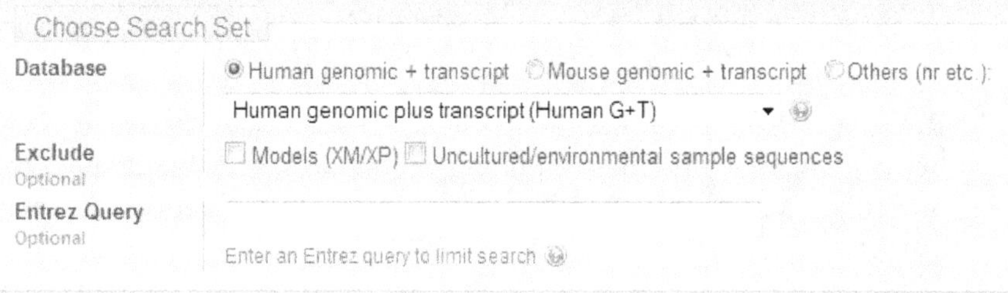

Algorithm for nucelotides

(i)   Megablast

(ii) BlastN

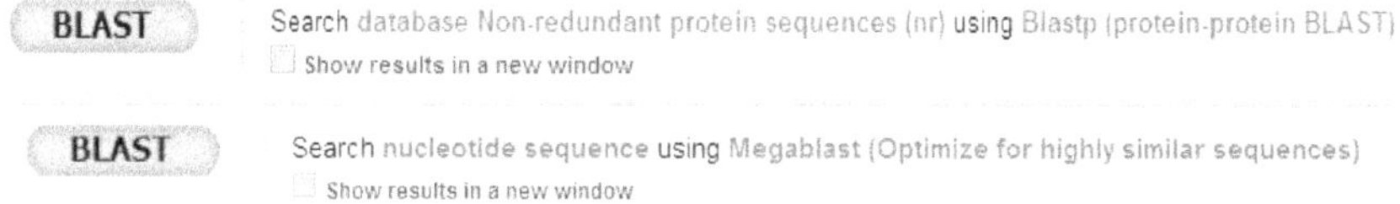

8. Select general parameters

(a)   Maximum target sequence

(b)   Expected threshold

(c)   Word size

(d)   Matrix

(e)   Gap costs

(f)   Filter and masks

9. Finally click on "BLAST" button.

10. Result page can be viewed to analyze the alignment.

Result will be displayed in the following format

(a)   Details of sequences along with program type can be viewed.

(b)   Below that graphical summary in colour code format for the alignment will be present.

(c)   Dot matrix plot follows the graphical summary.

Seq 1: gi 15489265, AAH13734, Prostaglandin-endoperoxidase synthase 2 (prostaglandin G / H synthase and cyclooxygense) [Homosapiens]

Seq 2: gi 38045924, AAR08907, Prostaglandin-endoperoxidase synthase 1 (prostaglandin G / H synthase and cyclooxygense) [Homosapiens]

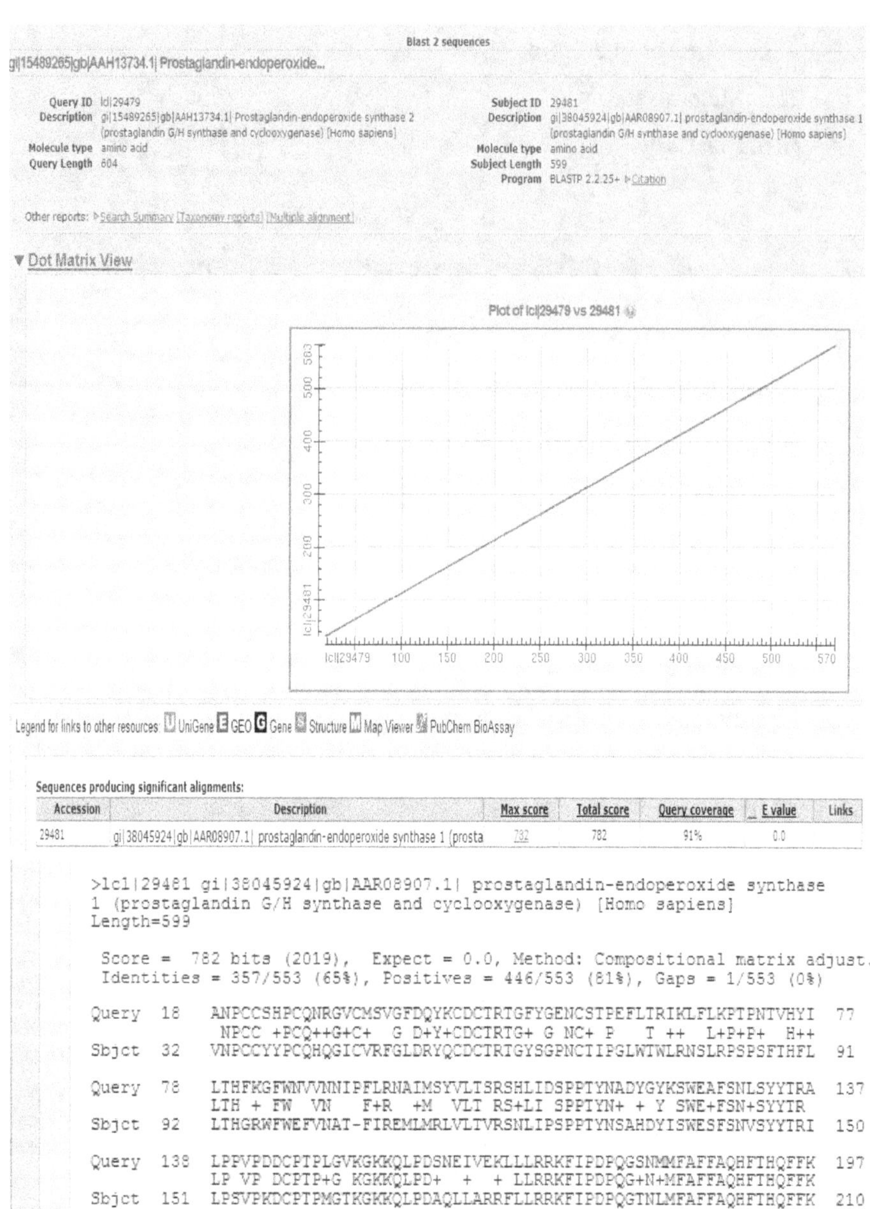

Sequences producing significant alignments:

Accession	Description	Max score	Total score	Query coverage	E value	Links
29481	gi|38045924|gb|AAR08907.1| prostaglandin-endoperoxide synthase 1 (prosta	732	782	91%	0.0	

```
>lcl|29481 gi|38045924|gb|AAR08907.1| prostaglandin-endoperoxide synthase
1 (prostaglandin G/H synthase and cyclooxygenase) [Homo sapiens]
Length=599

 Score =  782 bits (2019),  Expect = 0.0, Method: Compositional matrix adjust.
 Identities = 357/553 (65%), Positives = 446/553 (81%), Gaps = 1/553 (0%)

Query  18   ANPCCSHPCQNRGVCMSVGFDQYKCDCTRTGFYGENCSTPEFLTRIKLFLKPTPNTVHYI   77
            NPCC +PCQ++G+C+   G D+Y+CDCTRTG+ G NC+ P   T ++  L+P+P+  H++
Sbjct  32   VNPCCYYPCQHQGICVRFGLDRYQCDCTRTGYSGPNCTIPGLWTWLRNSLRPSPSFTHFL   91

Query  78   LTHFKGFWNVVNNIPFLRNAIMSYVLTSRSHLIDSPPTYNADYGYKSWEAFSNLSYYTRA   137
            LTH + FW VN   F+R +M VLT RS+LI SPPTYN+ + Y SWE+FSN+SYYTR
Sbjct  92   LTHGRWFWEFVNAT-FIREMLMRLVLTVRSNLIPSPPTYNSAHDYISWESFSNVSYYTRI   150

Query  138  LPPVPDDCPTPLGVKGKKQLPDSNEIVEKLLLRRKFIPDPQGSNMMFAFFAQHFTHQFFK   197
            LP VP DCPTP+G KGKKQLPD+  +  + LLRRKFIPDPQG+N+MFAFFAQHFTHQFFK
Sbjct  151  LPSVPKDCPTPMGTKGKKQLPDAQLLARRFLLRRKFIPDPQGTNLMFAFFAQHFTHQFFK   210
```

23.6 Interpretations

1. Blast version number, sequence database and query sequence can be identified.

2. References for that particular sequence can be viewed in result page.

3. Below this graphical representation will be displayed

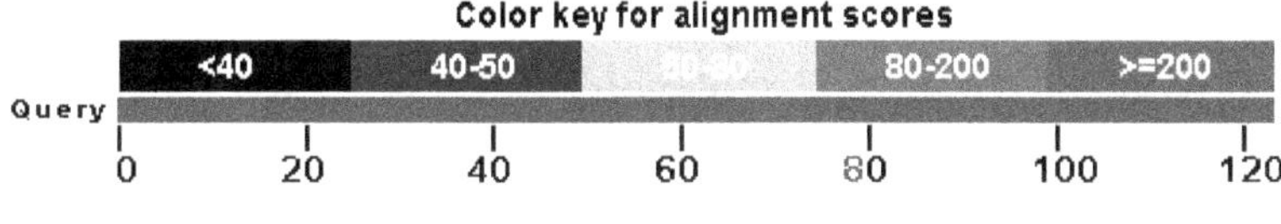

(a) Query sequence on the top

(b) Each bar appears below that represents the portion of another sequence similar to query sequence

1. Red bar – most similar sequence

2. Pink bar – similarity is there

3. Green bar – not impressive at all

4. Black / blue bar – bad score.

4. The score of database sequences in bits and expectation value (E value) of alignment.

5. Lower the E value, higher the significance in similarity.

An assessment of their statistical significance, based upon the extreme value distribution, called E values and it dependents on length of the query sequence, size of the database and raw score.

6. Gapped alignment between query and subject sequence are shown

7. Bits = (λ X raw score – ln k) / Ln 2, % identity, % positive and % alignment also seen.

8. As a general rule more than 25 % identity over a stretch of 100 residues can be considered to be good evidence of common ancestry for two sequences.

23.7 EMBOSS – Pairwise Alignment Tool

EMBOSS is "The European Molecular Biology Open Software Suite". EMBOSS is a free Open Source software analysis package specially developed for the needs of the molecular biology (e.g. EMBnet) user community. The software automatically copes with data in a variety of formats and even allows transparent retrieval of sequence data from the web. Also, as extensive libraries are provided with the package, it is a platform to allow other scientists to develop and release software in true open source spirit. EMBOSS also integrates a range of currently available packages and tools for sequence analysis into a seamless whole.

23.7.1 Advantages

- A properly constructed toolkit for creating robust bioinformatics applications.
- A comprehensive set of sequence analysis programs.
- All sequence and many alignment and structural formats are handled.
- Extensive programming library for common sequence analysis tasks.
- Additional programming libraries for many other areas including string handling, pattern-matching, list processing and database indexing.
- It is free-of-charge and an open-source project.
- It runs on practically every UNIX, MS Windows and MacOS.
- It integrates other popular publicly available packages.

23.7.2 Applications

1. Sequence alignment.
2. Rapid database searching with sequence patterns.
3. Protein motif identification, including domain analysis.
4. Nucleotide sequence pattern analysis.
5. Codon usage analysis for small genomes.
6. Rapid identification of sequence patterns in large scale sequence sets.
7. Presentation tools for publication.

23.8 Experimental Procedure for Pairwise Alignment Program (EMBOSS)

23.8.1 Steps

1. Open the URL page http://www.ebi.ac.uk/emboss/align/ for emboss program.
2. Copy protein / nucleotide sequence in any format from http://www.ncbi.nlm.nih.gov/ and place in a given box or we can enter the sequence manually or it can be uploaded.

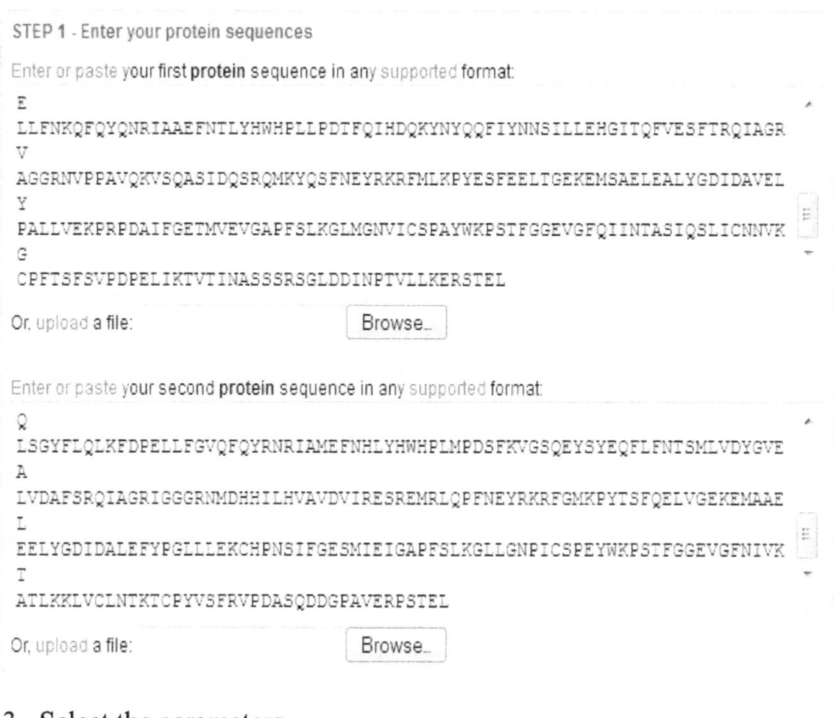

3. Select the parameters.

   (a) Method

   (b) Gap penalty

   (c) Matrix

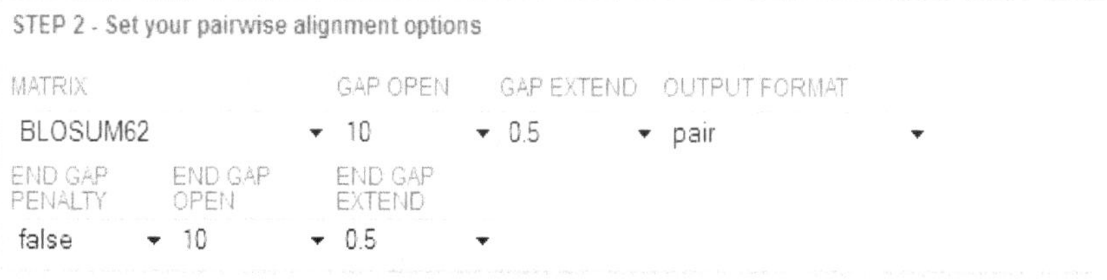

4. Finally click "Submit" to run the emboss program

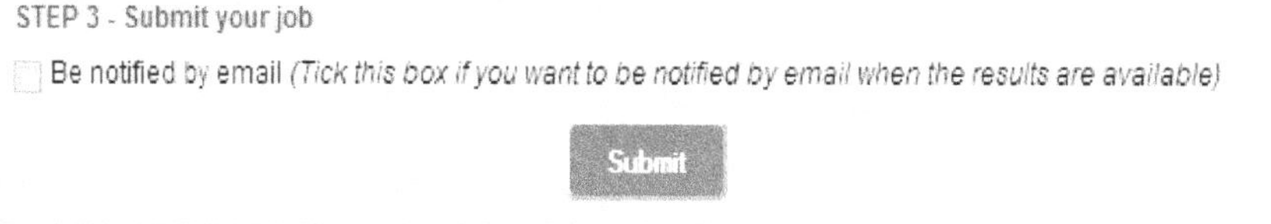

5. View the result page and perform the interpretations.

```
#
# Aligned_sequences: 2
# 1: AAH13734.1
# 2: AAR08907.1
# Matrix: EBLOSUM62
# Gap_penalty: 10.0
# Extend_penalty: 0.5
#
# Length: 620
# Identity:      372/620  (60.0%)
# Similarity:    465/620  (75.0%)
# Gaps:           37/620  ( 6.0%)
# Score: 2039.5
```

```
AAH13734.1        1 MLARALLLCAVLAL---------------SHTANPCCSHPCQNRGVCMSV     35
                    ::|:|||..:|.|               ....||||.:|||::|:|:..
AAR08907.1        1 -MSRSLLLRFLLFLLLLPPLPVLLADPGAPTPVNPCCYYPCQHQGICVRF     49

AAH13734.1       36 GFDQYKCDCTRTGFYGENCSTPEFLTRIKLFLKPTPNTVHYILTHFKGFW     85
                    |.|:|:|||||||:.|.||:.|...|.::..|:|:|:|:..|::|||.:.||
AAR08907.1       50 GLDRYQCDCTRTGYSGPNCTIPGLWTWLRNSLRPSPSFTHFLLTHGRWFW     99

AAH13734.1       86 NVVNNIPFLRNAIMSYVLTSRSHLIDSPPTYNADYGYKSWEAFSNLSYYT    135
                    ..| |..|:|..:|..|||.||:||.||||||:.:.|.|||:|||:||||
AAR08907.1      100 EFV-NATFIREMLMRLVLTVRSNLIPSPPTYNSAHDYISWESFSNVSYYT    148

AAH13734.1      136 RALPPVPDDCPTPLGVKGKKQLPDSNEIVEKLLLRRKFIPDPQGSNMMFA    185
                    |.||.||.|||||:|.||||||||:..:..:.|||||||||||||:|:|||
AAR08907.1      149 RILPSVPKDCPTPMGTKGKKQLPDAQLLARRFLLRRKFIPDPQGTNLMFA    198

AAH13734.1      186 FFAQHFTHQFFKTDHKRGPAFTNGLGHGVDLNHIYGETLARQRKLRLFKD    235
                    |||||||||||||..|.||.||.||..|||||||.||||:.|.||.:|||||
```

23.9 Uniprot- Pairwise Alignment Tool

1. Open http:// www.uniprot.org and select align

2. Reterive and place FASTA format of sequences from protein databases

3. Press 'Align' button to run the alignment

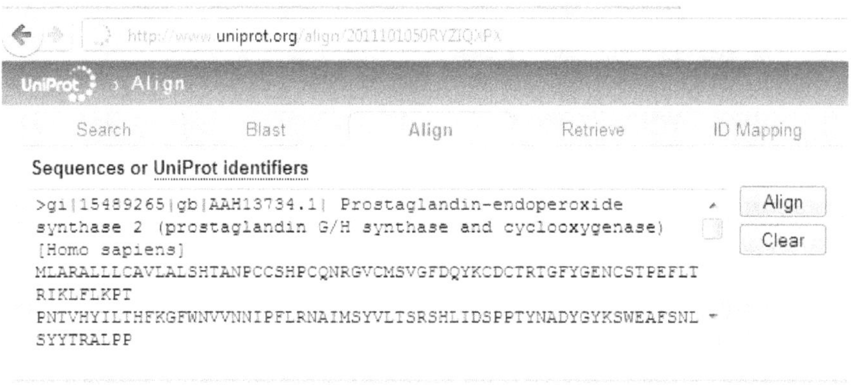

```
http://www.uniprot.org/align/2011101050RYZIQXPx

UniProt    Align

  Search        Blast         Align        Retrieve        ID Mapping

Sequences or UniProt identifiers

>gi|15489265|gb|AAH13734.1| Prostaglandin-endoperoxide          Align
synthase 2 (prostaglandin G/H synthase and cyclooxygenase)
[Homo sapiens]                                                  Clear
MLARALLLCAVLALSHTANPCCSHPCQNRGVCMSVGFDQYKCDCTRTGFYGENCSTPEFLT
RIKLFLKPT
PNTVHYILTHFKGFWNVVNNIPFLRNAIMSYVLTSRSHLIDSPPTYNADYGYKSWEAFSNL
SYYTRALPP
```

4. Result page will appear with alignment of two sequences

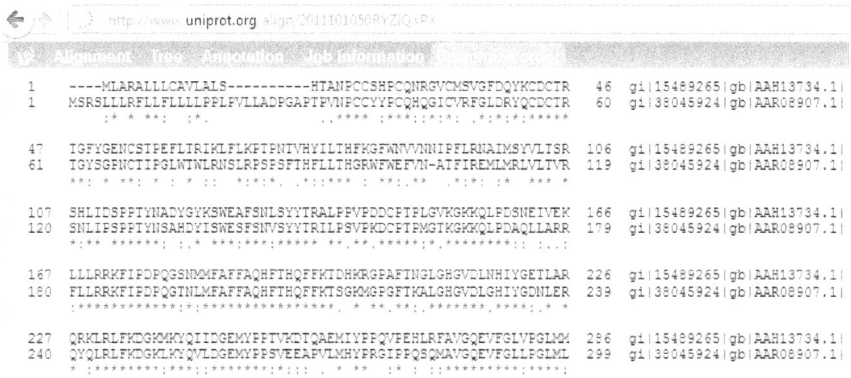

```
http://www.uniprot.org/align/2011101050RYZIQXPx

  Alignment   Tree   Annotation   Job Information

  1    ----MLARALLLCAVLALS----------HTANPCCSHPCQNRGVCMSVGFDQYKCDCTR    46   gi|15489265|gb|AAH13734.1|
  1    MSRSLLLRFLLFLLLLPPLPVLLADPGAPTPVNPCCYYPCQHQGICVRFGLDRYQCDCTR    60   gi|38045924|gb|AAR08907.1|
        :* * **:   :*.              ..**** :***::*:*: .*:*:*:*****

 47    TGFYGENCSTPEFLTRIKLFLKPTPNTVHYILTHFKGFWNVVNNIPFLRNAIMSYVLTSR   106   gi|15489265|gb|AAH13734.1|
 61    TGYSGPNCTIPGLWTWLRNSLRPSPSFTHFLLTHGRWFWEFVN-ATFIREMLMRLVLTVR   119   gi|38045924|gb|AAR08907.1|
        **: * **: * : * ::   *:*:*. .*::*** : **:.** .*:*: :* *** *

107    SHLIDSPPTYNADYGYKSWEAFSNLSYYTRALPPVPDDCPTPLGVKGKKQLPDSNEIVEK   166   gi|15489265|gb|AAH13734.1|
120    SNLIPSPPTYNSAHDYISWESFSNVSYYTRILPSVPKDCPTPMGTKGKKQLPDAQLLARR   179   gi|38045924|gb|AAR08907.1|
        *:** ******: :.* ***:***:***** **.**.*****:*.********:: :..:

167    LLLRRKFIPDPQGSNMMFAFFAQHFTHQFFKTDHKRGPAFTNGLGHGVDLNHIYGETLAR   226   gi|15489265|gb|AAH13734.1|
180    FLLRRKFIPDPQGTNLMFAFFAQHFTHQFFKTSGKMGPGFTKALGHGVDLGHIYGDNLER   239   gi|38045924|gb|AAR08907.1|
        :**********:*:**************** .* **.**:.*******.****:.* *

227    QRKLRLFKDGKMKYQIIDGEMYPPTVKDTQAEMIYPPQVPEHLRFAVGQEVFGLVPGLMM   286   gi|15489265|gb|AAH13734.1|
240    QYQLRLFKDGKLKYQVLDGEMYPPSVEEAPVLMHYPRGIPPQSQMAVGQEVFGLLPGLML   299   gi|38045924|gb|AAR08907.1|
        * :********:***::*******:*::: . * ** :*: : ::**********:****:
```

5. Amino acid properties option can be used to see the alignment of particular type of amino acids

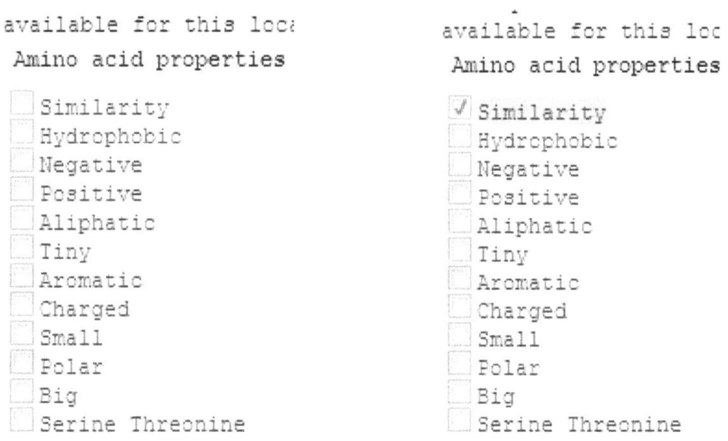

```
available for this loc              available for this loc
Amino acid properties               Amino acid properties

  [ ] Similarity                     [✓] Similarity
  [ ] Hydrophobic                    [ ] Hydrophobic
  [ ] Negative                       [ ] Negative
  [ ] Positive                       [ ] Positive
  [ ] Aliphatic                      [ ] Aliphatic
  [ ] Tiny                           [ ] Tiny
  [ ] Aromatic                       [ ] Aromatic
  [ ] Charged                        [ ] Charged
  [ ] Small                          [ ] Small
  [ ] Polar                          [ ] Polar
  [ ] Big                            [ ] Big
  [ ] Serine Threonine               [ ] Serine Threonine
```

```
     Alignment   Tree   Annotation   Job information   Customize order

  1    ----MLARALLLCAVLALS-----------HTANPCCSHPCQNRGVCMSVGFDQYKCDCTR    46   gi|15489265|gb|AAH13734.1|
  1    MSRSLLLRFLLFLLLLPPLPVLLADPGAPTPVNPCCYYPCQHQGICVRFGLDRYQCDCTR    60   gi|38045924|gb|AAR08907.1|
        :* * **:   :*.         ..**** :***::*:*: .*:*:*:*****

 47    TGFYGENCSTPEFLIRIKLFLKPTPNTVHYILTHFKGFWNVVNNIPFLRNAIMSYVLTSR   106   gi|15489265|gb|AAH13734.1|
 61    TGYSGPNCTIPGLWTWLRNSLRPSPSFTHFLLTHGRWFWEFVN-ATFIREMLMRLVLTVR   119   gi|38045924|gb|AAR08907.1|
       **: * **: * : * ::   *:*:*. .*::*** : **:.** .*:*: :* *** *

107    SHLIDSPPTYNADYGYKSWEAFSNLSYYTRALPPVPDDCPTPLGVKGKKQLPDSNEIVEK   166   gi|15489265|gb|AAH13734.1|
120    SNLIPSPPTYNSAHDYISWESFSNVSYYTRILPSVPKDCPTPMGTKGKKQLPDAQLLARR   179   gi|38045924|gb|AAR08907.1|
       *:** ******: :.* ***;***;***** **.**.*****:*.*********:: :..:

167    LLLRRKFIPDPQGSNMMFAFFAQHFTHQFFKTDHKRGPAFTNGLGHGVDLNHIYGETLAR   226   gi|15489265|gb|AAH13734.1|
180    FLLRRKFIPDPQGTNLMFAFFAQHFTHQFFKTSGKMGPGFTKALGHGVDLGHIYGDNLER   239   gi|38045924|gb|AAR08907.1|
       :***********:*:**************** * **.**:.*******.****:.* *

227    QRKLRLFKDGKMKYQIIDGEMYPPTVKDTQAEMIYPPQVPEHLRFAVGQEVFGLVPGLMM   286   gi|15489265|gb|AAH13734.1|
240    QYQLRLFKDGKLKYQVLDGEMYPPSVEEAPVLMHYPRGIPPQSQMAVGQEVFGLLPGLML   299   gi|38045924|gb|AAR08907.1|
       * :*********;***::*******;*:::  . * ** :* : ::**********:****:
```

23.10 Multiple Sequence Alignment (MSA)

Multiple sequence alignment (MSA) involves alignment of more than two biological sequences of DNA / RNA / protein. It is a valuable tool in the study of protein structure, function and phylogenetic study. MSA also helps in predict the conserved domain sites, motifs, similar regions, patterns and profile in sequence alignment. Understanding the structure, function and evolution of genes is fundamental in genome analysis.

23.10.1 Applications

1. Identification of highly conserved residues which are essential for the structure and function
2. Identification of evolutionary relationship of distantly related members of a family
3. Prediction of protein structure prediction and its possible function

23.10.2 Algorithms

Global alignment: It uses Needleman-Wunsch algorithm. The disadvantage of this method is it requires more time for alignment, which roughly proportional to the sequence length. ClustalW is the most widely used version of the MSA.

Local alignment: Useful in optional cases, where sequences share a similar region but are otherwise completely different.

Blast 3: Useful in finding proteins that share a region of only weak similarity.

Hidden Markov Model: Probabilistic model considers all possible combinations of matches, mismatches and gaps to generate an alignment of a set of sequences.

Genetic algorithm

23.10.3 Multiple Sequence Alignment Methods

1. Sum of pairs (SP) method

2. Progressive alignment method

3. Iterative alignment method

4. Profile alignment method

5. Multi dimentional dynamic program

Sum of pairs (SP) method: A well known scoring function of multiple sequence alignment and are deficient from an evolutionary perspective.

Progressive alignment method: First aligns two most alike sequences by pairwise method and further aligns 3rd sequence to the 1st one. The process continues until all the sequences are aligned and the scores obtained after alignment will be converted into distances. The distances are used in the construction of phylogenetic trees. CLUSTALW and CLUSTALX are the programs known for progressive alignment method.

Iterative alignment method: Iterative methods works similar to that of progressive methods, but repeatedly realign the initial sequences as well as new sequences. It reduces errors inherent in progressive method. PRRN / PRPP software supported with hill climbing is the program operates this kind of alignment. DELAIGN and MUSCLE are the other iterative programs

Profile alignment method: Alignment between profile to profile rather than sequence to sequence.

Multi dimentional dynamic program: Impractical in case of more number of sequences and the method is more time consuming.

23.10.4 Multiple Sequence Alignment Steps

In general MSA involves three important steps

- Search for homologous sequences

- Computation of sequence alignment for multiple sequences

- Interpretation of alignment

23.10.5 Multiple Sequence Alignment Programs

1. ClustalW

2. Align

3. Kalign

4. MAFFT

5. MUSCLE

6. T-Coffee

23.11 ClustalW

ClustalW is a general purpose multiple sequence alignment program for DNA or proteins. It produces biologically meaningful multiple sequence alignments of divergent sequences. It calculates the best match for the selected sequences, and lines them up so that the identities, similarities and differences can be seen. Evolutionary relationships can be seen via viewing Cladograms or phylogram.

Phylogram: A branching tree estimates and infers evolutionary relationship among the biological species based on the similarities in their genetic characteristics.

Cladogram: A branching tree of phylogeny estimate; where the branches are of equal length. This shows common ancestry, but do not indicate the amount of evolutionary time separating taxa.

23.12 Experimental Procedure for Multiple Sequence Alignment Program (CLUSTALW)

1. Open the URL page http://www.ebi.ac.uk/Tools/clustalw/

2. Select protein / nucleotide sequence in a FASTA format through http://www.ncbi.nlm.nih.gov/.

STEP 1 - Enter your input sequences

Enter or paste a set of Protein ▾ sequences in any supported format:

```
>gi|358439789|pdb|3RX2|A Chain A, Crystal Structure Of Human Aldose
Reductase Complexed With Sulindac Sulfone
MGSSHHHHHHSSGLVPRGSHMASRLLLNNGAKMPILGLGTWKSPPGQVTEAVKVAIDVGYRHIDCAHVYQ
NENEVGVAIQEKLREQVVKREELFIVSKLWCTYHEKGLVKGACQKTLSDLKLDYLDLYLIHWPTGFKPGK
EFFPLDESGNVVPSDTNILDTWAAMEELVDEGLVKAIGISNFNHLQVEMILNKPGLKYKPAVNQIECHPY
LTQEKLIQYCQSKGIVVTAYSPLGSPDRPWAKPEDPSLLEDPRIKAIAAKHNKTTAQVLIRFPMQRNLVV
IPKSVTPERIAENFKVFDFELSSQDMTTLLSYNRNWRVCALLSCTSHKDYPFHEE
>gi|46015262|pdb|1PWL|A Chain A, Crystal Structure Of Human Aldose
Reductase Complexed With Nadp And Minalrestat
MASRILLNNGAKMPILGLGTWKSPPGQVTEAVKVAIDVGYRHIDCAHVYQNENEVGVAIQEKLREQVVKR
EELFIVSKLWCTYHEKGLVKGACQKTLSDLKLDYLDLYLIHWPTGFKPGKEFFPLDESGNVVPSDTNILD
TWAAMEELVDEGLVKAIGISNFNHLQVEMILNKPGLKYKPAVNQIECHPYLTQEKLIQYCQSKGIVVTAY
SPLGSPDRPWAKPEDPSLLEDPRIKAIAAKHNKTTAQVLIRFPMQRNLVVIPKSVTPERIAENFKVFDFE
LSSQDMTTLLSYNRNWRVCALLSCTSHKDYPFHEEF
>gi|171848769|pdb|2PDK|A Chain A, Human Aldose Reductase Mutant L301m
Complexed With Sorbinil.
MASRILLNNGAKMPILGLGTWKSPPGQVTEAVKVAIDVGYRHIDCAHVYQNENEVGVAIQEKLREQVVKR
EELFIVSKLWCTYHEKGLVKGACQKTLSDLKLDYLDLYLIHWPTGFKPGKEFFPLDESGNVVPSDTNILD
TWAAMEELVDEGLVKAIGISNFNHLQVEMILNKPGLKYKPAVNQIECHPYLTQEKLIQYCQSKGIVVTAY
SPLGSPDRPWAKPEDPSLLEDPRIKAIAAKHNKTTAQVLIRFPMQRNLVVIPKSVTPERIAENFKVFDFE
LSSQDMTTLLSYNRNWRVCALMSCTSHKDYPFHEEF
>gi|93278511|pdb|1Z3N|A Chain A, Human Aldose Reductase In Complex With
Nadp+ And The Inhibitor Lidorestat At 1.04 Angstrom
GSHMASRILLNNGAKMPILGLGTWKSPPGQVTEAVKVAIDVGYRHIDCAHVYQNENEVGVAIQEKLREQV
VKREELFIVSKLWCTYHEKGLVKGACQKTLSDLKLDYLDLYLIHWPTGFKPGKEFFPLDESGNVVPSDTN
ILDTWAAMEELVDEGLVKAIGISNFNHLQVEMILNKPGLKYKPAVNQIECHPYLTQEKLIQYCQSKGIVV
TAYSPLGSPDRPWAKPEDPSLLEDPRIKAIAAKHNKTTAQVLIRFPMQRNLVVIPKSVTPERIAENFKVF
DFELSSQDMTTLLSYNRNWRVCALLSCTSHKDYPFHEEF
```

Or, upload a file: Choose File , No file chosen

3. Select the parameters.

    1. Protein / DNA weight Matrix
    2. Gap open and extension penalty
    3. Clustering type
    4. Output order

STEP 2 - Set your Pairwise Alignment Options

Alignment Type: ◉ Slow   ○ Fast

Slow Pairwise Alignment Options

Protein Weight Matrix   GAP OPEN   GAP EXTENSION

| BLOSUM ▾ | 10 | ▾ | 0.1 | ▾ |

BLOSUM
PAM
Gonnet
ID

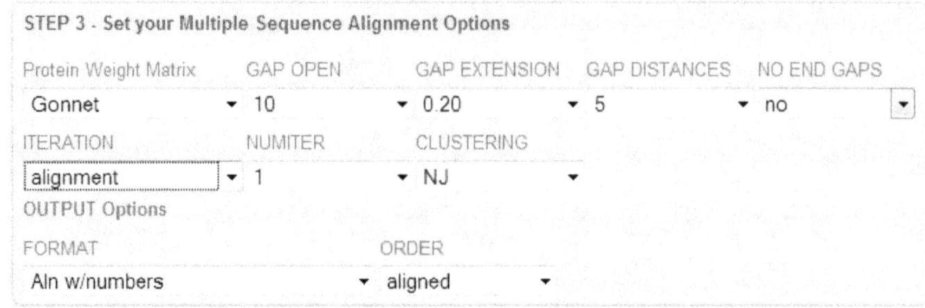

4. Finally click "Submit"

5. View the results page and interpret the results.

   Alignment of sequences

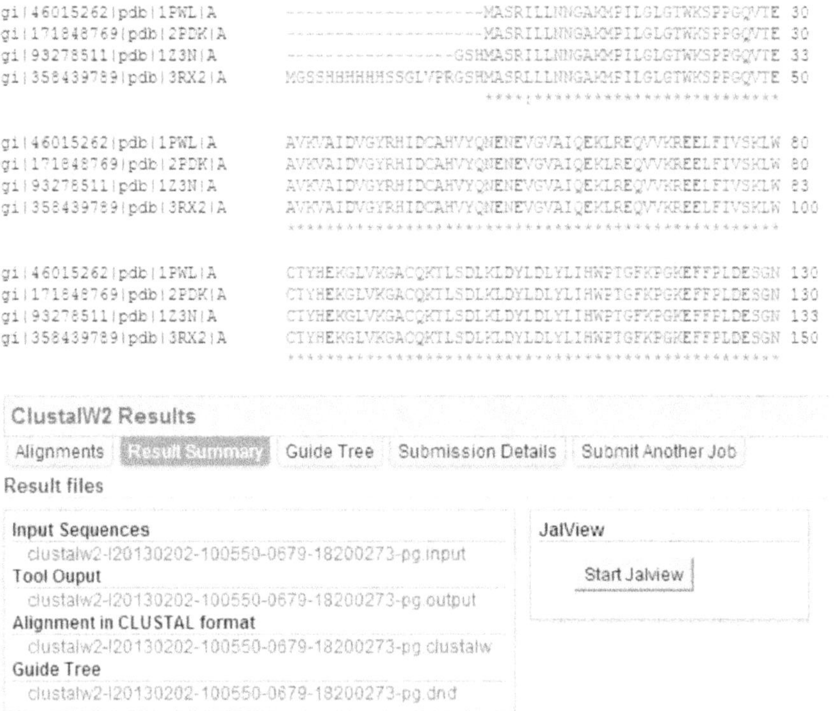

Scores Table

View Output File

SeqA	Name	Length	SeqB	Name	Length	Score
1	gi|358439789|pdb|3RX2|A	335	2	gi|46015262|pdb|1PWL|A	316	99.0
1	gi|358439789|pdb|3RX2|A	335	3	gi|171848769|pdb|2PDK|A	316	99.0
1	gi|358439789|pdb|3RX2|A	335	4	gi|93278511|pdb|1Z3N|A	319	99.0
2	gi|46015262|pdb|1PWL|A	316	3	gi|171848769|pdb|2PDK|A	316	99.0
2	gi|46015262|pdb|1PWL|A	316	4	gi|93278511|pdb|1Z3N|A	319	100.0
3	gi|171848769|pdb|2PDK|A	316	4	gi|93278511|pdb|1Z3N|A	319	99.0

File   Edit   Select   View   Format   Colour   Calculate   Help

```
                      10           20           30           40           50           60           70
gi|46015262|pdb|1PWL|A/1-316  · · · · · · · · · · · · · · · · · · MASRILLNNGAKMPILGLGTWKSPPGQVTEAVKVAIDVGYRHIDCAHVYQNEN
gi|171848769|pdb|2PDK|A/1-316 · · · · · · · · · · · · · · · · · · MASRILLNNGAKMPILGLGTWKSPPGQVTEAVKVAIDVGYRHIDCAHVYQNEN
gi|93278511|pdb|1Z3N|A/1-319  · · · · · · · · · · · · · · · GSHMASRILLNNGAKMPILGLGTWKSPPGQVTEAVKVAIDVGYRHIDCAHVYQNEN
gi|358439789|pdb|3RX2|A/1-335 MGSSHHHHHHSSGLVPRGSHMASRLLLNNGAKMPILGLGTWKSPPGQVTEAVKVAIDVGYRHIDCAHVYQNEN

Conservation     · · · · · · · · · · · · · · · · · · · · · · · · · ·

Quality

Consensus        · · · · · · · · · · · · · · · · · · · · GSHMASRILLNNGAKMPILGLGTWKSPPGQVTEAVKVAIDVGYRHIDCAHVYQNEN
```

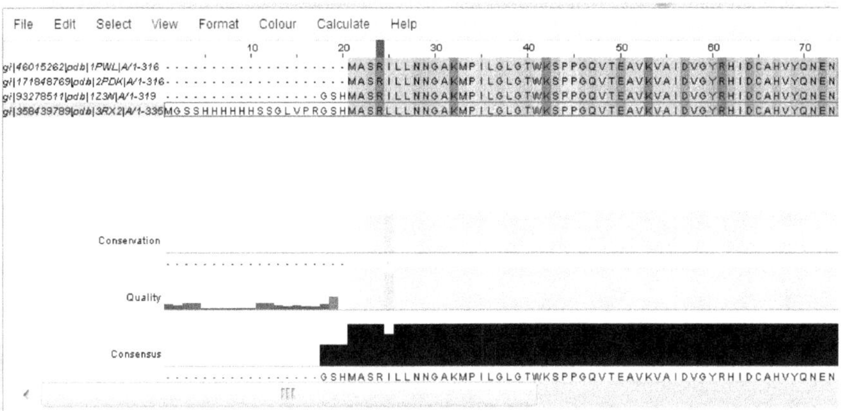

Phylogram

Show as Cladogram Tree   Show Distances

```
                                                          ─────────────────── gi|358439789|pdb|3RX2|A
       ┌ gi|46015262|pdb|1PWL|A
       │                          ───────── gi|171848769|pdb|2PDK|A
       └ gi|93278511|pdb|1Z3N|A
```

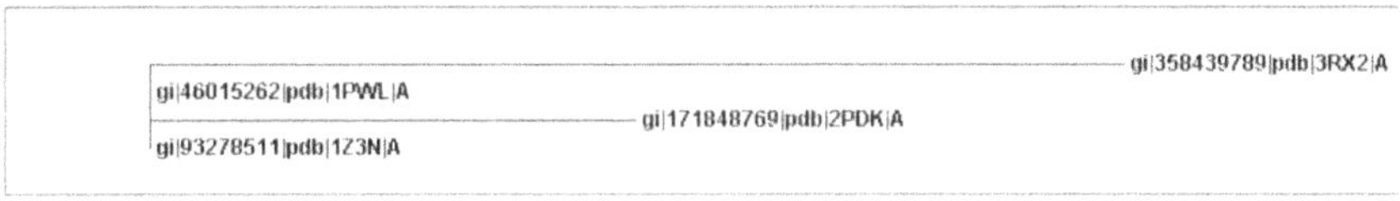

Cladogram

Show as Phylogram Tree   Show Distances

```
  ─────────────────────────────────────── gi|358439789|pdb|3RX2|A
  ─────────────────────────────────────── gi|46015262|pdb|1PWL|A
  ─────────────────────────────────────── gi|171848769|pdb|2PDK|A
  ─────────────────────────────────────── gi|93278511|pdb|1Z3N|A
```

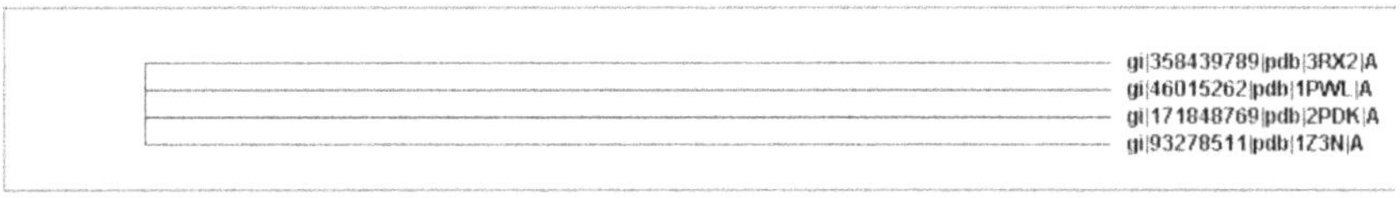

23.13 Interpretation

1. " * " indicates that residues or nucleotides are identical

2. " : " indicates conserved constitutions

3. " . " indicates semi conserved constitutions

4. When aln / GCG is selected as a output format, one can see the alignment in colur display, by clicking "show colour" button.

5. Graphical interfaces allow colouring or shading residues (amino acids or nucleotides) according to their chemical nature

6. Hydrophobic residues and hydrophilic residues can be visualized.

7. Colour code helps in interpretation of Multiple Sequence Alignment

8. Results obtained through CLUSTALW (EBI) can be viewed through Jalview.

## CHAPTER 24

PHYLOGENETIC ANALYSIS

MSA gives evolutionary relationship between sequences called as phylogenetic analysis. This can be studied by generating a phylogenetic tree. Study of evolutionary relationships, also known as "cladistics" Clade-greek word means set of descendants from single ancestor. Involves creating a branching structure, termed as phylogeny / tree, which illustrates the relationship.

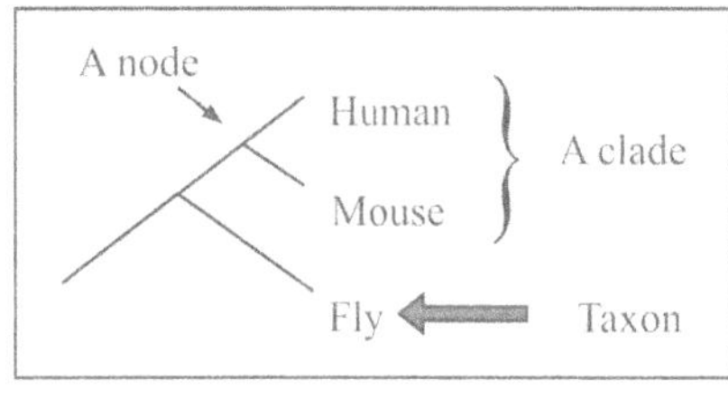

Unrooted tree

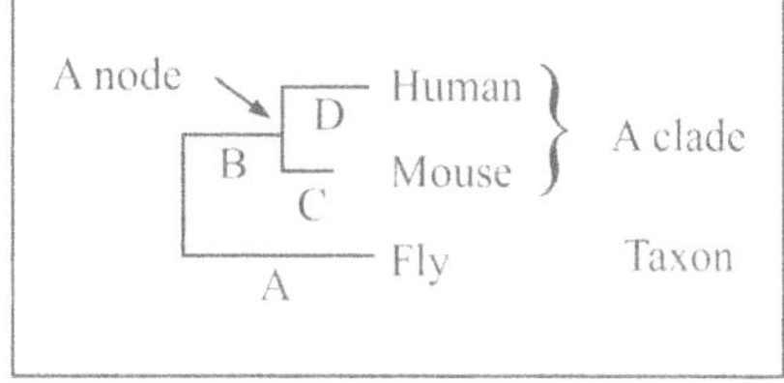

Rooted tree

Clade: Groups of organism for which evolutionary theory utilized

Taxon: Any named group of organism and evolutionary theory not necessarily involved.

24.1 Phylogentics Analysis Steps

- Alignment
- Determination of the substitution model
- Tree building
- Tree evaluation

24.2 Phylogenetics Methods

Broadly they are classified into phenetic method and cladistic method.

Phenetic method: Each organism is compared with every other for all characters, and number of similarities calculated. Most similar are grouped close together, more different are linked more distantly and No genetic evolutionary relationship.

Cladistic method: Relationship between taxa are clarified. Members of group share common evolutionary history are known as synapomorphies .

Phylogenetics also can be conveniently classified into

1. The visual methods
2. Computer algorithms
3. Distance matrix methods
4. Character based methods

24.2.1   The Visual Method - Dot Matrix Method

Two different sequences can be aligned without gaps. If gap occurs in one of the sequences, the alignment of diagonal will be shifted vertically or horizontally.

24.2.2   Computer Algorithms

Each residue of the sequence is compared with each residue of the other. Appropriate weight matrix will be used to score identity or similarities and penalize gaps.

24.3 Distance Matrix Method

Distance matrix method uses amount of dissimilarity between two aligned sequences to derive trees. It reconstruct the true tree if all genetic divergence events were recorded in the sequence. Subsequent mutations can make them reverse the methods available for this are

- UPGMA
- Neighbor Joining methods
- Transformed distance method
- Least squares methods
- Fitch Margoliash method
- Minimum evolution method

24.3.1 UPGMA – Unweighed Pair Group Method with Arithmetic Mean Simplest Method

Distance between (A,B), C   = Dist A,C + Dis BC / 2

                                   = 4 + 4 /2 = 8/2= 4

Distance between (A,B), D   = Dist A,D + Dis BD / 2

Distance between (A,B), E   = Dist A,E + Dis BE / 2

Distance between (A,B), F   = Dist A,F + Dis BF / 2

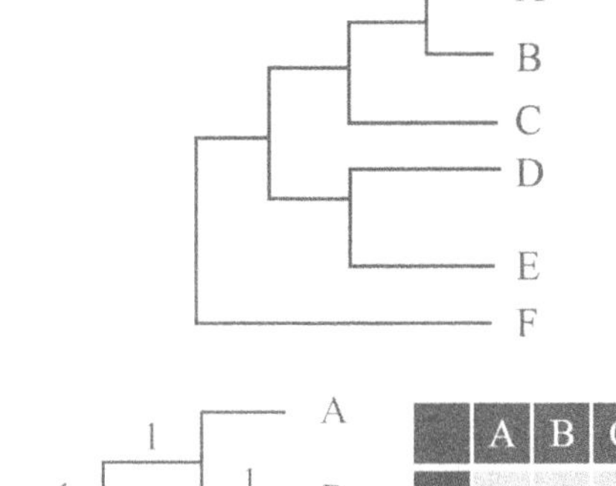

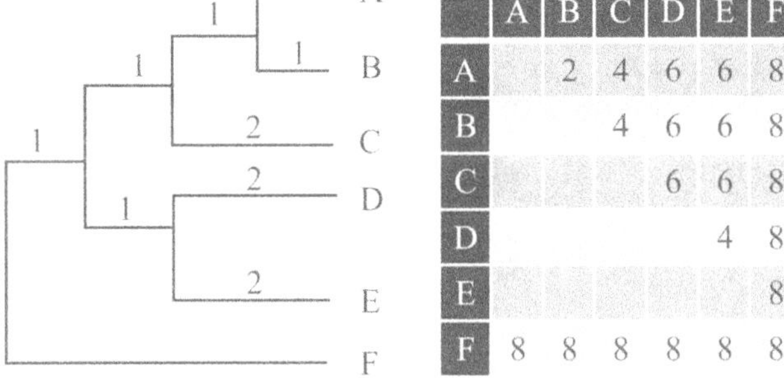

	A	B	C	D	E	F
A		2	4	6	6	8
B			4	6	6	8
C				6	6	8
D					4	8
E						8
F	8	8	8	8	8	8

24.3.2 Neighbor Joining (NJ) Method

Pairing those sequences that are the most alike and using that pair to join to next closest sequence programs. It performs through Clustalw, Phylip and Distnj. It is the most common algorithm and "Speedy-and-popular" method. Distance estimates the total branch length between a given two species/genes/proteins

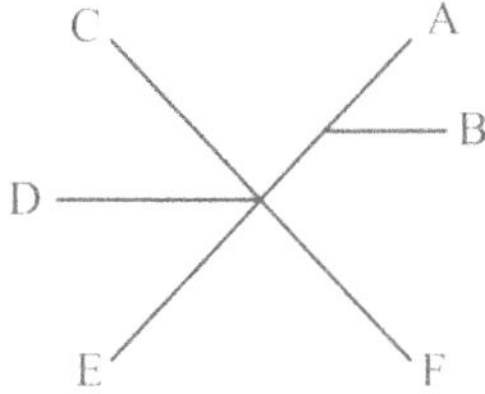

24.3.3 Advantages

- Fast and suited for large databases
- Permits correction for multiple substitutions

24.4 Character based Method

- Protein maximum liklihood
- Protein maximum parsimony

24.4.1 Maximum Parsimony

Simpler hypothesis are preferable for more complicated ones. It gives numerous trees that have the same score. In few steps it produces tree for observed variation in sequences (minimum evolution method).

24.4.2 Maximum Likelihood

It is useful when more variable sequences are under study. It produces trees and then sees if the data could generate that tree. It gives an estimation of the likelihood of a particular tree, given a certain model of nucleotide substitution.

## CHAPTER 25

GENE PREDICTION

Gene identification is the process of identifying the regions of genomic DNA (gene), that encode proteins. Gene prediction is statistical analysis of sequence in genome coding regions. Gene finding programs use sequence similarity search tools to identify protein coding genome region. This process involves the comparison of expanded sequence tags (ESTs) and known protein to the region of known genome. A comparison of codon frequency in a region of the genome of a species with the typical codon frequency in the same species may give an idea of the regions coding for a particular protein.

25.1 Pattern Recognition

It is the method of scanning sequence (DNA/protein) for short sequence patterns, which are responsible for function. The observation of pattern in target sequence, suggest their functional nature.

25.2 Gene Prediction Methods

1. Sequencing the fragments
   - Sangers method
   - Maxam Gilbert method
   - Automated sequencing
   - Shot gun sequences
   - Mass spectroscopy
   - Next generation DNA sequencing methods
2. Blotting methods
   - Southern blotting
   - Northern blotting
   - Western blotting

3. Polymerase Chain Reaction (PCR)

4. *In Situ* hybridization (ISH)

5. Open reading frames prediction (OPR)

25.2.1 Sequencing the Fragments

DNA sequencing promotes new discoveries of many disciplines such as molecular biology, genetics, and forensic sciences.

Sanger's sequencing (Chain terminating / dideoxy nucleotide method).

This method involves the DNA polymerase catalysed polymerization of deoxynucleoside triphosphate (dNTP) complementary to the template DNA. This method also involves base specific interruption of *in vitro* enzymatic synthesis of DNA by terminator nucleoside (dideoxynuceoside triphosphate-ddNTP). The polymerization continues until enzymes encounters the terminator nucleoside.

1. The reaction will be carried out in four tubes containing DNA template, DNA primer, DNA polymerase, deoxy nucleosides (dATP, dGTP, dCTP and dTTP) and one of the terminator nucleoside (ddATP, ddGTP, ddCTP and ddTTP).

2. Equivalent concentration of dNTPs and $1/10^{th}$ equivalent of ddNTP (controls the polymerase catalysed synthesis) will be used for polymerization.

3. Insertion of ddATP instead of dATP for T present in the template terminates the chain elongation.

4. The DNA fragments with various length formed will be resolved by polyacrylamide gel electrophoresis (PAGE) and the sequence can be visualised by auto radiography.

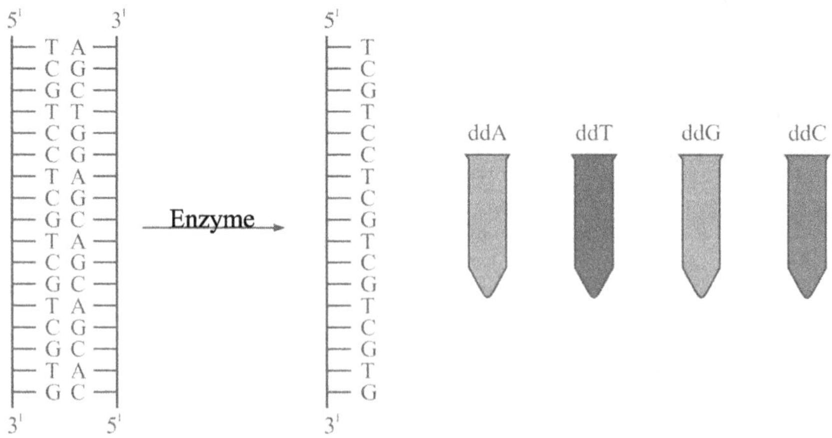

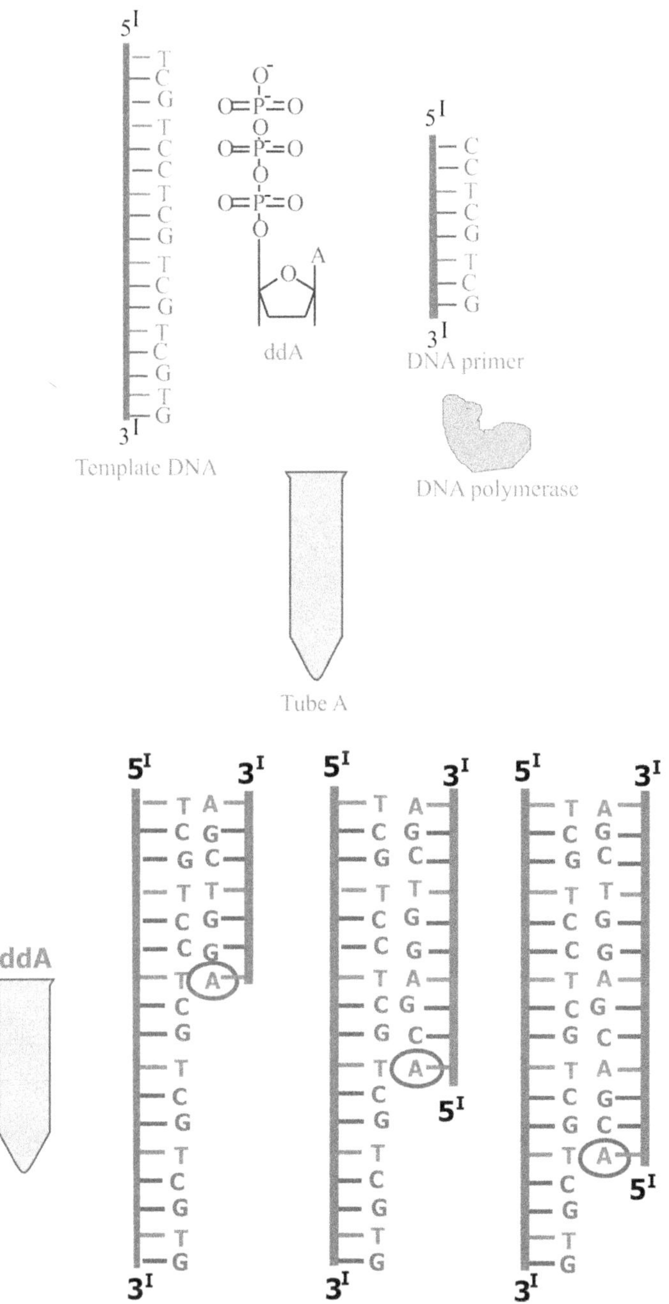

Fig. 25.1 The image depicts the process of elongation and termination of DNA synthesis.

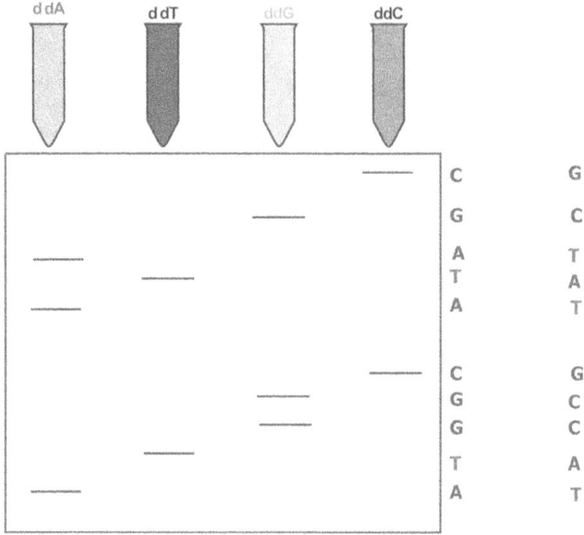

Fig. 25.2 The image depicts the auto radiography run.

Maxam-Gilbert sequencing

It involves base specific interruption of DNA template by base specific chemicals (cutter). Similar to sanger's method four different reaction with various base specific chemicals will be conducted for sequencing the DNA template.

Table 25.1 Some of the important base specific cutters.

Nucleotide	Base specific cutters
Adenine	Potassium tetrachloro palladium (K_2PdCl_4)
Thymine	0.5 M sodium boro hydride ($NaBH_4$) in H_2O at pH 8-10
	Osmium tertaoxide (OSO_4)
	1M spermine in H_2O + UV
Guanine	Dimethyl sulphate (($CH_3)_2SO_4$)
	Methylene blue
	0.5 % Dimethyl sulphate (($CH_3)_2 SO_4$) in formate buffer at pH 3.5
Cytosine	Hydrazine (NH_2NH_2) + 2M NaCl
	2-3 M hydroxyl amine HCl ($NH_2OH . HCl$) in H_2O at pH 6
	2-3 M hydrogen peroxide (H_2O_2) in carbonate buffer at pH 8.3 / 7.4

The concentration of chemicals should be adjusted to get optimum rate of fragmentation. These base specific cutters generates various length of fragments which can be resolved by gel electrophoresis (PAGE) and the visualised through auto radiography.

Automated sequencing

In case of Sanger's and Maxam-Gilbert methods use of primer with fluorescent dye (red, blue, green, yellow) at 5^1 ends generates characteristic fluorescence for the fragment. The fluorescent dye can be visualized with autoradiography.

Shotgun sequencing

This method suitable for DNA sequences longer than 1000 base pairs. In this method the target DNA is broken into random fragments (2-3 kb size) by sonication and nebulisation scission methods. These random fragments are cloned and then overlapping regions are reassembled and sequence can be deduced.

Mass spectroscopy

Matrix-assisted Laser Desorption Ionization – Time of light (MALDI-TOL) and Electrospray Ionization (ESI) are two mass spectrometry methods used in Sanger's DNA sequencing technique.

Next generation DNA sequencing methods

- Massively parallel signature sequencing (MPSS)
- Polony sequencing
- Pyro sequencing
- Illumina (solexa) sequencing
- Solid sequencing
- Ion semiconductor sequencing
- DNA nanoball sequencing
- Heliscope single molecule sequencing
- Single molecule real time (SMRT) sequencing

25.2.2 Blotting Methods

Southern blotting: dsDNA digested with restriction enzyme will be placed in wells in the surface of agarose gel placed on the sponge (in the tray of buffer). The nitro cellulose paper (filter) will be placed over the gel and covered with paper towels, they pull the buffer through the gel and filter. Gel electrophoresis will be employed to separate the fragments based on their size. Fragments will be denatured with alkali and then blotted on nitro cellulose paper (filter), move from gel to the filter. Alternatively depuration with hydrochloric acid can also be employed. The filter is then hybridised with radioactive probe and unbound probe is removed by washing. The bound probe can be viewed by placing the filter on X-ray film, it appears as band.

Northern blotting: The same procedure, when it is applied to RNA fragments is known as northern blotting.

Western blotting: The procedure, when applied to proteins is known as western blotting. This method is also known as immune blot.

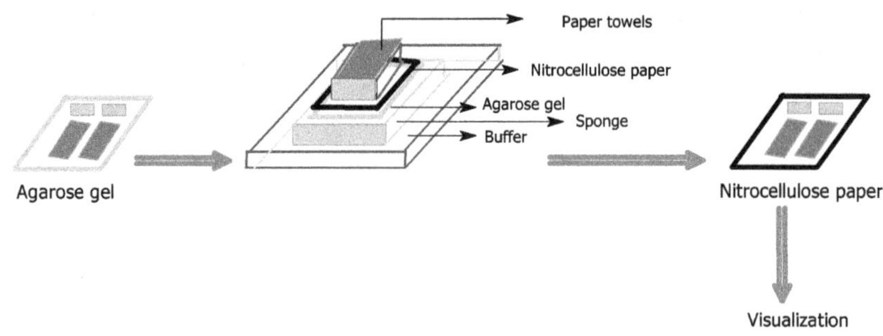

Fig. 25.3 Blotting technique.

25.2.3 Polymerase Chain Reaction

Polymerase chain reaction (PCR) amplifies DNA fragments, which are isolated from cloning. Reverse transcriptase polymerase reaction (RT-PCR) detects gene expression through the creation of cDNA transcripts from RNA. The cDNA will be amplified through PCR.

25.2.4 *In Situ* Hybridization

In Situ hybridization (ISH) uses a labeled cDNA / RNA strand (i.e., probe) to localize a specific DNA/RNA sequence. Fluorescent *In Situ* hybridization (FISH) is used to detect and localize the presence/absence of specific DNA sequences on chromosomes. FISH uses fluorescent probes that bind to only those parts of the chromosome with which they show a high degree of sequence complementarity. Fluorescence microscopy can be used to find out where the fluorescent probe is bound to the chromosomes.

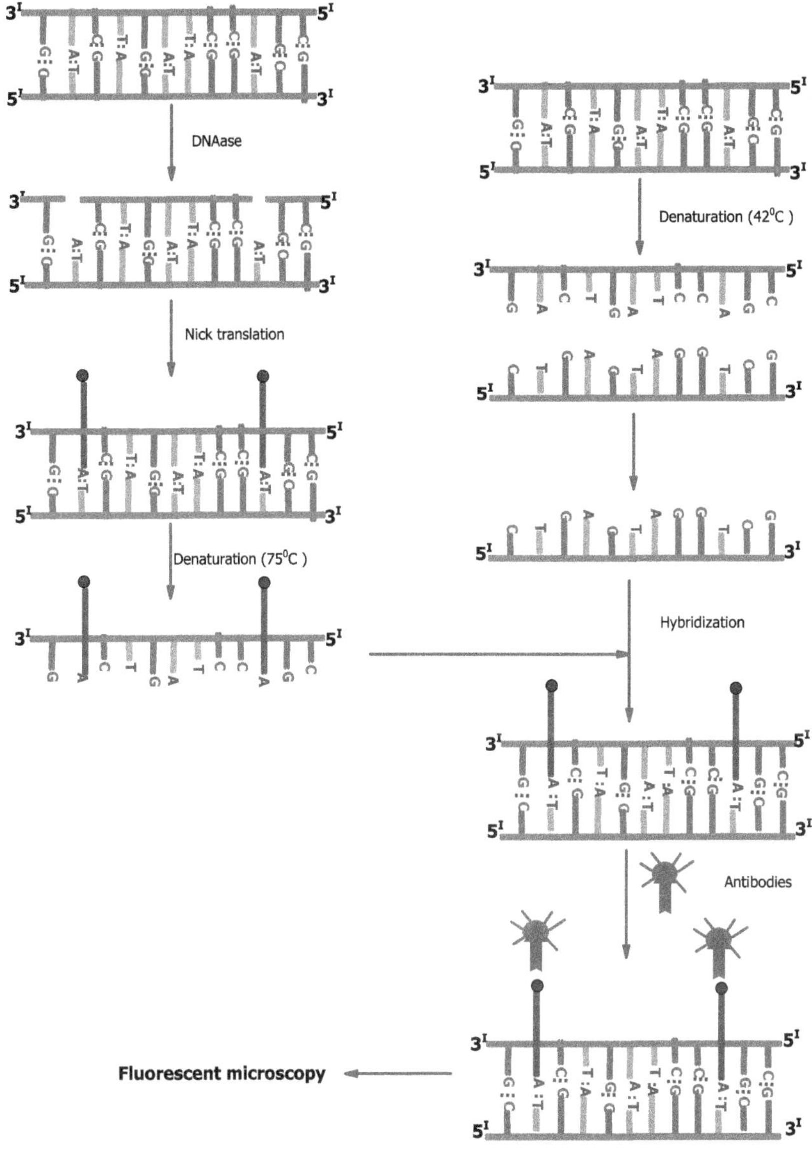

Fig. 25.4 Fluorescent in situ hybridization (FISH).

25.2.5 Open Reading Frames Prediction (ORFP)

An open reading frame (ORF) is the part of a reading frame that contains no stop codons. A stop-codon would be expected once every 21 codons. One common use of open reading frames is as one piece of evidence to assist in gene prediction.

25.3 Computational Gene Prediction Methods

Computational methods for finding genes in a genome has evolved significantly. They are more essential for the automatic analysis and annotation of large uncharacterised genomic sequences. They are grouped into two categories

1. Sequence similarity search
2. Gene structure and signal based search (Ab initio gene finding)

25.3.1 Sequence Similarity Approach

Sequence similarity search is based on finding similarity in gene sequences between ESTs, proteins and genomes to the input genome. The basis for this approach is that functional regions (exons) are more conserved than non-functional (introns). Once there is similarity between a certain genomic region and an EST, DNA and protein, the information can be used to infer gene structure or function.

25.3.2 Gene Structure and Signal based Search
(Ab initio gene finding)

Ab initio methods rely on signal sensors (short sequence motifs) and content sensors (patterns of codon). Coding sequences are distinguished from non-coding sequences by statistical detection algorithms. Dynamic programming, Linear discriminant analysis, Hidden markov model (HMM) and Neural networks are major algorithms. The most successful programs are base on the HMM.

25.4 Computational Gene Prediction Tools

1st generation tools: Testcode and GRAIL - These programs couldn't predict presice exon location

2nd generation tools: SORFIND and Xpound - It combines splice signal and coding region to predict potential exons.

3rd generation tools: GeneID, GeneParser, GenLang and FGENEH

4th generation tools: GENSCAN and AUGUSTUS - It offers improved accuracy and applicability.

Other tools: CSTfinder

25.5 Hidden Markov Model (HMM)

A markov process is a stochastic (probabilistic) model considers all possible combination of matches, mismatches and gaps to generate an alignment of a set of sequences. The symbols omitted by the system are observable, not the underlying random walk between the states thus prefix Hidden added. Hidden Markov Model represents protein families, sequence domain and patterns in DNA sequence guess of expected variation in each position of the MSA. MSA requires set of 20-100 sequences / more data to train the model. Trained model produces most probable alignment. Model is used to search sequence databases to additional member of a sequence family.

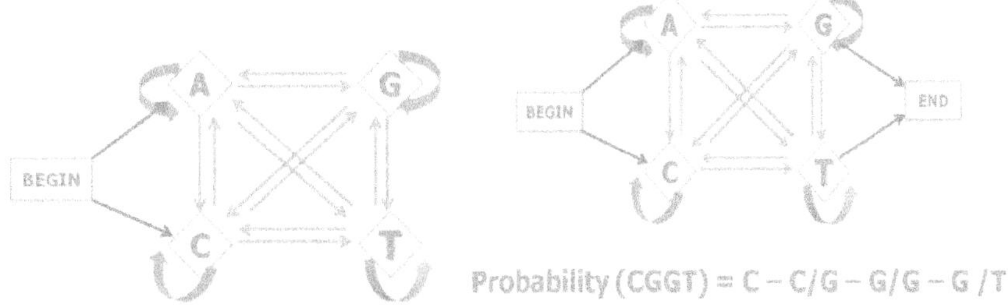

For DNA sequence   **For CGGT sequence**

In case of following sequences

NFLS   N - F L S
NFLS   N - F L S
NKYLT   NKYLT
QWT   Q - W - T

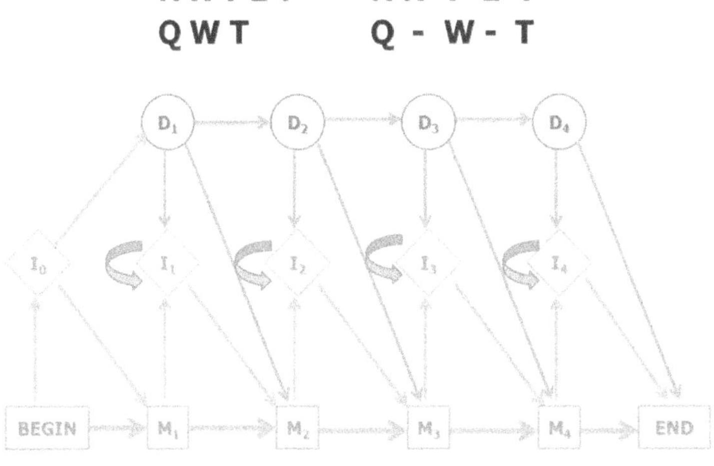

- There are 3 transitions from most states, the average value of a transition is 0.33

- But for M_4 and D_4 only 2 transitions, hence the average value of a transition is 0.5

- If a match state contains a uniform distribution across the 20 amino acid, the probability of any amino acid is 0.05

- Thus for the NKYLT probability is

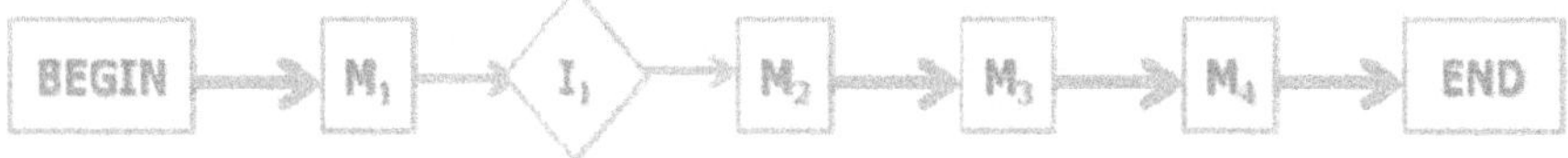

0.33 X 0.05 X 0.33 X 0.05 X 0.33 X 0.05 X 0.33 X 0.05 X 0.33 X 0.05 X 0.5 X 0.05 = 6.1 X10^{-10}

25.6 Hidden Markov Model Algorithms

- Viterbi algorithm / backward algorithm
- Forward algorithm
- Baum-Welch algorithm

25.6.1 Viterbi Algorithm / Backward Algorithm: A varient of the forward-backward procedure known as viterbi algorithm, which is similar to the profile alignment algorithm. Viterbi algorithm computes the negative logrithm of the probability of the single most likely path for the sequence.

25.6.2 Forward Algorithm: It is also known as process of filtering. It is close but distinct program from viterbi algorithm,.

25.6.3 Baum-Welch Algorithm: It helps in learning / training of models and used to find unknown parameters of HMMs.

25.7 HMM Advantages

- Strong statistical foundation
- Efficient learning algorithm
- Consistent treatment of insertion and deletion
- Wide range of application

25.8 HMM Applications

- HMM is used as an extensive sequence analysis tool.

- HMM predicts the location and orientation of alpha helices and beta strands present in transmemrane and helps in structure prediction.

- HMM is powerful tool in homology detection, it uses profiles of protein families in pairwise and multiple sequence alignment (normally BLAST will not consider).

- Enables gene identification, identification of G-protein coupled receptor (GPCR) and modeling protein domain.

- HMMs have been increasingly used in computational genomic annotations. It includes structural annotations for genes and other functional elements and functional annotations for assigning functions to the predicted functional elements.

- Important tool in data mining operations used in genetics.

25.9 HMM Softwares

HMMR: It produces profile hidden Markov models for homology search in a database.

SAM: A suite of tools for biological sequence analysis including homology detection, secondary structure prediction.

TMHMM: It models and predicts the location and orientation of alpha helices in membrane -spanning proteins.

HMMSTR: It predicts the structure and functions of proteins.

HMMSPECTR: A protein structure prediction tool.

COACH: A protein structure prediction tool.

## CHAPTER 26

SCORING SYSTEM

Alignment methods need methods to calculate score for matches and mismatches. Scoring system is used to estimate how well 2 residues of given types would match. The score is calculated from the frequency of occurrence of a match of 2 individual amino acids. Evolutionarily it has been observed that residues often get substituted / mutated (point or indel mutation) without causing any harm to the native structure and function of the protein. Identical and very frequently observed substitutions receive POSITIVE score. Matches that is unlikely and unrelated given NEGATIVE value. The highest score indicates the probability and lowest score indicates that they are unrelated. The scores for all positions in the alignment are then added to calculate a total score. Normalized sum of identity score is popularly quoted as "percentage identity". The scores are generally presented as log-odds matrices. Each score in the matrix is the logarithm of an odd ratio.

Mutated residues are considered to be similar. Substitution of isoleucine to valine and serine to threonine are considered to be mutations. Hydrophobic isoleucine and valine gets positive score and their functional role remains similar because of their similar chemical nature. The interaction pattern and biological function remain same because of their hydrophobicity. But hydrophobic isoleucine and hydrophilic cysteine receives negative score. The highest score indicates the possibility of evolutionary relationship between two amino acid sequences aligned. Evolutionary unrelatedness of the sequences are indicated by their lowest score.

Following is the example illustrates how optimal alignment between 2 sequences can be achieved. Moving the one of sequence in either side until maximum identical characters are observed, that is maximum score is obtained.

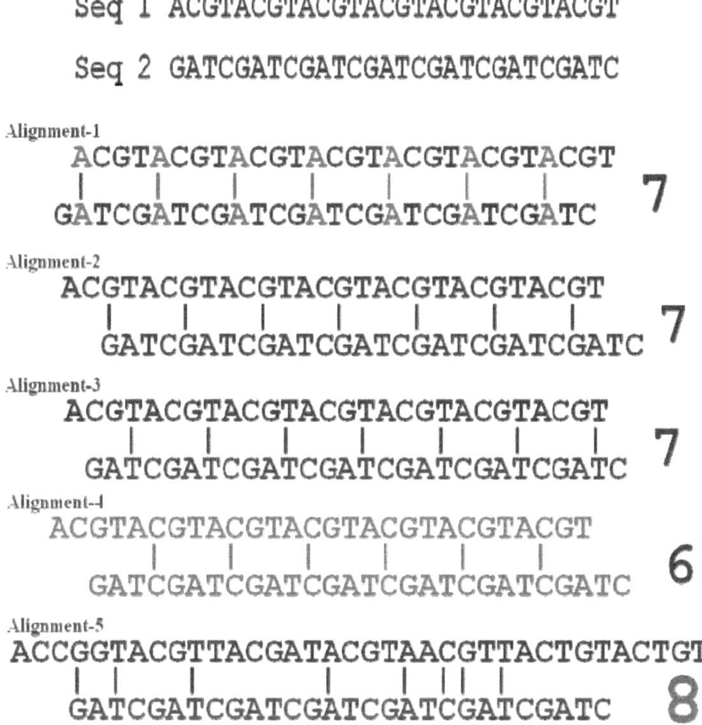

26.1 Gap Penalties

As sequences evolve and diverge they often accumulate insertion and deletion (INDEL mutation). To account this kind of mutational possibilities gap penalties are assigned.

26.1.1 Why Gap Penalties?

Gap penalties increase the quality of an alignment and will not allow non-homologous sequences to be aligned. It produces optimal alignment of two similar sequences and it

- Maximizes the number of matches
- Minimizes the number of gaps

In case of two sequences

Seq 1 = G A A T T C C G T T A

Seq 2 = G G A T C G A

Match: +5,   Mismatch = -3, Gap Opening = -4, Gap Extension = -1

When no gaps are introduced

$$
\begin{array}{l}
\mathtt{G\ A\ A\ T\ T\ C\ \mathit{C}\ G\ T\ T\ A} \\
\mathtt{|\ \ \ |\ |} \\
\mathtt{G\ G\ A\ T\ C\ G\ A}
\end{array}
$$

Score = 15

When gaps are introduced but gap extension is not considered

$$
\begin{array}{l}
\mathtt{G\ A\ A\ T\ T\ C\ \mathit{C}\ G\ T\ T\ A} \\
\mathtt{|\ \ |\ |\ \ |\ \ |\ \ \ \ |} \\
\mathtt{G\ G\ A\ T\ \_\ C\ \_\ G\ \_\ \_\ A}
\end{array}
$$

Score = 17

When gaps are introduced and gap extension is considered

$$
\begin{array}{l}
\mathtt{G\ A\ A\ T\ T\ C\ C\ G\ T\ T\ A} \\
\mathtt{|\ \ |\ |\ \ \ \ |\ |\ \ \ |} \\
\mathtt{G\ G\ A\ T\ \_\ \_\ C\ G\ \_\ \_\ A}
\end{array}
$$

Score = 20

26.1.2 Types of Gap Penalties

Two kinds are gap penalties are given and are

Gap creation penalty / gap opening penalty: Application of the negative scoring penalty to the substitution matrix for the first residue in a sequence alignment gap.

Gap extension penalty: Application of the negative scoring penalty to the substitution matrix for every additional residue in a sequence alignment gap.

26.1.3 Method of Calculating Penalty

Linear gap penalty score: $g(g) = -\,gd$

Affine gap penalty score: In tandem repeats it leads to heavy penalty

$$g(g) = -\,d - (g-1)\,e$$

where $g(g)$ = gap penalty score of a gap of length g

d = gap opening penalty

e = gap extension penalty

g = gap length

26.2 Scoring Matrix

Scoring matrices are also known as amino acid substitution matrices / symbol comparison tables. It is a two dimensional (2D) matrix containing all possible pair-wise alignment. Certain amino acid substitutions commonly occur in related proteins from different species. Often these substitutions are for a chemically similar amino acid, but are relatively rare. The most likely amino acid changes during evolution can be predicted by assessing the ancestor relationship among a group of proteins. The probability of changing amino acid A into B is always assumed to be identical to the reverse probability of changing B into A.

- The wealth of information accumulated in the gene/protein banks was utilised with dynamic programming procedure.

- Matrices for DNA are rather similar as there are only two options purine and pyrimidine and match and mismatch. But matrices of proteins are much more complex and the number of option is significant.

26.2.1 Types of Matrices
- PAM matrix
- BLOSUM
- GONNET matrix

26.3 PAM – Dayhoff PAM

PAM can be expanded as Percentage of Acceptable point Mutation / Point Accepted Mutation / Percent Accepted Mutation. It is also known as Mutation Data Matrix (MDM). It examines the kind of mutations that occur in closely related protein i.e at short evolutionary time. PAM is more suitable for studying quite distant proteins. Liklihood of change from one amino acid to another in homologous protein sequences during evolution can be tracked by PAM matrix. Amino acid substitution in a protein sequences are viewed as a markov model.

PAM matrices are usually converted into log odd matrices. The odd score represents the ratio of the chance of amino acid substitution by two different hypotheses.

1. Change represents an authentic evolutionary variation

2. Change occurred because of random sequence variation of no significance

Odd ratios are converted to logarithms to give log odds score for convenience in multiplying odd scores of amino acid pair in an alignment by adding the logarithms.

Many PAM matrices are available and can be utilised depending upon the situation. PAM matrices are denoted with numbers and the number with matrix refers to the evolutionary distance.

PAM 1 = Reflects an amount of evolutionary change that yields 1% of the residues undergone mutation

PAM 100= (PAM 1)^{100} = 100 % = 100 accepted mutations per 100 residues

PAM 250= (PAM 1)^{250} = 250 % = an average of 2.5 accepted mutation per residue (250 point changes per 100 amino acids)

PAM 250 = Used for sequences that are 20% similar

PAM 120 = Used for sequences that are 40% similar

PAM 80   = Used for sequences that are 50% similar

PAM 60   = Used for sequences that are 60% similar

Amino acids present in the proteins are grouped based on their chemical nature to facilitate the scoring operation.

1. (C) Sulfhydryl

2. (STPAG)-Small hydrophilic

3. (NDEQ) Acidic

4. Acid amide and hydrophilic

5. (HRK) Basic

6. (MILV) Small hydrophobic

7. (FYW) Aromatic

Scoring matrices: Percent Accepted Mutation

	C	S	T	P	A	G	N	D	E	Q	H	R	K	M	I	L	V	F	Y	W
C	12																			
S	0	2																		
T	-2	1	3																	
P	-3	1	0	6																
A	-2	1	1	1	2															
G	-3	1	0	-1	1	5														
N	-4	1	0	-1	0	0	2													
D	-5	0	0	-1	0	1	2	4												
E	-5	0	0	-1	0	0	1	3	4											
Q	-5	-1	-1	0	0	-1	1	2	2	4										
H	-3	-1	-1	0	-1	-2	2	1	1	3	6									
R	-4	0	-1	0	-2	-3	0	-1	-1	1	2	6								
K	-5	0	0	-1	-1	-2	1	0	0	1	0	3	5							
M	-5	-2	-1	-2	-1	-3	-2	-3	-2	-1	-2	0	0	6						
I	-2	-1	0	-2	-1	-3	-2	-2	-2	-2	-2	-2	-2	2	5					
L	-6	-3	-2	-3	-2	-4	-3	-4	-3	-2	-2	-3	-3	4	2	6				
V	-2	-1	0	-1	0	-1	-2	-2	-2	-2	-2	-2	-2	2	4	2	4			
F	-4	-3	-3	-5	-4	-5	-4	-6	-5	-5	-2	-4	-5	0	1	2	-1	9		
Y	0	-3	-3	-5	-3	-5	-2	-4	-4	-4	0	-4	-4	-2	-1	-1	-2	7	10	
W	-8	-2	-5	-6	-6	-7	-4	-7	-7	-5	-3	2	-3	-4	-5	-2	-6	0	0	17
	C	S	T	P	A	G	N	D	E	Q	H	R	K	M	I	L	V	F	Y	W

26.4 Blocks Substitution Matrix (BLOSUM)

BLOSUM is useful for more conserved proteins of domains contain sequence at all different evolutionary distance. Different kinds of BLOSUM are available and are

1. BLOSUM 62 - Sequences greater than 60 % are clustered
2. BLOSUM 80 - Sequences greater than 80 % are clustered
3. BLOSUM 30 - used to comparing highly diverged sequences
4. BLOSUM 90 -for very close sequences

26.5 Choosing the Best Matrices

Amount of similarity between sequences mayn't be known by using the series of PAM matrices and then to choose the best alignment score.

- Low PAM are well suited to finding short but strong similarities
- High PAM are well suited to finding long regions of weak similarities
- BLOSUM 32 is widely used

BLOSUM matrices are more effective in detecting homologous proteins BLOSUM -62 and BLOSUM -50 are superior in detecting weak homologies. BLOSUM 32 is also used widely.

- BLOSUM 62 uses only 62 % of the repeats on one column and thereby reduces the relative weight given to those substitutions in the matrix
- BLOSUM 62 is more suitable for protein database similarity searches than PAM 250 matrix
- BLAST programs uses BLOSUM 62 scoring matrix
- BLOSUM 50 is more suitable for FASTA and SSEARCH programs

CHAPTER 27

3D STRUCTURE PREDICTION USING SWISS MODEL

Swiss-Model can be accessed through http://swissmodel.expasy.org. Three different modeling modes are available in swiss-model.

1. First approach mode

2. Alignment mode

3. Project mode

First approach mode: It requires only an amino acid sequence of target protein and server will automatically select suitable templates. Upto five template structures can be specified and modeling will start with template having more than 50 % sequence identity with target sequence.

Alignment mode: In the alignment mode the modeling procedure starts after submitting the sequence alignment of target and template. Target and template should be specified. The server will build the model based on the given alignment.

Project mode: This method uses DeepView project file, it contains the superposed template structures and the alignment between target and template.

Modeling procedure includes the following steps

1. Identification of Target and Template

2. Target-template sequence alignment

3. 3D structure prediction for target (Model building)

4. Model Evaluation

27.1 3D Structure Prediction using Alignment Mode of Swiss Model

27.1.1   Step 1: Identification of Target and Template

1. Open **http://www.ncbi.nlm.nih.gov/protein** and select target protein sequence

2. Run BLAST program to identify template protein for the target.

3. Retrieve FASTA format of target and template protein sequences.

27.1.2   Step 2: Target-template Sequence Alignment

1. Open **http://www.ebi.ac.uk/Tools/msa/clustalw2/**

2. Paste FASTA format of target and template sequences (Step-1)

3. Change the title of target and template protein sequences into > **Target** and > **Template** respectively

4. Change Aln W / Numbers to PIR mode in **Step 3 FORMAT option**

5. Click submit

6. Copy alignment file

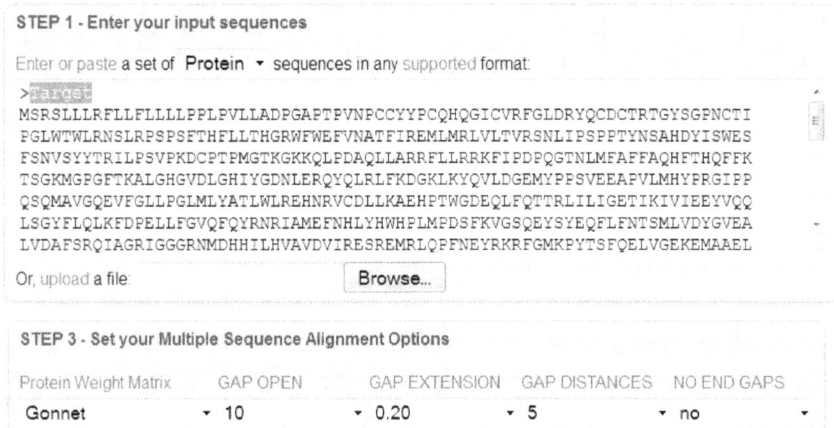

27.1.3   Step 3: 3D Structure Prediction for Target

1. Open **http://swissmodel.expasy.org/**

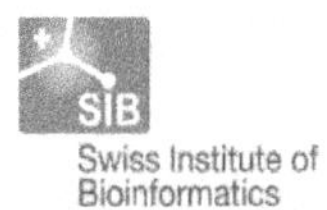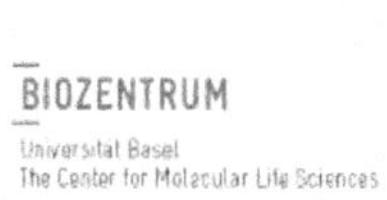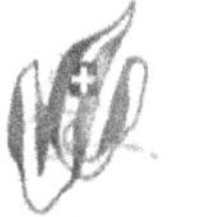

SWISS-MODEL is a fully automated protein structure homology-modeling server, accessible via the ExPASy web server, or from the program DeepView (Swiss Pdb-Viewer). The purpose of this server is to make Protein Modelling accessible to all biochemists and molecular biologists worldwide.

SWISS-MODEL Team
Torsten Schwede: Project Leader
Florian Kiefer: SWISS-MODEL Repository
Lorenza Bordoli: Method Development and user support
Konstantin Arnold: SWISS-MODEL Workspace

2. Select alignment mode of modeling tool

3. Paste target-template alignment file (Clustal W2)

4. Remove P1; from both target and template sequences

SwissModel Alignment Mode

Email:
Project Title:

Alignment Input Format: FASTA

Cut & paste your Target-Template Alignment:
> 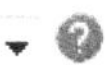Target

```
MSRSLLLRFLLFLLLLPPLPVLLADPGAPTPVNPCCYYPCQHQGICVRFGLDRYQCDCTR
TGYSGPNCTIPGLWTWLRNSLRPSPSFTHFLLTHGRWFWEFVNATFIREMLMRLVLTVRS
NLIPSPPTYNSAHDYISWESFSNVSYYTRILPSVPKDCPTPMGTKGKKQLPDAQLLARRF
LLRRKFIPDPQGTNLMFAFFAQHFTHQFFKTSGKMGPGFTKALGHGVDLGHIYGDNLERQ
YQLRLFKDGKLKYQVLDGEMYPPSVEEAPVLMHYPRGIPPQSQMAVGQEVFGLLPGLMLY
ATLWLREHNRVCDLLKAEHPTWGDEQLFQTTRLILIGETIKIVIEEYVQQLSGYFLQLKF
DPELLFGVQFQYRNRIAMEFNHLYHWHPLMPDSFKVGSQEYSYEQFLFNTSMLVDYGVEA
LVDAFSRQIAGRIGGGRNMDHHILHVAVDVIRESREMRLQPFNEYRKRFGMKPYTSFQEL
VGEKEMAAELEELYGDIDALEFYPGLLLEKCHPNSIFGESMIEIGAPFSLKGLLGNPICS
```

Or upload an alignment file   Browse_

5. Submit alignment

6. Select target and template appropriately, enter template PDB ID and submit alignment

Workunit: P017663
Title:
Status: submission
back

Please select sequences from your alignment:

Target Sequence   Target ▼
Template Sequence   1CQE_A ▼   PDB-Code: 1CQE   Chain-ID: A
                       Target
                       1CQE_A

[submit alignment]

7. Submit alignment

   (Alignment file will be generated for target and template sequences)

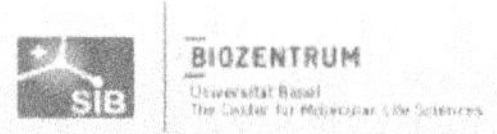
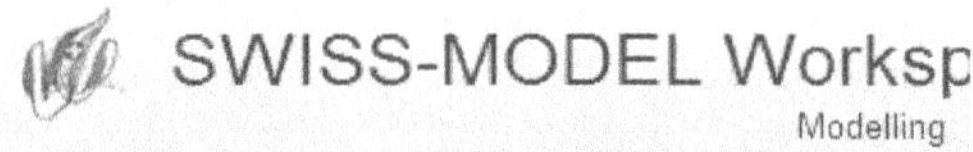

BIOZENTRUM
Universität Basel
The Center for Molecular Life Sciences

SWISS-MODEL Worksp
Modelling

[myWorkspace]

Workunit: P017663
Title:
Status: submission
back

Before submission, please ensure that the alignment has been interpreted correctly:

```
CLUSTAL W(1.81) multiple sequence alignment


Target/1-582        MSRSLLLRFLLFLLLLPPLPVLLADPGAPTPVNPCCYYPCQHQGICVRFGLDRYQCDCTR
Template/1-552      -----------------------------PVNPCCYYPCQHQGICVRFGLDRYQCDCTR
                                                 ****************************


Target/1-582        TGYSGPNCTIPGLWTWLRNSLRPSPSFTHFLLTHGRWFWEFVNATFIREMLMRLVLTVRS
Template/1-552      TGYSGPNCTIPEIWTWLRTTLRPSPSFIHFLLTHGRWLWDFVNATFIRDTLMRLVLTVRS
                    ***********:*****,:******* ********:*:********; *********
```

```
Target/1-582     ATLWLREHNRVCDLLKAEHPTWGDEQLFQTTRLILIGETIKIVIEEYVQQLSGYFLQLKF
Template/1-552    ATIWLREHNRVCDLLKAEHPTWGDEQLFQTARLILIGETIKIVIEEYVQQLSGYFLQLKF
                  **:********************************:************************


Target/1-582     DPELLFGVQFQYRNRIAMEFNHLYHWHPLMPDSFKVGSQEYSYEQFLFNTSMLVDYGVEA
Template/1-552    DPELLFGAQFQYRNRIAMEFNQLYHWHPLMPDSFRVGPQDYSYEQFLFNTSMLVDYGVEA
                  *******,*************:************:**,*:********************


Target/1-582     LVDAFSRQIAGRIGGGRNMDHHILHVAVDVIRESREMRLQPFNEYRKRFGMKPYTSFQEL
Template/1-552    LVDAFSRQPAGRIGGGRNIDHHILHVAVDVIKESRVLRLQPFNEYRKRFGMKPYTSFQEL
                  ********.*********:************:***.:***********************


Target/1-582     VGEKEMAAELEELYGDIDALEFYPGLLLEKCHPNSIFGESMIEIGAPFSLKGLLGNPICS
Template/1-552    TGEKEMAAELEELYGDIDALEFYPGLLLEKCHPNSIFGESMIEMGAPFSLKGLLGNPICS
                  .******************************************:****************


Target/1-582     PEYWKPSTFGGEVGFNIVKTATLKKLVCLNTKTCPYVSFRVP
Template/1-552    PEYWKASTFGGEVGFNLVKTATLKKLVCLNTKTCPYVSFHVP
                  *****,***********:*********************:**
```

[submit alignment]

8. Submit generated alignment for modeling.

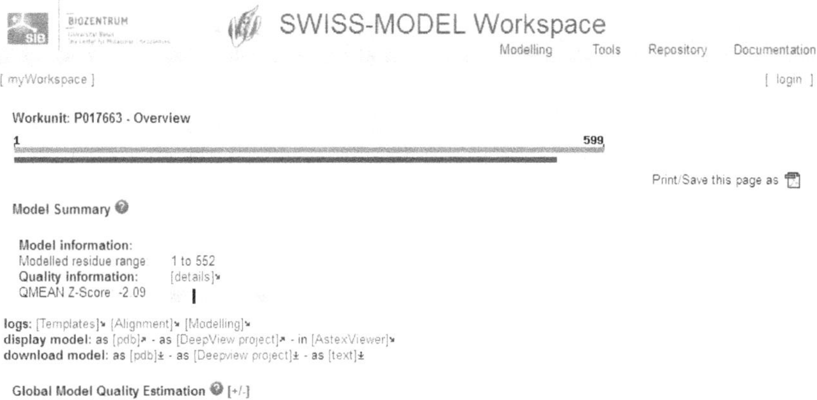

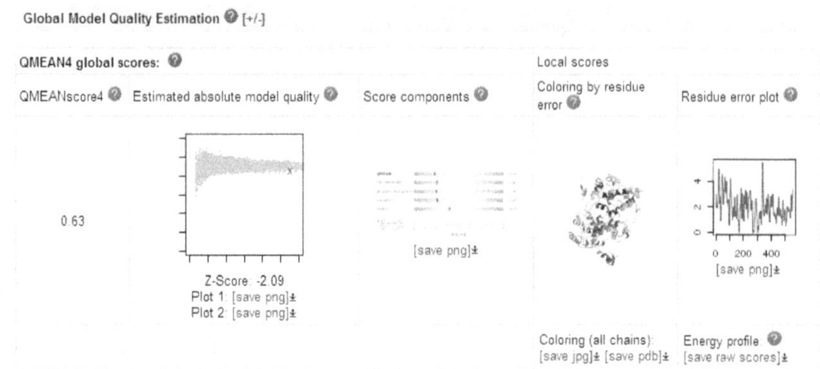

27.1.4 Model Evaluation

Quality of the model is more important for the applications. QMEAN, ANOLEA and GROMAS are three independent methods available in swiss model to assess the model quality. DeepView helps in visualising and analysing the model. WhatCheck and ANOLEA of SWISSMODEL assess the quality of model.

27.2 Ramachandran Plots

The scatter plot of φ (phi) and Ψ (psi) angles (dihedral angles- between N and C_α and C_α and C_β) for all residues in aprotein is called as Ramachandran plot. It shows the relationship between φ and Ψ angles of all residues present in protein. It provides simple view of molecular conformation. The φ and Ψ angles cluster into distinct regions in the plot, each region corresponds to particular secondary structure. Hence this can be used to verify the quality of the 3D structure. Glycine residues (contains no branch) are separately identified by triangles as these are not restricted to the regions of the plots.

27.2.1 Software Tools for Generating Ramachandran Plot

Downloadable

- PROCHECK
- PDBSUM
- WEBMOL
- VMD 1.9.1
- DeepView- SWISS PDB Viewer

Online server

- RAMPAGE
- STAN server
- MolProbity
- Ramachandran plot 2.0

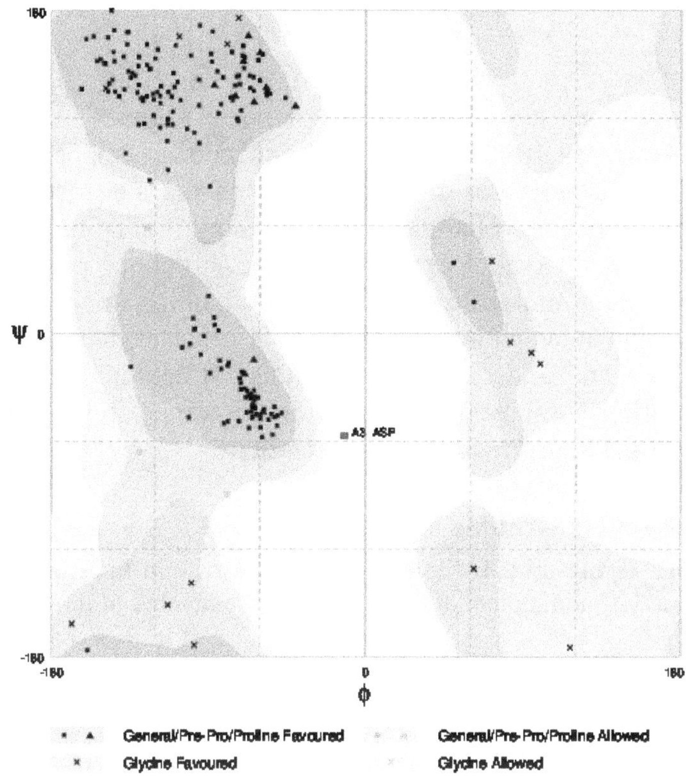

Fig. 27.1 RAMPAGE Ramachandran plot for PDB 1W3R.

The shading on the plot represents the different regions, the darkest area correspond to the 'core ' region which represent the most favorable combinations of φ and Ψ values. 90 % of residues in 'core' region is the measure of stereochemical quality.

## CHAPTER 28

MOLECULAR VISUALIZATION

Molecular visualization is of tremendous importance for understanding processes that are relevant in fields such as material sciences, genetics, pharmacy, immunology, and biology and chemistry in general. Research into the structural properties of small and large molecules is increasingly gaining importance. The function and interaction of molecules is often primarily analyzed based on an understanding of this structural information. Visualizations are created by blending (parts of) the molecule shown in different structural representations.

28.1 Molecular Graphic Models

1. **Wire frame model:** Molecule appears as a thin lines, coloured by atom type and indicating bond type via the number of lines.

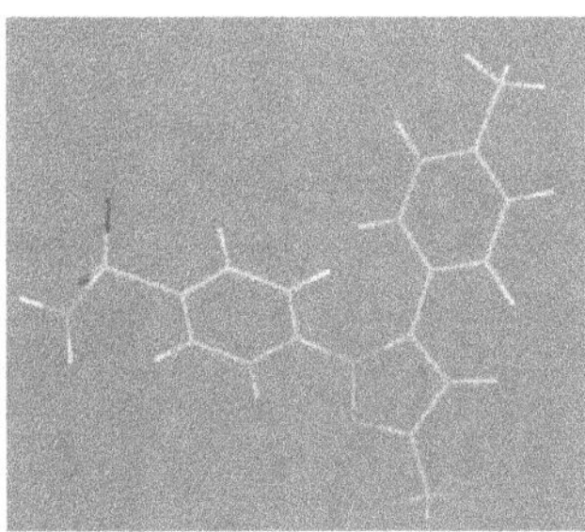

2. **Ball and stick model:** This molecular model displays 3D arrangement of atoms and bonds present in the molecule. The atoms are typically represented by spheres and rods connecting them represents bonds. Two and three curved rods are used to depict double and triple bonds respectively. This model does not provide a clear insight about the space occupied by the model.

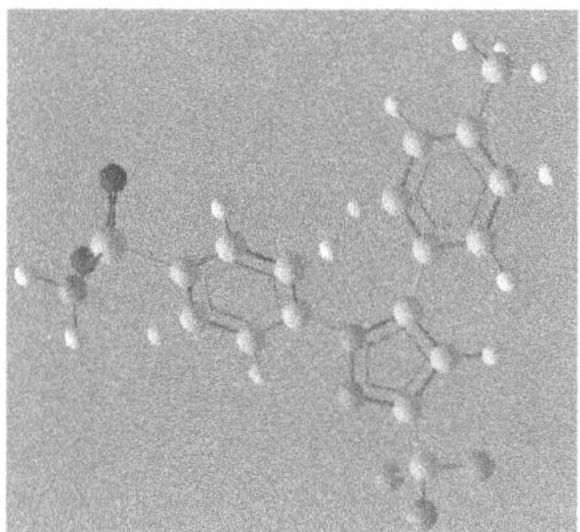

3. **Space filling/calotte model:** Space-filling model (Calotte model) provides occupied space and relative dimensions of the molecule but not the bonds. This model is also known as CPK model after the scientists Corey, Pauling and Koltun who pioneered this.

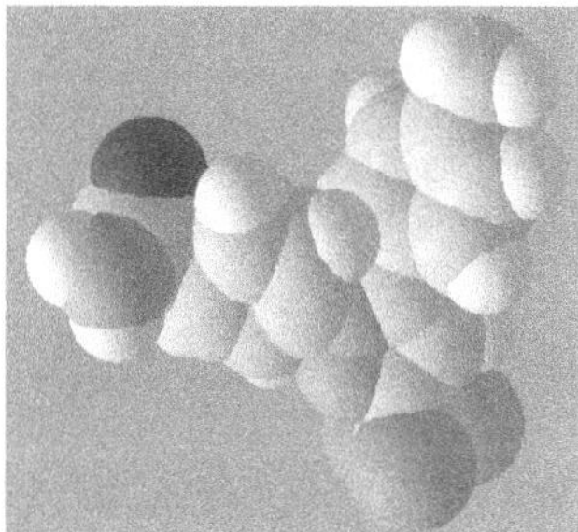

4. **Tube model:** Molecule appears as tube with no indication as bond type, coloured by atom type.

5. **Ribbon/Richardson model:** It traces the back bone of the protein. It highlights the secondary structural features of protein. Cylinders denote α-helices, arrows denote β-sheet and tubes represents coils and turns present in the protein.

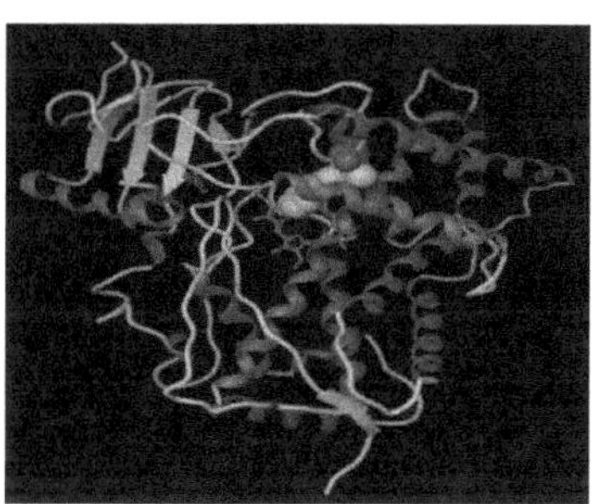

28.2 Molecular Visualization Tools

1. Preteopedia
2. Cn3D macromolecular structure viewer
3. Rasmol
4. Chimera
5. Discovery studio visualizer
6. Marvin space
7. Molgro molecular viewer
8. Pymol

## CHAPTER 29

RECEPTORS

Regulatory proteins (enzymes, hormones, carrier proteins and ion channels), mucopolysaccharides and nucleic acids (RNA and DNA) are the functional elements of the cell and acts as a targets / receptors of molecules and produce biological response. The interaction of the drug with component of cell (receptor / target) initiates series of biochemical reactions which results in biological response. Many receptors are structural units of the cell membrane and it consists of bio molecular layer of lipids (25 Å) held in between protein. These proteins adopt different conformations in bio-phase depending upon the environment and acts as receptor. These receptors through chemical communications (biochemical reactions) coordinate the functions of different cells. This process is known as signal transduction.

The amino acid side chains (constituents of cell membrane) in fixed positions forms specific interactions with molecules (endogenous and exogenous). Most drugs elicit its effect by binding on or within the surface of cells. The interaction of molecules to the amino acid side chains of the protein induces structural changes as well as physical properties (biological activity) of the target protein. Similarly, drug interactions may leads to no change in the configuration of the receptor and results in no response (blocking effect).

29.1 Components of Receptors

All most every receptors has got two different components in it and are

- Recognition component: It recognises the specific molecules.
- Amplification component: It initiates the biological response after binding results.

29.2 Classification of Receptors

1. G-protein coupled receptors (GPCRs)
2. Ion channels
3. Catalytic receptors
4. Nuclear / cytoplasmic receptors
5. Orphan receptors
6. Hijacked receptors

29.2.1 G-protein Coupled Receptors (GPCRs)

These receptors will have guanine nucleotides (GTP and GDP) as its structural components and are grouped into four classes

- G_s: Stimulates adenylyl cylcase activity and activates Ca^{2+} channels

- G_i: Inhibits adenylyl cyclase activity and activates K^+ channels

- G_q: Stimulates phospholipase activity

- G_{12}: Modulates Na^+/H^+ exchanger

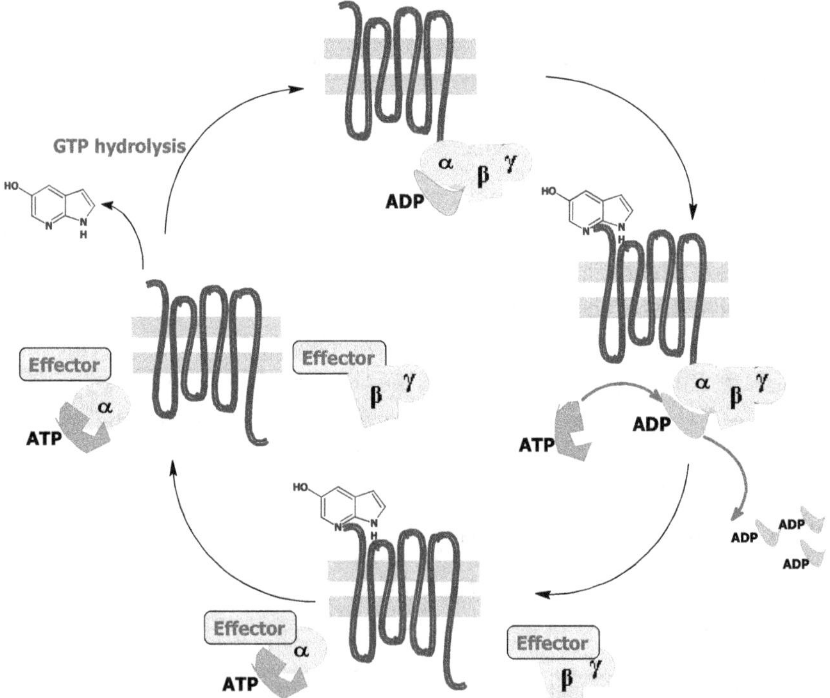

Fig. 29.1 GPCR activation.

GPCRs are made up of α, β and γ subunit and are anchored to the membrane through prenylation reaction. Guanine nucleotide (GTP) binds to α subunit and β, γ subunits remains as βγ complex. α subunit catalyses the conversion of GTP in to GDP and GDP binded α subunit exists as αβγ trimer in resting state. When GPCR agonist molecule binds to the receptor, it induces GDP dissociation expulsion and the same will be replaced with GTP (GDP / GTP exchange). The binding of GTP to αβγ trimer is responsible for the dissociation of trimer into α-GTP and βγ. α-GTP binds to the target and activates it by phosphorylation which requires hydrolysis of GTP into GDP. cAMP activates protein kinases, which in turn triggers dissociation of regulatory subunits.

29.2.2 Ion Channels

Ion channels are responsible for the movement of ion through the specified channels. It includes:

1. Ligand (transmitter) gated ion channels (LGIC)

2. Second messenger gated ion channels (SGIC)

3. Voltage gated ion channels (VGIC)

Ligand gated channels: Nicotinic acetyl choline receptor is the best characterised LGIC. It consists 5 subunits (two α, β, γ and δ). The binding of acetylation to two α subunits (binding site) induces conformational change and sodium selective ion channel. LGICs are also known as ionotropic / metabotropic receptor. GABA, glutamate, NMDA, AMPA, glycine ad serotonin receptors are some of the well known LGICs.

Second messenger gated ion channels: Second messengers cAMP, cGMP, IP_3 and DAG influences the opening and closing of channels. Ca^{2+} and K channel opening is regulated by these second messenges.

Voltage gated ion channels: Changes in membrane (chemical) potential regulates the opening of the channels. Voltage gated ion channels open, when cell membrane is depolarised. eg: Na, K, and Ca channels. Depolarization caused by the opening of Na^+ influx initiates the opening Ca^{2+} channels. This kind of channel opening is short-lasting even if the depolarisation is maintained. It produces influx of Ca^{2+} and oxidative phosphorylation.

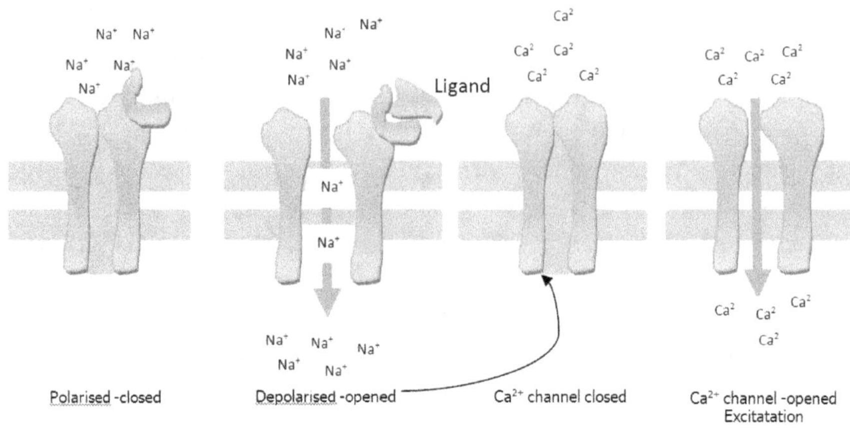

Fig. 29.2 Opening of Ligand gates and voltage gated ion channels.

29.2.3   Catalytic (kinase linked) Receptors

This kind of receptors mediates the actions of protein mediators (growth factors and cytokines) and hormones (insulin and leptin). Growth factor receptors are also known as "tyrosine kinases". Catalytic receptors contain extracellular ligand binding domain and intracellular effector domain. Ligand binding leads to dimerization of pairs of receptors (*i.e* association of extracellular domain). This association allows autophosphorylation of tyrosine and this serve as high affinity binding sites for intracellular proteins, which initiates signal transduction process. These adapter proteins are known as "SH2 domain" proteins. The phosphorylated receptors binds to "signal transducers and activators of transcription" (STATs), which translocates into nucleus and initiate gene transcription. These SH2 domain proteins (Grb2 and Jak) proteins involve in the control of cell growth, cell division and cell differentiation.

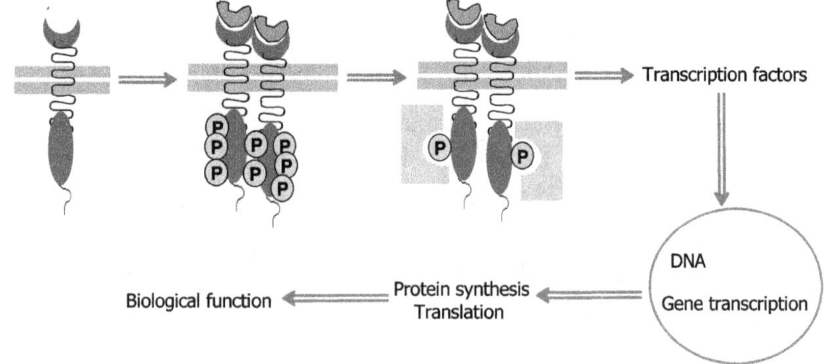

Fig. 29.3 Functioning of catalytic receptor.

29.2.4 Nuclear Receptors

The nuclear receptors regulate DNA transcription by steroid and thyroid hormones. These receptors are located in the nucleus and the ligands are all liphophilic, which can readily cross the cell membrane. The nuclear receptors contain ligand binding domain and DNA binding domain. Steroid molecules change the conformation of nuclear receptors, which facilitates the dimerization process. These dimers bind to specific sequences of the nuclear DNA known as "hormone responsive elements". This element increases the RNA polymerase activity and initiates the production of specific mRNA. Retinoic acid bind to nuclear receptor and facilitates the embryonic development.

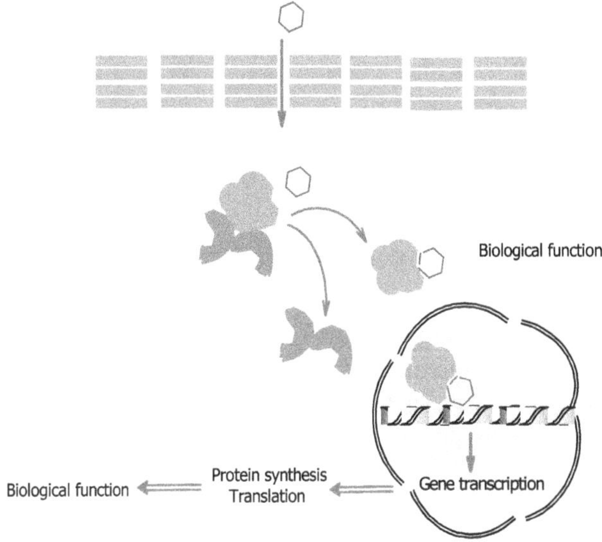

Fig. 29.4 Functioning of nuclear receptor.

29.2.5 Orphan Receptors

The receptors with no defined pharmacological activity is known as orphan receptor.

29.2.6 Hijacked Receptors

The receptor for known ligand and physiological function will bind with another kind of ligand. Most viruses gain cellular entry through this mechanism.

29.3 Drug Receptor Interactions

The drug-receptor interactions are key for biological responses. The attraction between receptor and ligand due to their affinity results in drug-receptor interaction. The ability of the molecules to produce biological response is termed as efficacy or intrinsic effect. Based on the efficacy the molecules are broadly classified into two groups

1. Agonists: Ligands, which have affinity for the receptor and activates it for the regular physiological function are called as agonists.

    (a) Full agonist: A ligand with same strength of pharmacological potential as that of natural ligand.

    (b) Partial agonist: A ligand with similar pharmacological activity, but less potential irrespective of their concentration.

    (c) Full inverse agonist: A ligand with affinity for the receptor, but produces opposite activity. [eg: diazepam (inhibition) and β-carboline (excitation)]

    (d) Partial inverse agonist: A ligand, which produces lesser pharmacological activity (< 100 %) compared to that of an inverse agonist.

2. Antagonists: Ligands, which have affinity for the receptor without activating them are called as antagonists.

    (a) Competitive antagonist: A ligand binds to the binding site of the receptor with similar affinity as that of the natural ligand. But it will activates the receptor and hence no biological response results by blocking the binding of natural ligand (agonist).

    (b) Non-competitive antagonist: A ligand binds to the allosteric binding site of the receptor (where natural ligand will not bind) and induces the conformational change. The newly induced conformation will not favour the binding of natural ligand (agonist) and produces no biological response.

In most cases drug-receptor interactions are reversible and drug dissociates from its receptor as soon as its concentration decreases in extracellular region. Drugs binding to receptors through electrostatic interactions may obey this, whereas covalently binding drugs will not.

1. Covalent bonding
2. Non-covalent bonding

    (a) Ionic

        • Electrostatic interaction
        • Ion-dipole interaction

- Dipole-Dipole interaction

- Hydrogen bonding

(b) Van der walls interaction

(c) Hydrophobic interaction

29.3.1 Covalent Bonding

It is the strongest bond involved in the drug-receptor interactions and are most important in biology. One atom from ligand and one from receptor share pair of electrons and form covalent bond. Bond energy associated with this kind of bond is 50-150 kcal/mole and are irreversible in nature. Tthis leads to complete destruction of the receptor. In selective cases, such as a anti-bacterial and anticancer drugs long lasting and irreversible effects are required and are produced by forming covalent bon with its receptor. Arsenicals and mercurials forms covalent bond with sulphhydryl group present in receptor. Penicillins produces antibacterail effects by acetylating the bacterial cell wall (covalent binding). Full recovery of cellular function is possible only through the synthesis of new receptors. It is a time taking process and thus produce extremly prolonged duration of block.

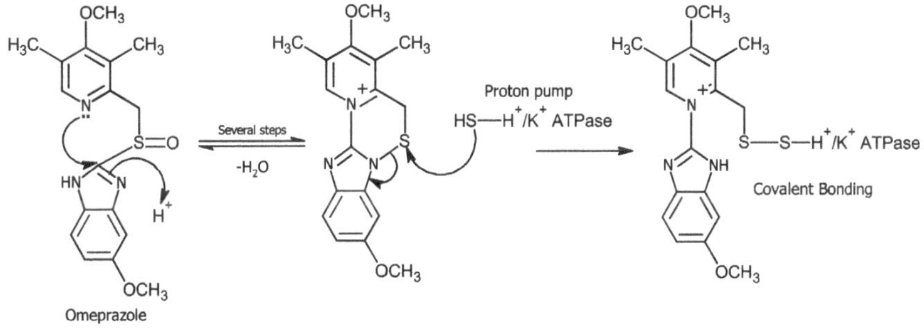

Fig. 29.5 Covalent interaction between omeprazole and proton pump.

29.3.2 Non-covalent Bonding

Non-covalent bonds are much weaker (10-100 times) interactions than covalent bonds.

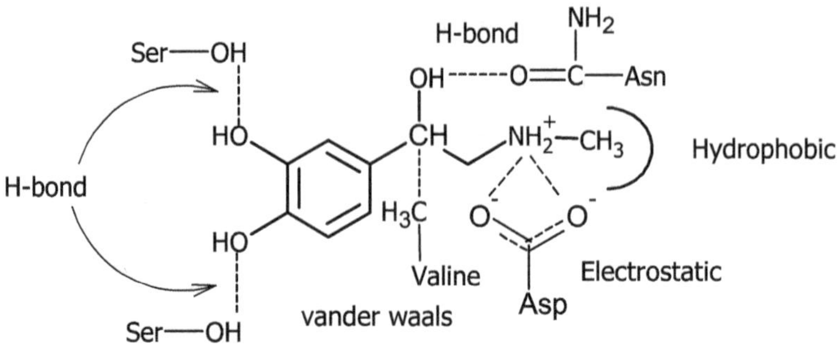

Fig. 29.6 Non-covalent interactions between acetylcholine and its receptor.

Ionic bond

Electrostatic interactions: Atoms with opposite charges are attracted to each other and results in electrostatic interaction. One atom from ligand and another from receptor forms this kind of bond. The bond strength of this type is 5-10 kcal/mole and is distance dependent.

Dipole moment: Dipole moment is due to the movement of electrons along the bond. In a molecule higher electro negativity atoms draws electrons towards it from other atom (which is being utilized for bond formation). This introduces polarity in molecule and such molecules are known as polar.

Van der waals force: this results when two uncharged atoms approach very closely due to their temporary polarizaibility. The strength of this kind of bond is inversely proportional to the 7th power of distance and normally in the range of 0.5-1 kcal/mole. Though the individual bond is weaker, in high molecular weight molecule summation of these forces provides significant bonding.

Hydrophobic interactions: Association of non-polar regions of drug molecule and biological receptors results through hydrophobic interactions. A non-polar region of the molecule can't be solvated by water, hence water molecules in this region associate to form quasi crystalline structure (ice-bergs). Thus non-polar segment of molecule produce high degree of atom.

29.4 Receptor Theories

The difference in the biological potential of molecules is well explained through different hypothesis-theories. These theories suggest how a drug molecule binds to receptor and the kind of binding it makes for their bioactivity potential. The more important drug receptor theories are

1. Side chain theory
2. Occupancy theory
3. Ariens-Stephenson theory
4. Rate theory
5. Induced fit theory
6. Macromolecular-perturbation theory
7. Activation-aggregation theory

29.4.1 Chain Theory

Paul-Ehrlich suggested that side chains of cells through specific groups binds to particular molecule and elicit characteristic biological response. These side chains are latter identified as amino acids and collectively known as receptor. This theory is called as 'side chain theory".

29.4.2 Occupancy Theory

Occupancy theory states that the characteristic biological response of molecule is directly proportional to the number of receptors occupied. The structural feature of the drug molecule decides the affinity towards receptor and initiates the pharmacological response. This is well explained through "dose response curve". The number of drug-receptor complexes (results by drug receptor interaction), which is concentration dependent is responsible for the observed biological response. The association of drug to receptor initiates the biological effect and the dissociation of drug from receptor ceases the response.

29.4.3 Ariens-Stephenson Theory

Agonist and antagonist molecules possess structural features complemantarity to receptor and have desirable affinity for it. However agonists alone produce intrinsic-stimulant action, whereas antagonists retain zero intrinsic effect. In fact antagonists possess great affinity, but still produce no biological response (due to its inability to induce conformational change). In case of agonists, difference in their binding affinity towards receptor is reason for their biological potential variation (agonist and partial agonist vary in their response).

29.4.4 Rate Theory

It explains that activation of receptor by drug is proportinal to the rate of drug-receptor association in unit time thus the rate of association and dissociation of drug-receptor complex rather than number of receptors occupied is responsible for the observed pharmacological response. In case of agonist dissociation is rapid compared to association. Whereas association is rapid and dissociation is slow with antagonists.

29.4.5 Induced Fit Theory

A receptor will undergo conformational change as the ligand approaches it. In the induced conformation receptors will expose catalytic groups for binding to drug. Thus the receptor will initiate the biological response and returns to its original conformation once the drug is released.

29.4.6 Macromolecular Perturbation Theory

Ligand interaction with macromolecule produce specific conformational perturbation (SCP) and non-specific conformational perturbation (NSCP) in receptors. SCP favours the binding of certain molecules having intrinsic activity (agonists). NSCP favours the binding of molecules with no intrinsic activity (antagonists). A partial agonist will induce both SCP and NSCP.

29.4.7 Activation-Aggregation Theory

Even in resting state receptors will exhibit dynamic equilibrium between active and inactive form. Agonists bind to active form and produce biological response. Antagonists binds to inactive form and inhibits the biological effect. Partial agonists binds to both the forms, but shows preferential binding to active form and produce mixed response (less biological response).

29.5 Receptor Promiscuity

Molecules (agonists, inverse agonists, antagonists) exhibit entirely different biological response in different bio-phase, even though the binding receptor is same. This phenomenon is called as receptors promiscuity and can be exemplified by the action of H1 and H2 blockers on histamine receptors in different locations of the biological system.

29.6 Stereochemical Aspects of Drug Activity

Relative effectiveness of various molecules with defined structural features enabled the better understanding of stereo chemical properties of the receptor as well as the molecules. Spatial arrangement of atoms present in molecules decides its affinity for receptors and thus its pharmacological response.

Enantiomers: Enantiomers will show altered affinity for receptors, different binding energies and chemical properties. Muscarinic receptor is highly streospecific, it makes binding interaction with L(+) isomer of muscarine In L(+) muscarine 5-methyl and 2-CH_2-N $(CH_3)_3$ groups are cis in orientation and 4-OH group exist in trans orientation.

Muscarine

An enantiomer with potent activity is termed as "eutomer" and less potent isomers as "distomer". The ratio between the eutomer and distomer is known as 'eudismic ratio'. When streogenic centre is present in the pharmacophore it gives high eudismic ratio. High eudismic ratio refers that eutomer is having therapeutic potential because of their high receptor complementarity. Distomer for the one pharmacological effect may be eutomer for the secondary pharmacological effect.

Distomers with undesirable side effects are named as "isomeric ballast". The S-isomeric form of hypnotic and sedative drug thalidomide is typical example of isomeric ballast, as it produces teratogenic effects.

Thalidomide

A compound having two pharmacological potential through different molecular mechanism are termed as 'hybrid drugs'. Propronolol in levo (-) form produce local anesthetic potential and anti-hypertensive potential through different mechanism. An S(+) enantiomer of ketoprofen is non-steroidal anti-inflammotry agent, where as R(-) is useful in the treatment of peridontal disease.

Propronolol

Ketoprofen

Multiple isomeric forms differ in their receptor affinity and produce different biological effect are known as 'pseudo hybrid drug'. Labetalol in R,R isomeric form shows selectivity for β-receptor and produce antogonistic effect. Similarly S,R form of the drug produce α-receptor blocking effect.

Labetalol

Marketing single enantiomeric form of the racemate drug is called as 'recemic switch' or 'chiral switch'. Esomerazole [(S)-omeprazole-anti-ulcer], Escitalopram [(S)-citalopram-antidepresant], Levocetrizine [(R)-cetrizine-antihistamine] and Levalbuterol [(R)-salbutamol-antiasthmatic] are some of the examples for chiral switch approch.

Geometrical isomers: Triprolidine, antihistaminergic drug is active only in Z (cis, H/Pyridyl) configuration. In this isomeric form triprolidine inter nitrogen distance (4.8 ± 0.2 Å) is close to histamine inter nitrogen distance (4.55 Å). Diethyl stilbesterol, a synthetic analogue of oestogen is active in E (trans) isomeric form. Two benzene rings are twisted out of plane by alkane group. In the resulted conformation the angular methyl group and ring D of oestradiol are comparable. The E isomeric form, minimal steric interference offers same plane for two aromatic rings. The distance between two hydroxyl group are 14.5 Å, which is comparable to oestradiol.

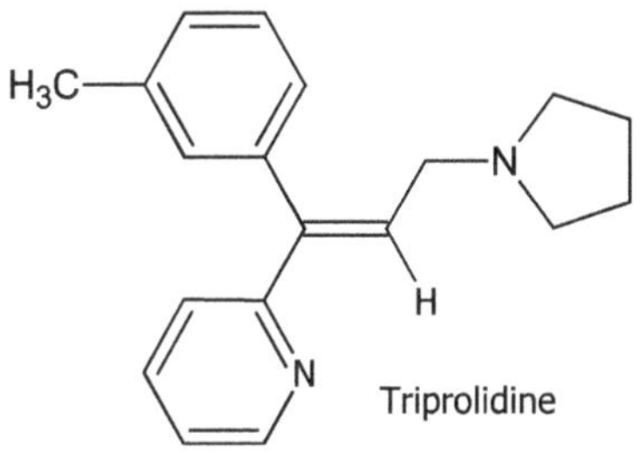

Triprolidine

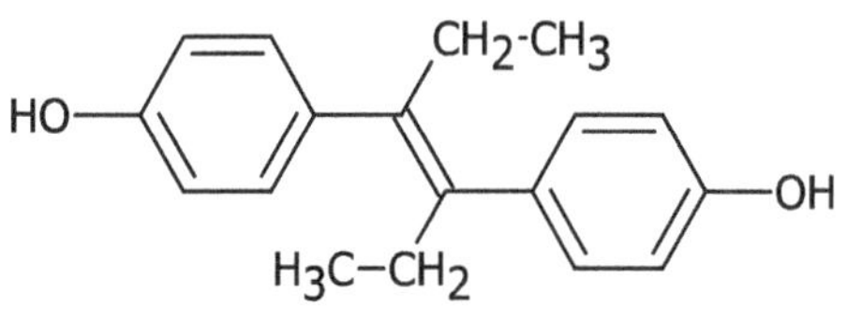

Diethyl stilbesterol

Three point attachment-Easson-stedman hypothesis: In asymmetric molecule (-) epinephrine, the quaternary nitrogen, aromatic group and alcoholic hydroxyl groups are involved in the receptor binding. The p and m hydroxy groups (catechol hydroxy) determines the intensity of attachment through metal binding. whereas (+) epinephrine alcoholic hydroxy group is in opposite orientation to that of (-) epinephrine. The presence and correct orientation of beta hydroxy group results in higher adrenergic activity.

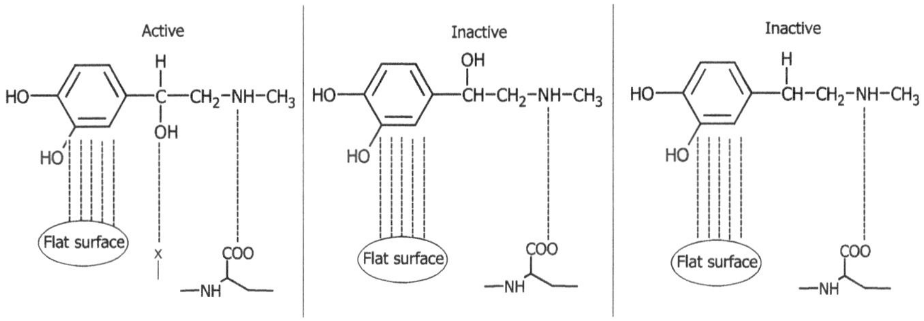

Fig. 29.5 Three point attachment of epinephrine to the receptor.

GLOSSARY

- **Analogous:** Similar sequences in same organism derived from convergent evolution.

- **Antibody Directed Enzyme Prodrug Therapy (ADEPT):** An antibody raised against a particular tumor cell line is conjugated with the enzyme that is needed to activate an antitumor prodrug.

- **Antisense technology:** Antisense technology is a rational drug design tool useful in discovering more specific treatments for diseases. It is recognised to be efficient for the identification of gene expression in a sequence-specific way.

- **Auxophore:** The atoms / groups present in the structure essential for the integrity of the molecule and may interfere with the pharmacophore in binding pattern.

- **Barcodes:** Information carrying graphical patterns designed for easy and reliable automatic retrieval. It is an optical machine-readable representation of data, provides detailed up-to-date information quickly with more confidence.

- **Basic Local Alignment and Search Tool (BLAST):** Basic Local Alignment and Search Tool is used alignment of protein / nucleotide sequences and helps to detect related proteins and to study the relationship between the sequences.

- **Bibliographic database:** The specialized database designed for handling bibliographic references. They are also known as personal information systems, bibliographic reference managers, or personal bibliographic software.

- **Bio-assay:** Bio assays measures the potency of the new or chemically undefined substance. This also evaluates the toxicity profile of the test molecule and determines the specificity of the substance to receptors.

- **Bioinformatics:** A management information system, searches biological databases, compares sequences, predicts structure of the protein and (homololgy modeling).

- **Bio-isosterism:** Bioisosterism is a special process of molecular modification applied in rational drug design strategy.

- **Biological database:** Biological databases are large organized body of persistent data from genomics, proteomics, metabolomics, phylogenetics. They are the important tool for the understanding of the biological phenomena from the structure of the biomolecules and their interactions.

- **Biological response:** The interaction of the drug with component of cell (receptor / target) initiates series of biochemical reactions which results as biological response.

- **Bio-PERL:** A popular tool-kit developed as a collection of integrated PERL modules for transforming and manipulating sequence data and annotations, accession remote databases and parsing output from programs such as BLAST, FASTA etc.

- **Bioprecursor prodrug:** A bioprecursor prodrugs produce their effects after *in vivo* bio-chemical modification in to new compound. They rely on oxidative and reductive activation where as prodrugs requires hydrolytic activation.

- **Bipartate prodrug:** A prodrug in which active drug is attached to the carrier and get released in *in vivo* enzymatic hydrolysis.

- **BLOcks SUbstitution Matrix (BLOSUM):** BLOSUM is a scoring matrix useful for more conserved proteins of domains contain sequence at all different evolutionary distance.

- **Chemical reaction informatics:** Chemical reaction informatics enable a chemist to explore synthetic pathways, quickly design and record completely new experiments using reaction databases.

- **Cheminformatics:** An integral part of the drug discovery process, from lead identification through lead development. It deals with the storage, retrieval and analysis of the immense amount of molecular data.

- **Cladogram:** A branching tree of phylogeny estimate; where the branches are of equal length. This show common ancestry, but do not indicates the amount of evolutionary time separating taxa.

- **Clinical studies:** Study of drug effectiveness, it involves battery of tests to generate safety and efficacy data for the drugs, diagnostics, devices and therapy protocols.

- **ClustalW:** ClustalW is a general purpose multiple sequence alignment program for DNA or proteins. It produces biologically meaningful multiple sequence alignments of divergent sequences.

- **Consensus docking**: This technique improves the probability of finding a correct solution by combining multiple scoring functions in docking procedures.

- **Databases:** The database system is a collection of related information and can be accessed through database management systems.

- **Database management system (DBMS):** Database management involves creating, modifying, deleting and adding data in files and using this data to generate reports or answer the queries. The software allows to perform these functions easily are called as database management system.

- **Data mining:** Data mining is the process of discovering valid, novel, understandable and potentially useful patterns in data.

- **Distomer:** An enantiomer with less potent activity is termed as ditomer.

- **Docking:** The process of fitting molecule into a model receptor binding site to predict possible ligand receptor interaction. This approach helps in predicting the binding pattern compounds to the target using computer programs.

- **DNA databank:** A DNA databank is essentially a storage facility that maintains DNA extracted from a variety of sources including blood, saliva, hair, skin, muscle and liver, etc. DNA databanks can serve a variety of purposes that include screening for disease gene- genetic diseases, paternity testing, identity matching for criminal investigations, genetic fingerprinting for criminology and research-related studies.

- **DNA Database of Japan (DDBJ):** DNA data bank in Japan, established by National Institute of Genetics, Japan. It includes the functions of EMBL and NCBI through the collaboration (international databank collaboration). Public gene expression database CIBEX is available through DDBJ.

- **Dot plots analysis:** A method after comparing two sequences and tries to locate possible alignment of characters between the two sequences. One sequence will be placed in X-axis and other in Y-axis, whenever there is a match found between two sequences a dot will be placed in the corresponding position.

- **Drug design:** Designing molecules with more complementarity for the active sites of the receptor protein is called as drug design. It involves mainly the identification of target, ligand and its 3D structural studies.

- **Drug development:** Drug development process involves optimization of lead molecules, generation of analogs and formulation development. Its main aim is to improve pharmacokinetic (ADME) properties, increase potency and to decrease toxicity associated with parent molecule.

- **Drug discovery:** Traditional drug discovery process involves the identification of compounds from chemical libraries and natural products, mostly through serendipitous discovery. Modern drug discovery utilises high throughput screening and computer aided drug design to design and discover drug candidates.

* **Drug information:** Drug information is the provision of unbiased, well-referenced and critically evaluated up-to-date information on any aspect of drug use.

* **Drug-likeness:** A delicate balance among molecular properties affecting pharmaco-dynamics and pharmacokinetics of molecules which ultimately affects their absorption, distribution, metabolism, and excretion in human body.

* **Dynamic programming (DP):** A computational method used to align two protein or nucleic acid sequences, compares every pair of characters and generates best or optimal alignment.

* **Energy minimization:** The calculation of the total energy $[E_{total}]$ of the molecule using the values of the relevant parameters together with the initial atomic coordinates by the force field equation. The goal of the energy minimization is to reduce the energy of high energy coordinates by optimizing the geometry.

* **Eudismic ratio:** The ratio between the eutomer and distomer is known as eudismic ratio.

* **European Molecular Biology Open Software Suite (EMBOSS):** EMBOSS is a free Open Source software analysis package specially developed for the needs of the molecular biology (e.g. EMBnet) user community. The software automatically copes with data in a variety of formats and even allows transparent retrieval of sequence data from the web.

* **Eutomer:** An enantiomer with potent activity is termed as eutomer.

* **FAST Approximation (FASTA):** FASTA is a powerful tool for scanning databases to find sequences that are similar to a query sequence. Generally best to make protein-protein

comparisons but can also compare DNA sequence to DNA databanks.

- **FASTA sequence format:** FASTA format is a text-based format for representing protein and nucleotide sequences using standard IUB / IUPAC single- letter codes. A sequence in FASTA format begins with > symbol followed by single line description. In case of single-letter code lower-case letters are accepted and are mapped into upper-case. A single hyphen or dash represents a gap in the sequence.

- **Ferguson principle:** Ferguson related the biological activity to their thermodynamic property. The biological potency of nonreactive gases and vapours can be controlled by an equilibrium between the agonist in gas phase and agonist in receptor phase.

- **Foreign key:** A field in a table that refers to parent records in another table. It need not have unique values in the referencing relation.

- **Gene Directed Enzyme Prodrug Therapy (GDEPT):** GDEPT involves delivering the gene encoding prodrug-activating enzyme through liposomes. The prodrug gets activated by the enzyme expressed by the gene delivered previously.

- **Genetic Prodrug Activation Therapy (GPAT):** GPAT uses known transcriptional differences between normal and tumor cells to drive the selective expression of a drug-metabolizing enzyme which converts nontoxic prodrug into a toxic moiety.

- **Genome informatics:** Genome informatics analyzes and extracts biologically relevant information from the rapidly growing biological databases.

- **Global alignment:** Global alignment method compares two sequences over their entire lengths and maximizes region of similarity and minimizes gaps.

- **Hard drugs:** Biologically active and non-metabolizable compounds, which resists bodily biotransformation thus generates no toxic metabolites.

- **Health information technology (HIT):** Health information technology is most promising tool for improving the overall quality, safety and efficiency of the health delivery system. HIT uses both computer hardware and software for storage, retrieval, sharing and use of health care information, data and knowledge for communication and decision making.

- **Hidden markov model:** A markov process is a stochastic (probabilistic) model considers all possible combination of matches, mismatches and gaps to generate an alignment of a set of sequences. The symbols omitted by the system are observable, not the underlying random walk between the states thus prefix Hidden added.

- **Homologous:** Genes from different organisms having similar sequences because of the common ancestor gene.

- **Homology modeling / comparative modeling:** Homology modeling predicts the 3D structure of the target, when crystal structures of proteins are not available. A combination of homology modeling and docking is effective virtual screening tool in ligand identification and ligand optimization.

- **Immunoinformatics:** Immunoinformatics facilitates the understanding of immune function by modeling the interactions among immunological components.

- **Lead identification:** The identification of the lead (hit) compounds with desirable pharmacological effect through random screening of natural products and chemical libraries. High through put screening of chemical libraries and *in silico* screening of virtual libraries are the current lead identification technologies.

- **Lead optimization:** It involves in the improvement of pharmacokinetic (ADME) properties to increase absorption, potency and to decrease toxicity associated with parent molecule.

- **Library catalogue:** A library catalogue is a register of all bibliographic items found in a library or network of libraries.

Library catalogue gives access to physical items (books, CDs, etc) and electronic resources.

- **Local alignment:** Local alignment compares two sequences over particular length.

- **Microarrays:** Microarrays assess gene and protein expression and validates at the targets at the tissue and cell levels (tissue and cell micro arrays).

- **Molar refractivity (MR):** Molar refractivity is the measure of steric factors and bulkiness of the molecule and it shows a strong correlation with ligand binding.

- **Molecular graphics:** Molecular visualization tools helps viewing 3D structure data and to explain their structural features. It illustrates catalytic binding process of macromolecules with the aid structural biology.

- **Molecular mechanics:** Molecular mechanics finds stable, low-energy conformations of molecules by changing their geometry at $0°$ K, assists in drug receptor interaction analysis and 3D visualization (bioactive conformation) of molecules.

- **Molecular modelling:** Molecular modeling helps understanding the types, nature and bonds involved in the atoms. Key aspect of molecular modeling studies involves the calculation of the energy of conformations and its interactions.

- **Mutual prodrugs:** A mutual prodrug is bipartate / tripartate prodrug in which the carrier acts as a synergistic drug.

- **NMR spectroscopy:** NMR spectroscopy is a powerful tool for the structure determination of a protein-ligand complex. It explains the exact intermolecular interactions and thus helps in the identification of best fit molecule.

- **Normalization:** A critical part of database architecture, which ensures data integrity and avoids data redundancy. It decomposes data into two dimensional tables, eliminates any relationship in which table data does fully depend upon the primary key of a record and contains transitive dependencies.

- **Normal forms:** The series of guidelines developed by database community is called as normal forms.

- **Orthologous:** Similar sequences in different organisms, which have arisen due to speciation event and it retains their functionality throughout evolution.

- **Overton and Meyor theory:** The narcotic effects of group of structurally non-specific compounds parallels the partition coefficient (lipophilicity in cell). Higher the liphophilicity drug absorption will be more due to more affinity.

- **Pairwise alignment:** Identifation of the regions of similarity that may indicate functional, structural and evolutionary relationship between two biological sequences (protein/DNA).

- **Paralogous:** Similar sequences in same organism, due to gene duplication with divergent function.

- **Partition coefficient:** A free energy related parameter which expresses the relative free energy change occurring on movement of compound from one phase to another.

- **PAM [Dayhoff PAM/]:** PAM can be expanded as Percentage of Acceptable point Mutation / Point Accepted Mutation / Percent Accepted Mutation. It is also known as mutation data matrix (MDM) and examines the kind of mutations that occur in closely related protein at short evolutionary time.

- **PERL –Practical Extraction and Report Language:** PERL is a high level but easy to use programming language and available for most operating systems. PERL is preferred for processing sequence analysis and database management.

- **PFAM:** A database of multiple alignments of protein domains / conserved protein regions and profiles Hidden Markov Model (HMM). Profile HMM is useful in determination of the protein family and deals sensibly with multi domain protein.

- **Pharmacoinformatics:** An informatics based discipline, concerned with the information on drugs and related substances, discovery and development of drugs using high performance computing and graphic tools.

- **Pharmacophore:** A functional group(s) / nucleus present in a molecule that interfere with a receptor and produce the biological activity.

- **Primary key:** A field in a table whose value uniquely identifies each record and defines relationship within a database.

- **Prodrugs:** Chemically modified inert drug precursor which upon biotransformation liberates the pharmacologically active parent compound. It is useful in optimization of clinical application of drug and corrects a flaw in a drug candidate.

- **PROSITE:** Prosite is the database of biologically significant sites and patterns. It determines the function of proteins transcribed from genomic or cDNA sequence. It contains as many biologically meaningful patterns and profiles as possible and are highly specific.

- **Protein crystallography:** Purified proteins (targets) will be subjected for crystallization and it yields 3D structure by X-ray crystallography. Complexed structure reveals major / minor conformational changes of the protein and is useful in the designing of newer molecules.

- **Protein Data Bank (PDB):** PDB is developed by Brookhaven National Laboratories and is managed by the Research Collaboratory for Structural Bioinformatics (RCSB). It contains information regarding all 3D structures of proteins, nucleic acids, carbohydrates and a variety of other complexes experimentally determined by X ray crystallography and NMR spectroscopy.

- **Proteome informatics:** Proteome informatics include identification and validation of targets and natural protein therapeutics, drug candidate selection, mode of action studies and discovery of diagnostics.

- **Protein Information Resource (PIR):** PIR is established by National Biochemical Research Foundation (NBRF) and provides protein database and analysis tools on molecular evolution, functional genomics and computational biology.

- **Phylogram:** A branching tree estimates and infers evolutionary relationship among the biological species based on the similarities in their genetic characteristics.

- **Quantitative Structure Activity Relationship (QSAR):** Quantitative structure activity relationship uses parameters assigned to the various functional groups and modifies the structure of a compound. These parameters (also known as descriptors) are a measure of the potential contribution of its group to a particular property of the parent drug.

- **Quantum mechanics:** Quantum mechanics involves in the calculation of molecular orbital energies and molecular geometry, energy, vibrational spectra, and electronegativity.

- **Random screening:** The biological activity testing of compounds (natural / synthetic) without considering their structure.

- **Rational drug design:** Rational drug design utilises knowledge on physiological and chemical properties of target and its interactions with molecules to design newer ligands.

- **Receptor:** Regulatory proteins (enzymes, hormones, carrier proteins and ion channels), mucopolysaccharides and nucleic acids (RNA and DNA) are the functional elements of the cell and acts as a targets / receptors of molecules and produce biological response.

- **Receptor promiscuity:** Molecules (agonists, inverse agonists, antagonists) exhibit entirely different biological response in different bio-phase, even though the binding receptor is same.

- **Recombinant DNA (rDNA) technology:** To understand a complex biological process, a biochemist isolates and studies the individual components *in vitro*. rDNA involves isolation and manipulation of DNA to make chimeric molecules and making identical copies (cloning).

- **Redundancy:** Database systems with repeated field in two or more tables leads to data anomalies and corruption.

- **Richet rule:** The narcotic actions of group of compounds are inversely proportional to their water solubility.

- **Search algorithms:** Algorithms are deeply concerned with the process of sorting and searching the data, which provides an ideal framework for the application to information retrieval.

- **Serendipity:** Serendipity in drug discovery implies the finding of one observation during the other research program. Most of the drug discoveries are result of a false hypothesis or due to chance observation.

- **Signal transduction:** Chemical communications (bio-chemical reactions) through which receptors coordinate the functions of different cells.

- **Soft drugs:** Soft drugs are active isoelectric-isoelectronic analogues of a lead compound that are deactivated in a predictable and controllable way into inactive non-toxic species after excerting their therapeutic effect.

- **Solvent effect:** Solvent energy is the energy released due to attractive dispersion and electrostatic forces and entropy of water. It plays pivotal role in the qualitative understanding of the drug-receptor interaction and ranking of ligands.

- **SwissProt:** The curated protein sequence database established by department of Medical Biochemistry of the University of Geneva [Swiss Institute of bioinformatics (SIB)] and the EMBL data entry library. It provides a high level of annotations such as functions, domain structure, post transitional modifications (PTMs), variants of the proteins.

- **Targeted prodrug design:** Prodrugs can be designed to target specific enzymes by considering enzyme-substrate specificity in order to overcome various undesirable drug properties.

- **Target identification:** Target identification is the process of identifying new targets (protein or DNA/RNA) whose modulation might inhibit or reverse disease progression Target identification finds best interaction mode between the potential target candidates and small molecule probes.

- **Target validation:** Target validation is the process of finding the importance of target in the specific disease. New drug target validation provides insight into the pathogenesis of target related diseases.

- **Toxicoinformatics:** It helps in the prediction of the toxicity of chemical molecules in biophase.

- **Tripartate prodrugs:** The prodrug linkage in bipartate prodrugs is too labile or to stable and renders it ineffective. A tripartate prodrug overcomes this problem. In a tripartate prodrug the carrier is not connected directly to the drug, but rather to a linker that in turn attached to the drug.

- **Virtual screening:** Virtual screening uses computer-based methods to discover new ligands on the basis of biological structures.

- **Virus Directed Enzyme Prodrug Therapy (VDEPT):** VDEPT uses viral vectors for efficient delivery of "suicide gene" encoding an enzyme, which converts non-toxic prodrug to cytotoxic agent.

- **Xenologous:** Similar sequences due to horizontal transfer of genetic material through symbioses and virus-induced transduction between unrelated organisms (don't share evolutionary origin).

G

H

K

L

M

T